Culpeper's Medicine

Graeme Tobyn is a member of the National Institute of Medical Herbalists and a practising qualified herbalist. He is a translator of medieval astrological texts and teaches for the Company of Astrologers in London.

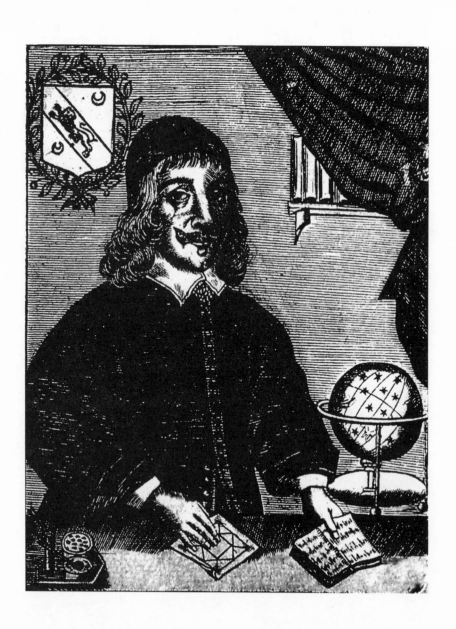

Culpeper's Medicine

A PRACTICE OF
WESTERN HOLISTIC MEDICINE

Graeme Tobyn

ELEMENT

Shaftesbury, Dorset • Rockport, Massachusetts
Brisbane, Queensland

© Element Books Limited 1997
Text © Graeme Tobyn 1997

Published in the USA in 1997 by
Element Books, Inc.
PO Box 830, Rockport, MA 01966

First published in Great Britain in 1997 by
Element Books Limited
Shaftesbury, Dorset SP7 8BP

Published in Australia in 1997 by
Element Books Limited
for Jacaranda Wiley Limited
33 Park Road, Milton, Brisbane 4064

Cover design by Mark Slader
Design by Roger Lightfoot
Typeset by Bournemouth Colour Press
Printed and bound in the USA by Courier Westford, Inc.

British Library Cataloguing in Publication
data available

Library of Congress Cataloging in Publication
data available

ISBN 1-85230-943-1

CONTENTS

List of Tables

List of Figures

List of Plate Illustrations

1 Winter
2 Spring
3 Summer
4 Autumn
5 The four temperaments
6 Zodiac man
7 A doctoral diploma in medicine from Padua, 1618
8-25 Medicinal herbs
8 Elecampane
9 Rue
10 Sage
11 Violets
12 Garlic
13 Liquorice
14 Parsley
15 Hyssop
16 Spinach
17 Borage
18 Wormwood
19 Betony
20 Centaury
21 Eyebright
22 Fumitory
23 St John's Wort
24 Deadnettle
25 Hops

Picture Credits

The author and publishers wish to thank the following for permission to reproduce works from their collection:

Bayerische Staatsbibliothek, Munich: plate 7.

British Library: figures 8 (30.g.9), 12 (C.123.K.28), 14 (718.I.15), plate 6 (Egerton 2572, fol.51^{v}), plates 18, 19, 20, 21, 22, 23, 24, 25, 26 (all 36.h.8).

Österreichische Nationalbibliothek, Vienna: plates 1–4, 9–17.

Uppsala Universitetsbibliotek: plate 8.

The Wellcome Institute Library, London: figures 1, 2, 3, 13, 16.

Geoffrey Cornelius: figure 12.

Acknowledgements

I would like to thank Geoffrey Cornelius, Patrick Curry, Michael McIntyre and Vernon Wells for kindly looking over the text and offering criticism and advice. I am indebted to Maggie Hyde for introducing me to Culpeper's astrology all those years ago, and to Chris Hedley and Elisabeth Brooke for their tuition, support and inspiration in herbal medicine. Finally I owe much gratitude to my wife and children for tolerating me while I struggled to put together *Culpeper's Medicine*.

This book is dedicated to my parents, Bill and Margaret.

Notice

The practical information in this book on dietary and herbal approaches to the treatment of disease is intended for the interested herbalist or other medical practitioner. In addition to any such practical application, I hope that the topics discussed will be of much interest to the general reader.

It is not at all the purpose of this book to replace the guidance of medical practitioners and anyone who believes he or she is ill should seek their professional advice. The use of any information presented in this book should be undertaken only with their co-operation.

INTRODUCTION

Why Read Culpeper Today?

Nicholas Culpeper, the 17th-century English herbalist and astrologer, remains the best-known advocate of Western holistic medicine. His medicine was the medicine of the famous Greek physicians Hippocrates and Galen, and had been used traditionally throughout Europe for 1400 years.

However, before Culpeper appeared on the scene, knowledge of the medicine was only available to learned medics. Culpeper sought instead to communicate this system of holistic healing to his fellow countrymen and women both by writing original works of his own and by translating those of the leading medical practitioners from Latin into English. During his lifetime Culpeper's books were immensely popular, and his popularity continues today: *Culpeper's Herbal* is still in print after over 300 years. Despite the fact that the book retains its author's 17th-century medical language, without any explanatory notes, the sales of the book show that the substance of his words is just as relevant today as it was then, founded as it is upon principles of health still observed by millions of people. This book therefore aims to uncover these principles and to describe Culpeper's practice of Western holistic medicine so that the applicability of this medicine will be apparent to today's reader.

Historians of medicine are now revising their opinion of Culpeper. In the last few decades, he has been rehabilitated from the 'vituperative quack' who practised medicine illegitimately and irritated the august Royal College of Physicians in the process, to a much more significant figure. As F N L Poynter, former Director of the Wellcome Institute for the History of Medicine, observed:

> If our concern is the history of medicine as it was professed and practised, then Culpeper is a figure of outstanding importance, for he had a far greater influence on medical practice in England between 1650 and 1750 than either Harvey or Sydenham [the

discoverer of the circulation of the blood and 'the English Hippocrates' respectively]. His writings reflect faithfully the orthodox medicine of his own time, and his translations of the leading European medical writers of his age gave to English doctors for the first time a comprehensive body of medical literature in their own tongue which represented the best contemporary authorities.[1]

A few years ago, the first full-length biography of the man appeared. This work on the English herbalist and astrologer, written by Olav Thulesius,[2] reveals Culpeper to be an early scientist of the modern school, for his time particularly knowledgeable about anatomy, paediatrics and materia medica. Thulesius, however, denies Culpeper the authorship of several works, notably his *Treatise of Aurum Potabile*, in which he explains the philosophy he followed, and has reduced Culpeper's medical astrology to, in the words of a reviewer, a 'simplistic discussion'.[3] Moreover, he fails to give a satisfactory explanation for Culpeper's failure to accept Harvey's discovery of the circulation of the blood. Yet, despite these errors of comprehension (as I see them), I am indebted to Thulesius for adding to my knowledge about the details of Culpeper's life and I refer the reader to his biography in several places in the text.

This book is not intended to be a new biograpy of Culpeper, although Part 1 will introduce the reader to the known facts of his life and work. Rather, it will be an exposition of Culpeper's holistic practice of medicine. In the expanding world of holistic medicine today, much attention and credit is being paid to traditional systems of healing in which the emphasis is on the functioning of the human mind and body together, both in respect to their separate organs or parts and also with regard to the operation and integrity of the whole being. Mind, body and spirit are one unity and health is defined as wholeness. This is contrasted with modern Western medicine which treats the mind and body as separate, as parts of a machine, with the focus on what has gone wrong with the machine. The emphasis here is not so much on physiology, function and relationship, but on pathology, a knowledge derived from the dissection of dead and spiritless bodies. Treatment is directed towards reversing or halting cellular changes or to replacing the parts. As Kerry Bone, a respected herbalist, commented:

An excessive focus on pathology will lead to a medical system which is interventionist and directed towards compensating for the physiological deficiencies and imbalances which arise in disease, without seeking a greater understanding of how they arose in the first place. The basic strategy will be superficial and short term. This is increasingly the orthodox medical system which we have today. While it is a very useful system for advanced pathologies and life-threatening states, it is incomplete.[4]

So-called natural systems of healing are becoming recognized for their ability to complete or complement this medicine, by virtue of their holistic orientation, particularly with cases of chronic functional complaints and less advanced diseases. Indeed, with the overuse of chemicals and antibiotics – and the subsequent creation of resistant 'super-bugs' – the case for the inclusion of natural medicines in orthodox treatment is strong. This is especially so when it is remembered that 80 per cent of people die, not in intensive care or on the operating table, but from chronic illnesses. If these people had been treated by a holistic practitioner at an earlier stage in the disease process, many of them might have had a very different lease of life.

Such 'energetic' systems of healing were once widely available in the West, as they are today in China and India. As the herbalist David Frawley stated:

> Systems which organize medicines and diseases according to prime elements, energies and biological humours reflect the language of nature and are more effective in transmitting nature's healing power … Such systems did exist in ancient and medieval Western medicine. Fragments of them endured into the early part of this century. Though once common, their traces have largely been eradicated and discredited by allopathic medicine. Now that the limitations of allopathy are clear to many of us, the validity of these traditional systems is again becoming apparent.[5]

Culpeper's Medicine is my contribution to the rediscovery of traditional Western medicine. I intend to show that the philosophies and principles of this energetic system of medicine are just as relevant and applicable today, and I propose to do this by looking closely at the medicine which Culpeper practised and the philosophy underpinning its concepts.

Such principles did not stand by themselves as generalities but were part of an integrated approach to health and disease. My aim therefore is to introduce the reader to the fundamentals of

Culpeper's medicine and to set it into its context so that the knowledge contained in Culpeper's writings, particularly his *Herbal*, will be more comprehensible and so open to further examination.

Although traditional Western medicine has suffered a break in transmission, it is of far more cultural relevance to Europeans and their descendants than the energetic systems of Chinese, Indian or Tibetan medicine. Descriptions such as sanguine, melancholic and phlegmatic, for example, still convey much of their former meaning and are more readily comprehensible to a European than the terminology of Eastern systems.

The consideration given to diet also shows just how relevant the principles of Western holistic medicine are today. A recent paper[6] suggested that advances in the understanding of the effects of free radicals on the body, which has brought the latest trend of antioxidant therapy and underlined the importance of fruit and vegetables in the diet, may lend more credibility to toxaemia theories and to the restoration and promotion of eliminative functions in the sick advocated by naturopaths, herbalists and osteopaths over the last century and more. It should be apparent, reading this book, where those ideas came from.

The discrediting of traditional Western medicine from a modern point of view focuses on two points in particular: the lack of knowledge of the circulation of the blood at the time, and of bacteria as the causes of infections. In the Western tradition, the heart was the organ from which the vital faculty arose. The vital spirits, by which every part of the body is made alive, were reckoned to be elaborated in the heart from breath, or pneuma, and blood. The spirits flowed along the arteries, their force creating a pulse. It was believed that blood could pass from one side of the heart to the other through passages in the walls of the chambers. The heart was thus whole, as the faith in a unified cosmos was wholehearted. However, Harvey's discovery – that blood must be pumped from one side of the heart through the lungs and entire body in order to move to the other side – showed that the heart was divided. The psychotherapist James Hillman wrote of this discovery as the moment of birth of the 'dead heart' in Western consciousness. For the heart, with an impassable wall down its middle, was reduced to a machine part, a mere pump and no longer the courageous heart of a lion. Hillman noted that 'the evisceration of tradition takes place when the heart loses its relation with organic nature, its empathy with all things, when the core of our breast moves from an animal to a mechanical imagination.'[7]

The heart as machine then became a tyrant, he went on, and heart and circulatory diseases were now 'the number one killers': 'It cannot be trusted; we cannot have faith in the very organ which once was the source of faith. The heart has become my enemy, my killer, my death.'

Without the knowledge of bacterial infection, physicians of the past concerned themselves with the maintenance of health more than with fighting the 'war against disease'. In fact, as medical historian Roy Porter pointed out,[8] until antibiotics were pioneered in the 1930s there was no medicine for curing lethal diseases. However, whilst many lives have been saved by antibiotics which may otherwise have been lost, these drugs and other potentially harmful chemicals are now frequently prescribed for many non-life-threatening infections. Regarding infections, as a case in point, Kerry Bone compares traditional and orthodox treatments:

> The traditional approach is to support immunity and to fine tune the normal physiological responses to infection such as fever In contrast the orthodox approach is to suppress the fever and kill the bacteria with antibiotics, thereby compensating for weakened or overloaded bodily defences. The latter approach has life-saving value, but will not prevent infections from recurring. The traditional approach may see a higher rate of failure in acute situations, although this is debatable, but will lead to improved immunity and a reduced rate of recurrent infections.[9]

The reapplication of this gentler approach could, therefore, complement and balance the undoubted and impressive achievements of modern emergency medicine. Thus, in Bone's words, 'clearly, an important complementary role for traditional medicine can be argued'.

Culpeper's medicine, however, was not confined to the practice of Western holistic medicine alone. An integral part of the medicine he practised was the use of astrology. He used it throughout his work, in diagnosis, prognosis and prescription. In Culpeper's time the unity of the cosmos, of heaven and earth, was generally accepted, so it seemed quite conceivable that connections existed between the planets and stars above and human life below. As Jim Tester remarked:

> The acceptance [of astrology] as a learned and scientific study was a
> common, if not the normal, attitude to it down to the 18th century,
> and it is impossible to understand men like Kepler and Newton
> unless astrology is seen for what the Greeks made it, a rational
> attempt to map the heavens and to interpret that map in the context
> of that 'cosmic sympathy' which makes man an integral part of the
> universe.[10]

Indeed the attractions of astrology are still prevalent today and
the art has had high-profile supporters in the 20th century. In
1928 Rudyard Kipling, addressing the Royal Society of Medicine,
made an earnest plea for the restoration of astrological medicine:

> Suppose, then, at some future time when the bacteriologist and the
> physicist are for the moment at a standstill, wouldn't it be interesting
> if they took their problem to the astronomer and in modern scientific
> language, of course, put to him Nicholas Culpeper's curious question
> 'What was the aspect of the heavens when such and such phenomena
> were observed?'[11]

Generally, however, the acceptance of astrology among scientists,
doctors and educated people began to wane in the decades
following Culpeper's death in 1654. For Culpeper, there were
social, political and religious reasons behind his stance but a new
enlightenment, which revealed the human body as a machine
and distanced it from the heavens and from the soul, was being
propagated in place of the holistic embrace of all that cosmic
sympathy implied. In the early part of the 17th century, one
opponent of astrology, a Northamptonshire physician by the
name of John Cotta, conceded that astral forces might exist but
said they were mediated by other less remote factors more
amenable to action by a doctor. This was no rejection of astrology
but a choice about emphasis, about what was to be considered
more important. However, alongside the more recent
reacceptance of traditional medicine, astrology is enjoying a
sustained resurgence in popularity. I intend therefore to clarify
Culpeper's application of astrology to medicine so that readers
can make that choice for themselves.

While the reapplication of astrology to medicine may be
controversial, the demise of the use of Culpeper's medicine is
recent and partial. Hakim G M Chishti has noted that:

Many people may be unaware that herbal medicine served as the primary mode of medical practice in the United States until almost 1935 ... Of course, this practice did change as chemical medicine burst on the scene with penicillin. Yet prior to 1935 – for perhaps two thousand years prior to that date – all physicians accepted and adhered to the humoral basis of both human and herbal constitution.[12]

Humoral medicine has always had its supporters. Henry Sigerist, the famous historian of medicine, pointed out that:

Every medical theory is based on observation and reasoning, and every period thinks with the concepts available at the time. The humoral theory was the result of many brilliant and correct observations. It was logical, explained many phenomena of health and disease, and gave valuable guidance to the medical practitioner.[13]

Hans Eysenck also seems to be positive about the Doctrine of the Four Temperaments when he says that 'the highly successful typology thus established all those years ago was based on careful observation and provided a paradigm for scientific investigation that has lasted over two thousand years and may still have something to teach us'.[14]

I believe that, in the pages which follow, the reader will find this to be true.

PART 1

A Student of Physick and Astrology:
The Life and Death of Nicholas Culpeper
1616–1654

Nicholas Culpeper was born on 18 October 1616 a little after noon, probably at Ockley in Surrey,[1] and was baptized there, in St Margaret's Church, on 24 October. His father, also named Nicholas Culpeper and the rector of Ockley, 'a most eminently pious Minister, and much reverenced for his virtuous Qualities',[2] had been buried in that same churchyard just 19 days earlier.[3] Sudden death at the age of 36 had denied him the joy of seeing the birth of his first child and had deprived the infant Nicholas of a father. His mother, Mary Attersoll, stricken with grief and required to vacate the vicarage at Ockley, returned with her baby son to her father, the Reverend William Attersoll, rector of the parish of St Margaret's at Isfield in Sussex.

The Culpepers were a prolific and at one time ubiquitous family, originating, as far as can be traced, from Kent. The earliest mention of the Culpeper name is that of Thomas de Colepeper who was a Justice of the Great Assize in the reign of King John.[4] A century later his descendant Thomas Culpeper was keeper of Leeds Castle in Kent, a property which the Hollingbourne branch of the family came to own in Nicholas Culpeper's lifetime. The family coat of arms is first borne by a Culpeper in 1327 and its similarity to the coats of arms of other distinguished families in Kent may suggest that the Culpepers 'rose to their high position by a wealthy alliance and … acquired their coat armour with their property'.[5]

As generation followed generation, so several branches of the Culpeper family were formed. Nicholas Culpeper belonged to that part of the family whose seat was Wakehurst Place in Sussex. This property was obtained when Culpeper's great-great-grandfather, also named Nicholas, together with his brother Richard, abducted with offence and then married with honour the two Wakehurst heiresses, Margaret and Elizabeth, who had been placed in the charge of Sir John Culpeper of Bedgebury. The fortunes of the Culpepers of Wakehurst reached its climax in the latter part of the 16th and first half of the 17th centuries, followed by a disastrous downfall before 1700.

In the long line of Culpepers there were many illustrious individuals and even a Queen of England. For Catherine Howard, the fifth wife of Henry VIII, was the daughter of a Culpeper of the Oxenhoath branch. She was beheaded in 1542 aged 21, after only 18 months of marriage to the King, having been found guilty of adultery with her cousin Thomas Culpeper who was also executed for his crime. Their liaison, conducted with particular indiscretion, had been an open secret at court, the King being the last to find out.

Another family story concerns Sir Thomas and Walter Culpeper, sons of Thomas Culpeper, the keeper of Leeds Castle in Kent. The two were executed in 1321 for refusing Queen Isabella, the estranged wife and later enemy of King Edward II, admission to the castle. It is interesting to note that, although there is no satisfactory explanation of the origin of the name, Culpeper may be a nickname signifying the giving of offence or mischief-making, since the word 'pepper' symbolized this in popular understanding. Several Culpepers over the generations have 'got up the noses' of very important people, notwithstanding the likelihood of this for a distinguished and well-placed family. Nicholas Culpeper was to be no exception.

Two Culpepers were created baronets and as many as 12 members of the family were knighted, including Sir Edward Culpeper, the builder of Wakehurst Place (1590), and Sir Thomas Culpeper of the Hollingbourne branch, the first of the family to own Leeds Castle. This property was later purchased by Sir John Culpeper of the Wigsell branch who was MP for Kent in the Long Parliament, made Chancellor of the Exchequer in 1642, Master of the Rolls in 1643 and created Lord Culpeper in 1644. He was a loyal Royalist who accompanied Prince Charles (later Charles II) into exile in France and who returned with him to England at the Restoration of the Monarchy in 1660. Thomas, the second Lord Culpeper, was governor of Virginia in the Americas (1677–83) and his daughter Catherine married the fifth Lord Fairfax. The

Culpeper peerage became extinct in 1725 and the whole family died out.[6]

Nicholas Culpeper seems to have had little to do with his father's distinguished family[7] but was raised by his mother's family in the vicarage at Isfield. His grandfather, William Attersoll, had been appointed rector of the parish of St Margaret's in 1599. He had two degrees from Cambridge, wrote many theological books and was considered an important scholar in his day. A Puritan, serious, studious, and dissatisfied with the poor intellectual and financial rewards in his country parish,[8] he proved unpopular with his parishioners on account of his inability to inspire them from the pulpit and his unwillingness to socialize with them in daily life.[9] His library and his studies were his refuge.

William's daughter Mary was one of six children born to his wife Anne who died in 1624.[10] Mary Attersoll was no doubt influenced and aided by her father in her care for young Nicholas's education for 'she spent four hundred pounds on her said son, for his diet, schooling and his being at the University of Cambridge, where he continued some years, profited in all manner of learning, and gained the applause of the University whilst he remained there.'[11]

Culpeper attended a free-school in Sussex and went up to Cambridge in 1632[12] aged 16. His initial compulsory studies at Cambridge would have been Latin, in continuation of his schooling, together with some Greek. His mother and grandfather had then hoped that Nicholas would go on to study divinity and enter the church, as both he and the boy's own father had done. Nicholas clearly had other ideas. We learn that 'Mr Attersoll had formerly used his best arguments, though to no purpose to persuade him to embrace the Ministerial Function' and that 'he perceived contrary to his intention that Mr Culpeper bent his inclinations from the time that he was about ten years of age to … astrology and occult philosophy'.[13] Not that astrology and religion were incompatible,[14] for in that age many God-fearing persons believed that God had created the seven planets and the stars, set them in motion and ordered them so that they might reflect his will to those down below who had the knowledge to read the signs. And after all, where would he have read of astrology at the tender age of ten if not in books from his own grandfather's library? Yet Puritan ministers such as Attersoll, whilst they may well have possessed texts on such matters, would likely have followed Calvinist teaching in condemning it openly with great zeal.

Culpeper also seems to have shown an interest in medicinal herbs from an early age. Writing later in his famous herbal, he refers to the common names used in Sussex for some of them. We do not know, however, whether Culpeper had gone to Cambridge in order to study medicine or whether he simply intended to attend the lectures on medical subjects, while still engaged with Greek and Latin. It is not implausible that he intended to obtain a medical degree subsequently,[15] but he was young, no doubt impulsive and was enjoying himself at Cambridge. As it turned out, he never took a degree of any sort.

It was through an affair of the heart that providence stepped into Nicholas Culpeper's life and changed it forever. During his studies at Cambridge the young man was sufficiently in love with a lady to plan to elope with her in true Culpeper style; he meant to abandon his education and former life and to marry and to live in hiding until the parents were reconciled to the deed. The story is movingly told in a contemporary narrative:

> One of the first diversions that he has amongst some other smaller transactions and changes, none of his life proving more unfortunate, was, that he had engaged himself in the love of a beautiful lady. I shall not name her for some reasons. Her father was reported to be one of the noblest and wealthiest in Sussex. This fair lady after many generous treatments, as Mr Culpeper might clearly perceive, entertained the tenders of his service so far as to requite him with her entire and sincere affections. And though the strictness of parents have often too severe eyes over their children, yet where hearts are once united, lovers use to break through all difficulties. The riches of the lady, (which might have enchanted inferior spirits) in respect of the virtuous inclinations of her mind and person, had no power over him, so that like a true lover, the language of his eyes and his heart were the same, in so much that the languishing sincerities of these suffering inamoratos, put them to the extremity of the determination, some way to set a period to their martyrdoms. Mr Culpeper having then supplied himself with two hundred pounds from his mother, during his abode at Cambridge, his fair mistress and he by letters and otherwise, plotted secretly with the assistance of a gentlewoman that waited on her to pack up such rich jewels, and other necessaries as might best appertain to a journey, and so secretly to make their escape near to Lewes in Sussex, where they intended to marry; and afterwards for a season to live privately till the incensed parents were pacified. But this happiness was denied them by the malevolence of Mars, and some other envious planets, as you shall find in his nativity.

Not to vex the expectation of the reader any longer, but rather to epitomise so sad a story, Mr Culpeper hastes from Cambridge. His mistress with those that she durst trust were gone part of their way to meet him at the appointed place. But it pleased the great disposer of terrene affairs to order it otherwise. The lady and her servant being suddenly surprised with a dreadful storm, with fearful claps of thunder, surrounded with flames of fire and flashes of lightening, with some of which Mr Culpeper's fair mistress was so stricken, that she immediately fell down dead, exchanging of this life for a better, her marriage on earth for one in heaven. When the lady was stripped, all the marks that could be found on her fair body, was only a blue spot on her right side about the breadth of one's hand. The news of this sad accident met Mr Culpeper as he journeyed towards his dead to him, but otherwise a still living saint. At the instant when this direful mischance befell him, Sir Nicholas Astey his intimate acquaintance passing by, chanced to be an eye-witness to this sad disaster, who used the best rhetoric he had to comfort him in this his affliction. He took him up in his coach, and conveyed him to his mother, who not expecting then to have seen him, received him with a great deal of joy, till being truly sensible of his sorrow; she for that cause left that county, and afterwards fell into a fit of sickness which she was never rid of till her dying day.

It is impossible to express the sorrow of so true a lover as Mr Culpeper was, the strangeness of this misfortune being enough to shake the strongest resolutions of the most established person of the world. I shall only acquaint the reader with what I have heard of his best friends, that when that he was serious even to entertain the deepest melancholy that his frailty could suffer on earth, that then he would discourse at large the sad fate of his unfortunate mistress. This lady on whom this unhappy accident fell, had two thousand pounds in personal estate, and five hundred pounds a year. The loss of this jewel which Mr Culpeper valued above all worldly considerations, cast him into so deep a melancholy that he left the University of Cambridge, so that it was high time for his grandfather Mr William Attersoll whose care he was, to think of some seasonable way to divert this his extraordinary distemper.[16]

This calamitous event is likely to have taken place in the summer of 1634. By the autumn Nicholas, no doubt still numb with the awful shock of having lost his beloved in such a cruel way, was no longer of a mind to return to his studies at Cambridge nor to pursue any entry into the church. Then 'Mr Attersoll with the advice of friends, consulted how to dispose of Mr Culpeper, which was to send him to London where they placed him with Mr White, an apothecary near Temple Bar, to whom they gave with him fifty pounds. He not having been with him above a year and a half, Mr White failed, his necessities compelling him to go into Ireland with the loss of Mr Culpeper's money.'[17] After the departure of his master, Culpeper was helped to become apprenticed to another apothecary, Francis Drake, who lived in Threadneedle Street with his existing apprentice Samuel Leadbetter.[18] When Drake died, in February 1639, Leadbetter had just become a licensee of the Society of Apothecaries, or a 'master of the pestle', and was in a position to take over the running of his former master's shop. He and Culpeper had obviously struck up a friendship during their training because Culpeper agreed to set up in business with him at this time, though he had been 'turned over' to Mr Higgins, a warden of the Society, for the duration of his apprenticeship.[19]

At the time that Culpeper and Leadbetter went into practice together there was increasing opposition between the apothecaries and their overseers, the Royal College of Physicians, after an initial concord. Apothecaries, originally wholesale merchants and spice importers, had grown in number with the spread of retail trade and had become one of the fastest growing occupational groups in early modern England, with many shops in London and an increasing number in provincial capitals. As their numbers grew, the Royal College of Physicians became concerned about their powers.

The Royal College had been founded as a learned society by a royal charter of Henry VIII in 1518 and had gained statutory authority in 1523, by which the members of the College, now having the right to be sole practitioners of physick in London and within seven miles of the city, were granted juridical powers to hand down penalties on those infringing on this right. By an act of 1553 the college had further obtained the right to inspect the wares of apothecaries. Under James I the College had been able to exert considerable political influence, particularly through its Royal Physician, Sir Theodore de Mayerne, formerly the royal physician of the French King Henri IV, who had moved to the English court in 1610 and had accepted a fellowship of the College in 1616. During this period the College tried to separate the apothecaries from the Grocers' Company, one of the 12 great livery companies of London, and to give them separate status in imitation of the situation prevailing in France. This attempt had been met with fierce opposition from both the Grocers' Company and the City of London but finally proved successful in 1617 when the Worshipful Society of Apothecaries was formed by royal fiat. In the following year the College published an official pharmacopoeia which specified the drugs the apothecaries were allowed to dispense. The apothecaries as a result found themselves increasingly subordinated to the Royal College of Physicians. Only members of the Society could now practise the trade of apothecary, and their practice was restricted to selling medicines prescribed by physicians and to dispensing only medicines listed in the pharmacopoeia. In addition the College retained the right to inspect the drugs in their shops and to examine apprentices who wished to become members of the Society.[20]

The Royal College of Physicians sought to fine or imprison unlicensed practitioners or upstart apothecaries for practising any kind of medicine. Despite this the apothecaries continued to engage in general medical practice. They found themselves, as before, working alongside other practitioners of varying kinds who tried to meet the medical needs of a population too poor in most cases to afford a physician and too numerous for the numbers of physicians in London to attend individually. For there was roughly one licentiate of the Royal College of Physicians for every five thousand of the general populace.[21]

Among the other practitioners were the surgeons. The United Company of Barber-Surgeons had been formed in 1540, and its members were legally restricted to setting bones, healing outward sores and wounds with topical preparations, carrying out bleeding and undertaking operations such as amputations and 'cutting for the stone' (bladder stones). Herbalists, midwives and 'wise women' formed another group who tended the sick in their own communities. Those with 'the knowledge of the nature, kind and operation of certain herbs, roots and waters' had been given protection from prosecution by the physicians or surgeons by an Act of Parliament of 1542 (disparagingly known as the 'Quacks' charter'), but could only practise provided their treatment was given free of charge for certain specified conditions 'for the ease and comfort, succour, help, relief and health of the King's poor subjects'.[22] There were also travelling 'mountebanks', 'empirics' and 'quacks' who hawked their elixirs and panaceas in the villages and towns they entered.

The fact that the apothecaries, not content with their own

monopoly over the sale of drugs, were continuing to offer treatment in this general medical marketplace made the Royal College of Physicians increasingly angry. The College's censors tried to enforce the law and in 1634 clashed with the Society of Apothecaries over accusations that several of the Society's members were practising medicine. For their part, the Society entered a petition against the College during the Short Parliament of 1640 in response to further attacks on the activities of its members. The petition came to nothing as the parliament was soon dissolved by the King. Indeed, the rapidly changing and very volatile political situation at this time, on the eve of the Civil War, ruled out any early chance of resolving the College's predicament. After the Long Parliament was convened in 1641 (in perpetuity until it chose to dissolve itself), the College, seeing the way the wind was changing, became more concerned about its own security in the face of the imminent war than it was over the activities of unlicensed practitioners. Some of its members chose to go abroad for the duration, others kept a low political profile.[23] Such was the situation in which Samuel Leadbetter and Nicholas Culpeper set up their practice from their former master's shop in Bishopsgate.

Culpeper's association with Leadbetter continued until late 1643 or 1644. However, Culpeper never satisfactorily completed his training for the Society of Apothecaries and so was never a 'master of the pestle'. Moreover, on entering business with Leadbetter, he rather widened his approach, for we learn that 'for some space of time he studied physick' (medicine),[24] by which the writer means that Culpeper began to practise as an English physician. Leadbetter received two reprimands from the Society of Apothecaries concerning his unlicensed colleague. On 3 June 1643 he was 'ordered and warned to put away Nicholas Culpeper who so now employed in his shop', then on 22 September 'Mr Leadbetter is warned not to employ Culpeper in the making or administering of any medicine who promised to obey the same'.[25]

It is strange that Culpeper had not become a licensee of the Society of Apothecaries by this time. Details of Culpeper's life are few and far between and some reading between the lines is therefore necessary. It is possible that Culpeper's wholly illicit collaboration with Leadbetter, before completion of his apprenticeship, made him enemies at the Society and he was obstructed from sitting the examination. In fact Culpeper was imprisoned and tried for witchcraft on 17 December 1642, so it may well be that the opposition to his practice by high-ranking apothecaries, or perhaps by members of the Royal College of Physicians, became so fierce that this was engineered by false accusations. The offence of witchcraft carried the death-sentence but Culpeper was found not guilty and acquitted of the charge.[26]

A more likely reason could be that Culpeper's great desire to help the poor and needy of England in a direct and practical way, that compassionate concern for which he was later held in great regard, led him straight into illegal practice, not only as an apothecary but also as a physician. It would not have furthered his desire to help the poor, especially in the uncontrolled and calamitous times of the 1640s, to belong to an organisation that claimed a monopoly on the sale of medicines and charged high prices. On the contrary, Culpeper's heart-felt sympathy for the 'commonalty of England' in its poverty and deprivation eventually led him to adopt extreme political views. For not only was he for Parliament and the Commonwealth and against the Crown and the established Church, but he was a revolutionary who believed that the downfall of the King of England heralded the collapse of all nations and the establishment of a truly just and compassionate 'Fifth Monarchy' (ie the human approximation to the eternal reign of Christ, as foretold in the Bible by the Book of Daniel).

During the Civil War Culpeper fought for the Parliamentarians against the King, apparently without neglecting his medical practice all the while, and sometime in 1643 he received a gun-shot wound to the chest.[27] He also fought a duel during this period of which nothing is known except that 'he was forced to flee into France, remaining there a quarter of a year till the cure was perfected at his own expense'.[28] After the execution of King Charles I he waged a war of words against the crowned heads of all countries through the astrological prophecies contained in his yearly almanacs and foretold of the establishment of true democracy for the peoples of the world.

At the beginning of 1640, Culpeper must have had little to his name, but that was all to change in the course of a very eventful year. He not only entered practice with his colleague Leadbetter but now there were also changes for him in family life. His mother Mary had died a year earlier, in 1639, apparently never having recovered from the tragedy which befell her son and his intended bride on that fateful day five years before. Now Culpeper learned of the death of his grandfather, William Attersoll.[29] Again the contemporary biography provides us with one of Culpeper's choice turns of phrase in response to this event:

> Mr. Attersoll had formerly used his best arguments, though to no purpose, to persuade him to embrace the ministerial function, with an intention as it was supposed to after his decease to have settled his estate on him. Which, since he would not hearken to, he divided four hundred pounds a year amongst the rest of his grandchildren, and left him but a legacy of forty shillings, which was paid by the two executors at Nathaniel Brook his shop at the Angel in Cornhill. This small sum he received with a smile, and said, he had courted two mistresses that had cost him very dear, but it was not the wealth of kingdoms should buy them from him.[30]

The 'two mistresses' Culpeper refers to are Physick and Astrology. But these were not his only loves; another was to bring him much more than he was denied by his disapproving grandfather, as we discover when the story is resumed:

> ... though he was courted by his friends to alter the condition of his single life, he would admit of no such proffers, till like a skilful astrologer he had fixed his eyes upon the firmament, where Venus the star of his own affections governed, surrendering all the powers and faculties of his soul to the virtues and beauty of Mrs Alice Field ... whom it was his happiness afterwards to espouse at fifteen years of age. A gentlewoman who as she was of good extraction, so also, besides her richer qualities, her admirable discretion, and excellent breeding, she brought him a considerable fortune.

The money that marriage to Alice Field brought him was not important to Culpeper. Indeed Culpeper's mind and soul were fixed on such high aspirations that he cared little or nothing for his own material comforts. Brought up in a Puritan home, he was a 'despiser of the world' who 'was so far from covetousness that he cared not who was his purse-bearer, so long as he wanted not for necessary expenses, he durst trust God's providence with the rest. His mind was surprised with higher mysteries than to stoop to such worldly trifles.'[31] He was very free with his money, to the point of prodigality, at least from the time of his going up to Cambridge. He was known to say 'that the world was made for him to tread on, he would not stoop to fill his pockets with it'.

This applied just as much to possessions enjoyed by the mind. For, 'he had not many books, but those that he had were well selected. He was none of those that persuaded the world he was learned, by the getting together of a great library.'

However, Alice's dowry did mean that Culpeper could now afford to have his own home built. He was soon ensconced with his new wife in their new house in Spitalfields, outside the city walls of London, on Red Lion Street. The name Spitalfields derives from the priory and house of charity built there, 'St Mary Spittel without Bishopsgate'. This had been closed and pulled down by order of Henry VIII and the area had fallen into decay and squalor. Spital Square had been given to the Artillery Company and gunmen from the Tower of London used to practise firing their cannons in the open space there. In the year the Culpepers moved to Spitalfields, the Artillery Company found a new field for their gun practice in Finsbury. Later on in the century the district became known as the silk weavers' quarters, after the French immigrants who lived there and wove silk. It is quite characteristic of Culpeper that he should set up home in what was, and still is, an unfashionable and impoverished area of London.

When Leadbetter succumbed to pressure from the Society of Apothecaries to remove Culpeper from his shop, in later 1643 or 1644, Culpeper chose to set up his own practice at his home in Spitalfields. There he lived, practising astrology and medicine and writing his many works and translations until his death on 10 January 1654.

Culpeper 'acquired a high reputation among his patients in the East of London'.[32] He 'appears to have been as much of a philanthropist as illness and poverty allowed'.[33]

> Those that knew him rightly affirm that he was so charitable to his poor country-men, that the money that he received from rich persons, he spread upon the waters, laid it forth for the good of those that were in want, though through his charity he was sometimes necessitated [ie. without money himself]. He would not participate of any thing from the meaner sort of people, he only desired their prayers. I have heard those that rightly knew him say, that when he might have had a large sum to have gone to a rich person, he rather chose to go to one of his poor neighbours that hath been sick, where he hath given away his physick. Which some of his friends wondering at, he hath said, His conscience would not suffer him to do otherwise:

the Rich could not want help for their money, but the poor must perish if his charity did not relieve them.[34]

These testimonies show Culpeper to have been a very compassionate man who was most concerned about the welfare of his fellow countrymen. The legal status of the monopolies of the Royal College of Physicians over the treatment of disease in and around London, and of the Society of Apothecaries over the sale of medicines, meant nothing to him, especially when they acted against the interest of the poor and the sick in his community.

> Send for them [physicians] to a poor man's house who is not able to give them their fee, then they will not come, and the poor creature for whom Christ died must forfeit his life for want of money.[35]

Culpeper though did not expect physicians, surgeons and apothecaries to treat patients free of charge and at their own expense, as he often did, careless as he was of money. Instead he saw other and better ways of organizing medical provision:

> Physicians in Italy may not deny to go to any patient (if at leisure) that sends for them provided that they have their fee which (if they go alone) is about eighteen pence.[36]

This was far more affordable than the usual fee of an English physician who charged an 'angel', a gold coin to the value of 10 shillings, or the fee of an apothecary offering physick who would charge almost as much. In addition, the knowledge of medicine which such apothecaries enjoyed must have varied a lot and have been questionable in many cases. The continuing practice of writing medical books in Latin was intended to limit knowledge of medicine to the small group of learned physicians in the country. The *Pharmacopoeia,* or *London Dispensatory* as it was known, laid out the official medicines prescribed by the physicians that apothecaries were supposed to prepare. It was written in Latin, which must have posed many problems for them. It has been suggested that some of Culpeper's apothecary friends asked him, with his knowledge of Latin and Greek, to write his translation of the *Pharmacopoeia,* as he may well have been transcribing into English many of the formulae and prescriptions for them already.[37] It is certainly the case that he was asked to do it for we are told that he was 'so unexpectedly taken notice of, as to be put upon the Translation of the Doctors Dispensatory'.[38]

The publication of an English translation of the London

Dispensatory could hardly fail to have political ramifications and it is surely no coincidence that Culpeper's translation came into print in 1649, after the execution of Charles I in January that year. Those who had persuaded him into the project may have been apothecaries or they could have been staunch supporters of the new Commonwealth with a concern for the state of medical provision in England. In either case Culpeper's name was henceforth known far and wide throughout the land.

Needless to say, the appearance of *A Physical Directory or a Translation of the London Dispensatory* brought Culpeper much condemnation and abuse 'obviously inspired by political opponents and the societies whose monopolies Culpeper was charged with having infringed'.[39] One such attack appeared in the Royalist paper *Mercurius Pragmaticus*:

> The Pharmacopoeia was done very filthily into English by one Nicholas Culpeper who commenced the several degrees of Independence, Brownisme, Anabaptism. Admitted himself of John Goodwin's school of all ungodliness in Coleman Street. After he turned Seeker, Manifestation, and now he is arrived at the battlement of an absolute Atheist, and by two years' drunken labour hath 'Gallimawfred' the apothecaries book into nonsense, mixing every receipt therein with some scruples, at least, of rebellion or atheism, besides the danger of poisoning men's bodies. And to supply his drunkenness and lechery with a thirty shilling reward endeavoured to bring into obloquy the famous societies of apothecaries and chyrurgeons.[40]

A notable piece of abuse was penned by William Johnson, the College's new chemist:

> Pray let me not trouble your weak brains with a relation of a Gentleman and Scholar's censure upon your book, who perusing some passages in it in a Booksellers shop, asked whether Culpeper hath made Cul-paper, paper fit to wipe ones breech withall.[41]

Alongside such abuse came the criticism that the publishing of the pharmacopoeia in English would endanger lives by encouraging unskilled readers to meddle with powerful medicines. This was a standard form of attack made by the Royal College of Physicians on unlicensed practitioners at the time to reinforce their own threatened position and to try to re-establish the notion that medicine was safe only in the hands of university-trained and properly licensed physicians. Culpeper had already defended himself in the book in this way:

> All the ancient physicians wrote their own mother tongue and native language. Mesue, Avicenna, Rhazes, Serapio in Arabic, Galen and Hippocrates in Greek, Paracelsus in High Dutch. Did these do their countries good or harm, think ye? What reason can be given why England should be deprived of the benefit of other nations?

After the criticism which followed the first edition, he introduced a concluding statement to the next (and final) two editions of the original *London Dispensatory*, criticizing the College's regard for its own interests but nevertheless warning the reader that physic must be approached in a sober and serious way:

> I am not conscious to myself that I have justly given offence to any by translating this work. If any take offence, it is to be shrewdly suspected it ariseth from self-interests. Once more let me advise the ignorant not to be too busy with what they have no skill in. For as physick (as the never dying Hippocrates truly saith) was never ordained for disorderly and disobedient persons, so was the administration of it never ordained for dunces. Therefore let everyone that administers physick seriously consider the great accompt must be made another day, before God, and the Lord Jesus Christ, and the holy angels. And do nothing rashly, but upon serious consideration, as he desires it should fare well with him when the lord comes to make acquisition for blood.[42]

It was, anyway, beyond the powers of the College to succeed in taking legal action at this time against a man clearly in support of the new Commonwealth and of the common people. The King had been executed, the House of Lords abolished and the Long Parliament reduced to a tenth of its former number with only those who had supported the regicide remaining to conduct the business of government. The victorious Roundhead army represented the only restraint on this remnant or 'Rump' parliament and, in fact, the army leaders intended a complete dissolution of this ineffective parliament. In this political climate Culpeper's 'anti monarchical tenets and semisectarian religious opinions' found favour and his writings 'were welcomed by the parliamentary press'.[43] His call for the disbanding of the medical and legal professions and of the religious hierarchy was supported in the new Commonwealth:

> The Liberty of our Common-Wealth (if I may call it so without a solecism) is most infringed by three sorts of men, Priests, Physicians,

Lawyers; ... The one deceives men in matters belonging to their soul, the other in matters belonging to their bodies, and the third in matters belonging to their estates.[44]

Between 1651 and his death in January 1654, Culpeper promulgated his ideas for reform in the broad political arena through yearly almanacs. By means of the astrological interpretation of great conjunctions and annual ingresses, he deciphered the Will of God for such troubled times. The Civil War had its astrologers, who made predictions on the outcomes of battles and campaigns from the stars: George Wharton for the King's forces and, more successfully and famously, William Lilly for Cromwell and the Parliament. The same collapse of censorship over printed material which had allowed Culpeper to publish his translation of the College's pharmacopoeia had cleared the path for many others to enter into print on whatever subject was of concern to them. Many such writers of almanacs, broadsheets and pamphlets were astrologers and this 18-year period in the middle of the century saw a late flowering of English astrology.

Culpeper's first such publication, an *Ephemeris* (almanac) *for 1651*, came in the wake of the fame or notoriety he had gained as a result of publishing *A Physical Directory*. Interestingly, in the introduction to the ephemeris, dated 3 August 1650, Culpeper writes with apparent modesty that 'I peep out in print in this nature'. Perhaps he initially felt more tentative about such a publication especially as he included in the booklet the first printing of a short *Astrologo-Physical Discourse* so that the edition would still be serving the health needs of his fellow-countrymen. In justification, too, of such an almanac against the anticipated disapproval of many devout Presbyterians, Culpeper quoted the opening of *Psalm 19*: 'The Heavens declare the glory of God and the firmament sheweth forth his handiwork.' His meaning is that God set the planets in motion to rule over the elementary world, its changes and transformations. By his acceptance of the tenet of 'as above, so below', Culpeper could interpret signs in the heavenly perturbations of changes to come not only for the health or sickness of the microcosm which is the body of man but also, in the same sense, for the body politic. However, as Bernard Capp states:

Though stretching rather than breaking astrological laws, the political astrologers were clearly manipulating the stars into a party allegiance. It is impossible to discover how far this was a conscious process. Lilly's standards of professional ethics were by no means high. Men such as Wharton and Culpeper, however, displayed a passionate certainty concerning political issues of the nature of God's purpose on earth. They may well have believed that His message in the stars could be truthfully interpreted only in the way they have described. Astrological prophecy was thus akin to divine providence (epitomized in Cromwell's conviction that his victories were proof of divine support), and the possession of grace. All were controversial.[45]

Culpeper's 'passionate certainty' was more in evidence the following year in his publication of *Catastrophe Magnatum or The Fall of Monarchie. A Caveat to Magistrates, deduced from the eclipse of the Sunne, March 29th 1652. With a Probable Conjecture of determination of the Effects.* The pamphlet is addressed 'To the right Worshipful, Sir William Culpeper Knight and Baronet', Culpeper's relative, whom he had last seen around 15 years earlier and to whom he expressed the hope in his address that 'there is nothing in it unbeseeming the name of Culpeper'. This must have seemed unlikely, from the point of view of this high-ranking political figure, since Culpeper was now giving free rein to his hope of an imminent Fifth Monarchy for the fulfilment of which he 'predicted cheerfully the death and destruction of all the ruling heads'.[46] England had already achieved this, as the first step towards a new golden age.

> There was no republican astrologer to fill a role equivalent to that of Wharton. Most compilers accepted the Protectorate, and were even able to accommodate their millennial dreams within it. The most likely potential exception was Nicholas Culpeper, whose career was cut short by his early death in January 1654. His millenarian hopes had tended not towards a heroic conqueror but the withering away of states and rulers.[47]

The main celestial event under consideration in 1652 was the total eclipse of the sun on 29 March, which came to be known as 'Black Monday'. For Culpeper predicted in *Catastrophe Magnatum* that this would herald the invasion of the Turks, the fall of Kings and Popes, epidemic diseases and the establishment of a new order.[48] Other astrologers predicted similar calamities and the day was awaited with great trepidation.

There are reports of the rich fleeing from London, farmers driving livestock under cover, people laying in supplies of drinking water before it would be contaminated, sealing their windows with pitch and cowering in bed. Other accounts speak of deserted streets and abandoned markets, and even of breakdowns and suicides.[49]

Nothing characterized the inevitable anticlimax better than the fact that the eclipse was not total and there was no darkening of the sky. An anonymous pamphlet, *Black Munday Turn'd White* (sic), written days after the event, must have started the scorn and condemnation heaped on 'these great astrologers who by the help of tycho were able to guess at the time of the eclipse, yet could not tell whether the day would be clear or cloudy'.[50] This was followed by another pamphlet, presumably written in response to an astrologers' event organized for after the eclipse, for it was entitled *A Faire in Spittle Fields, where all the Knick Knack's of Astrology are Exposed to open Sale.*[51] It specifically attacked Culpeper, Lilly and Booker and captured in verse the most ignominious hour of these astrologers:

> ... the sun shone glorious, no Cummerian [Sumerian] shade
> made dark our dwellings, their predictions fail'd,
> their tales prov'd fables and the people rail'd
> against these jugglers whose prevarication's
> had filled their minds with such vain expectations.

No matter how correct any of the detailed predictions about the significance of the (partial) eclipse for England at that time may have turned out to be, 'Black Monday' must have represented a milestone. For by the end of the century, the widespread belief in astrology was increasingly rejected, particularly by the educated and scientific communities. Yet Culpeper's conviction about the validity of astrology would remain unshaken even if it were to transpire that his predictions were false. He discussed this possibility in the final chapter of the *Catastrophe Magnatum*, headed 'a fable for an epilogue':

> A few years will show whether what I have written be true or false. And he that carps at me before he knows that shows rather his own folly than my weakness.
>
> Imagine what I write be every word false, what harm will it do princes to prepare for the loss of a kingdom, though it never come? Is it not the way to teach them humility? I am sure they are proud enough. Were it not acceptable both before God and man that they would leave off their tyranny? Imagine such sicknesses never come to

the vulgar as I say this eclipse threatens. Will it do them any harm to make their peace with God, though they do not die? But most people send preparation for death before hand, and intend to overtake it on their death-beds.[52]

Culpeper accepts he may err like any other man in what he foresees, but he also takes into account human initiative as he does with medical astrology, which was his abiding concern. In the same way that the physician will struggle to preserve life and health despite all medical and astrological signs, he believed that a correct habit of body and moral rectitude can greatly benefit the health of a person or of a population; and it is in this spirit that his predictions for the nation seem to have been given, both here and again in his *Ephemeris for 1653*. This publication contained more dire predictions, notably for Londoners, of further outbreaks of plague, due to the conjunction of Mars and Saturn in Leo in both 1652 and 1654. The work is dedicated to his friend William Beal and addressed to the 'Reader that fears God'. In it he reiterates the axioms of astrology regarding fate and free will; that 'the wise man rules his stars, which can incline but not compel' and that 'the fates rule the foolish'. Finally, he says, 'he that is a wise man prepares his mind for every condition, and labours by art to increase what is good and mitigate what is bad'. Culpeper, by applying his astrological art to the health of the nation as a whole, tried to instruct his fellow countrymen on how to avoid what the signs of heaven foretold and what God might inflict on them if they did not mend their ways.

Culpeper write his *Ephemeris for 1653* 'from my house in Chesham in Buckinghamshire, August 20th 1652' where he had temporarily sought refuge. Culpeper had become sick and had been forced to consider his own health, leaving London to save himself from the plague he anticipated that summer in the city.

His attention in this period was focused primarily on medicine. In a second edition of his translation of the *Dispensatory*, published in 1650, Culpeper wrote: 'My pen (if God permit me life and health) shall never lie still, till I have given them the whole model of physick in the native language.[53] This was to be Culpeper's main project for the rest of his short life, while he had strength to continue. He would write medical texts in English, to be published at an affordable price for all his fellow countrymen to use in curing their ailments, in place of the physician they were unable to pay, and he would instruct them in the use of easily obtainable and inexpensive English herbs, they 'being the most fitted for English bodies':

> It is a base dishonourable unworthy part of the College of Physicians of London to train up the people in such ignorance that they should not be able to know what the Herbs in their Gardens be good for.[54]

To this end Culpeper republished his translation of the *Dispensatory* in 1651 with an additional section entitled '*Key to Galen and Hippocrates, their method of Physick*', and then included an '*Astrologo-Physical Discourse*' in the subsequent editions. The effect of this was to make the whole work a medical handbook of sorts. Culpeper also proceeded to write *Culpeper's Herbal* (1652); *A Directory for Midwives, or A Guide for Women, in their Conception, Bearing and Suckling their Children* (1651); and *Semeiotica Uranica, or An Astrological Judgement of Diseases from the Decumbiture of the Sick* (1651). He translated Francis Glisson's *Treatise of the Rickets* (1651), then the *Ars Medica*, which he entitled *Galen's Art of Physick* (1652), and produced a translation of John Vesling's *Syntagma anatomicum*, which he published as the *Anatomy of the Body of Man* (1653).[55]

Together these publications constituted the beginnings of an important body of medical knowledge in the English language. In *A Directory for Midwives* he delivered a blend of medical and commonsense advice on pregnancy, labour and nursing. Culpeper's mind focused particularly on such issues since he had witnessed over the years the deaths of six of his seven children. His wife Alice suffered from kidney disease which was aggravated during her pregnancies, endangering both mother and child.

It is quite likely that Alice Culpeper had several stillbirths or, if the child was born alive, it was poorly developed and lived only a short while.[56] We only hear mention of a sick, three-year old son[57] and a daughter, Mary, 'the true picture of her father' and the only one of Culpeper's children to outlive him. He was eager, therefore, to present his knowledge on these matters in a way that the common man or woman could understand so that they would be able to follow his advice and, hopefully, prevent such tragedies happening to them.

Culpeper's translation of Glisson's *Treatise of the Rickets* shows the breadth of Culpeper's learning and his spirit of questioning and innovation. Rickets was a new and pressing disease at this time and Culpeper's swift translation of the work shows his eagerness to accept and pass on new ideas. Culpeper had attended university in the time of Joseph Mede (1586–1638), the inspirer of the Cambridge Platonists or 'Latitudinarians' who 'transformed Cambridge thought by creating a philosophy which could accept the findings of modern science'.[58] Perhaps it was the exposure to this group of thinkers that had taught Culpeper how to be open to new ideas and advances while still maintaining the integrity of a traditional framework of holistic medicine. Certainly, he was no blind adherent to the traditional medicine of Galen and he often attacked 'tradition' in medicine and astrology:

> You know well enough, if the blind lead the blind, what will become of them both: Let every one, that desires to be called by the name of Artist, have his wits in his head (for that's the place ordained for them) and not in his books.[59]

And again:

> I cannot build my faith upon Authors' words, nor believe a thing because they say it, and could wish everybody were of my mind in this, to labour to be able to give a reason for everything they say or do. They say reason makes a man differ from a beast, if that be true, pray what are they that instead of reason, for their judgement, quote old authors? Perhaps their authors knew a reason for what they wrote, perhaps they did not, what is that to us, do we know it?[60]

In view of such comments it is remarkable that Culpeper nevertheless maintained his support for the basic theory and practice of Galenic medicine.

It is Culpeper's *Herbal,* however, which is his crowning achievement, the book for which he is most famous and through which his name lives on. This was printed in 1652 and was originally entitled *The English Physitian, or an Astrologo-physical discourse on the vulgar herbs of this nation. Being a compleat method of physick, whereby a man may preserve his body in health; or cure himself, being sick etc.* The herbal listed the medicinal uses of the plants in the common man's garden, hedge and field, indexed these to a list of typical illnesses at the end and used astrological, rather than Galenic categories to describe both diseases and drugs – and all this for three pence. Illustrations were omitted for the sake of cheapness, and Culpeper often also dispensed with descriptions, so familiar were the plants being discussed. The text was in

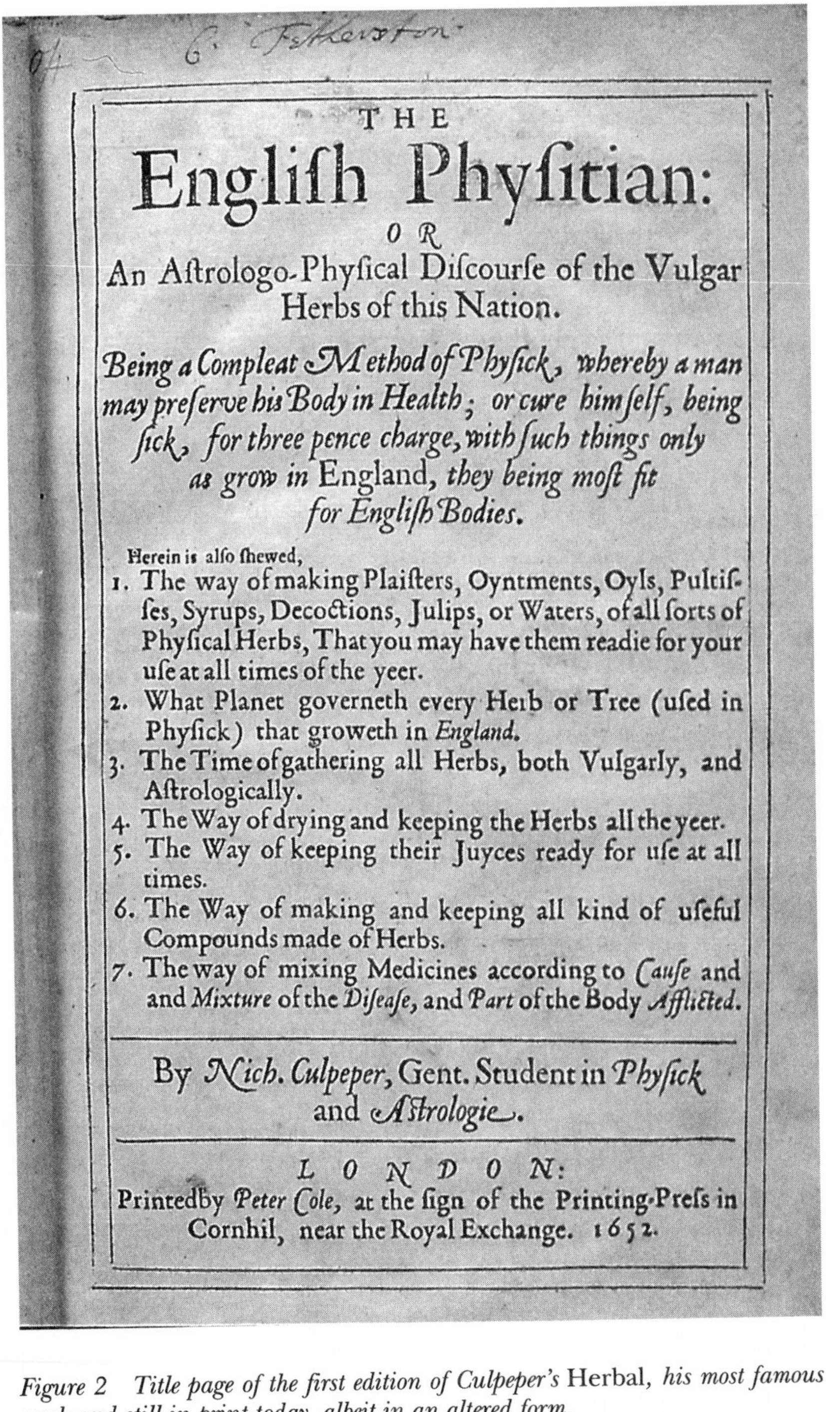

C. Fotheron

THE

Englifh Phyſitian:

O R

An Aftrologo-Phyſical Diſcourſe of the Vulgar
Herbs of this Nation.

*Being a Compleat Method of Phyſick, whereby a man
may preſerve his Body in Health; or cure himſelf, being
ſick, for three pence charge, with ſuch things only
as grow in* England, *they being moſt fit
for Englifh Bodies.*

Herein is alſo ſhewed,
1. The way of making Plaiſters, Oyntments, Oyls, Pultiſ-
   ſes, Syrups, Decoctions, Julips, or Waters, of all ſorts of
   Phyſical Herbs, That you may have them readie for your
   uſe at all times of the yeer.
2. What Planet governeth every Herb or Tree (uſed in
   Phyſick) that groweth in *England.*
3. The Time of gathering all Herbs, both Vulgarly, and
   Aftrologically.
4. The Way of drying and keeping the Herbs all the yeer.
5. The Way of keeping their Juyces ready for uſe at all
   times.
6. The Way of making and keeping all kind of uſeful
   Compounds made of Herbs.
7. The way of mixing Medicines according to *Cauſe* and
   and *Mixture* of the *Diſeaſe,* and *Part* of the Body *Afflicted.*

By *Nich. Culpeper,* Gent. Student in *Phyſick*
and *Aſtrologie.*

L O N D O N:
Printed by *Peter Cole,* at the ſign of the Printing-Preſs in
Cornhil, near the Royal Exchange. 1652.

Figure 2   Title page of the first edition of Culpeper's Herbal, *his most famous*
work and still in print today, albeit in an altered form.

Culpeper's direct and practical style, peppered with some humour, an admonition here and there or a point frankly made so that it was straightforward and easy to understand. Like the *London Dispensatory* it had an enormous sale in his lifetime and, out of all his other original works and translations is the only one still in print, albeit in an altered form.[61]

Culpeper was very aware that his life was drawing to a close by December of 1653. In his translation of the second, revised edition of the *Pharmacopoeia Londinensis* he wrote:

> I shall not trouble the reader further, being my self sick, and weak, no way fit for study or writing. But now pleasing my self in viewing those things that were written in my health, with this delightful thought, I shall do good to my countrymen; yea, them that are yet unborn; for their health (as well as the now living) I have lost my own. And could cheerfully (for the good of the English Nation) even cease to be.[62]

For some time he had been suffering from consumption, which perhaps originated from a wound to the chest he had received from a musket shot in the Civil War, but which was aggravated by some bad habits so that the disease continued unabated, 'wasting and consuming him by degrees, until it reduced him to a very skeleton, or anatomy'.[63] Culpeper's final hour upon the stage is told with suitable tenderness and no disguising of the truth.

> When Mr Culpeper's sickness stole upon him he was naturally consumptive for some years together; he was so truly sensible of his declination, as that he was often heard to say, that tobacco was the greatest enemy he had to his health, but he was too accustomed to it, to leave it. What Sir Theodore Mayern affirmed of the bad French wine, which he drank but a moderate quantity of at the Gilded Lion in the Strand, that it had killed him, as within few days afterwards was found too true, might be as certainly said of the destructive tobacco Mr Culpeper too excessively took, which by degrees, first deprived him of his stomach, and after other evil affects, in process of time, was one of the chief hasteners of his death.
>
> Mr Culpeper as hath been declared, for a long time perceiving his sickness to increase more strongly upon him, though he had held out the siege with his most studious endeavours to assist nature with his best art. Yet still finding as he made good one place to repair it, there was still a breach reinforced in another, battery upon battery. Seeing no remedy but that he must yield to the tyranny of the common enemy, the out-works being already taken in, though he knew with what inexpressible sorrow his wife must be afflicted to hear that

doleful news, that till then he had concealed from her. But finding, the approaches and infallible pangs of death to have already seized on him, taking her by the hand, as she stood by the bed-side in a most disconsolate condition, he breathed forth these his last words to her: Dearest, be not troubled, my peace I have already made with God. I am now going out of this miserable life, to receive a crown of immortality, after our so long continuance together, as Heaven hath thought fit, we must for the present part... He died in his own house in Spittle-fields the tenth day of January in 1654 in the thirty eighth year of his age. He was buried in the New Church yard of Bethlehem, where he desired to lie.[64]

Culpeper's moderate drinking of bad wine and excessive tobacco habit gives substance to the statement that 'he was a better Physician to others than he was to himself'. He was aware of these weaknesses although he may not have wished to admit them to himself. In an undated address to the reader at the front of his *Health for the Rich and Poor by Diet, without Physick,* published posthumously in 1656, he wrote:

> The reason of my pitching upon this subject and laying by other weighty study which groan for a deliverance, is my own want of health at present writing hereof. If my want come through intemperance which I am half afraid of, and it also make me unfit for study, oh what a student would temperance make me! I confess I am only ambitious that way, and if I have done so much being intemperate, oh what may I do, if I now turn temperate!

It is possible, however, that the consumption from which Culpeper died was a result of humoral imbalance. The physical description given of him in the posthumous biography in *Culpeper's School of Physick* (1659) accords to that of the choleric-melancholic temperament.

> Mr Culpeper was in his deportment gentle, pleasing and courteous. His complexion darkish and swarthy. His visage rather long than round. Of a pretence not so beautiful as amiable. His hair black and somewhat curling. His eyes piercing. His body a little above a medium, tending to tallness. Of a spare lean constitution. In his apparel not exceeding the moderation of one of his degree. Somewhat careless. He was of a clear and established judgement. Of an eloquent and good utterance. Of a quick spirit, full of swift thoughts and mounting. Of a sparkling ready wit, a gift which doth not always speak men fortunate. He was sometimes too much overtaken with deep speculations, though melancholy was somewhat

contrary to his nature, whatsoever he said otherwise of himself, so that it may rather be imputed to the crosses of his life, than to his own disposition.[65]

Culpeper was probably troubled with the 'adust choler' or 'bile burned black', a very hot and dry state of the body to which a person of this complexion is prone. The anger which reflected the 'furious and quarrelsome' side of such a temperament, by which he was judged by some to be surly and vindictive, appears to have been the embittered reaction of a sensitive soul. He once wrote, 'I have a very sympathetical spirit, and could either weep with Heraclitus or laugh with Democritus.' So, he outwardly displayed a righteous indignation against those he perceived to be taking advantage of the poor, the weak and the sickly, while he suffered stoically within himself the pain and grief of the tragedies or 'crosses of his life'. The sacrificing of his own health to benefit that of others was the outcome of such passion.

In keeping with the choleric-melancholic temperament, Culpeper 'was a person of so ready a mind, that he could more learnedly and suddenly dictate his papers for the press, than some that do take of the lamp and the oil more studiously to contrive them'. He displayed 'a nimble apprehension' and a wit that enlivened his writings, though he had occasion to apologize for his direct and uncompromising manner of address. As a man given over to study, he was learned and knowledgeable, yet for the practical purposes of educating his fellow countrymen he was straightforward and clear. He shunned the medical language of doctors, who sought to keep their patients in ignorance by using Greek and Latin terminology, on occasion even speaking entirely in the latter language. His was an inquiring and restless spirit, which stirred an incisive intellect and demonstrated a practical skill and knowledge. If he were not already inclined to be a little melancholy, perhaps his upbringing would have had the same result. He had 'spent his younger years is most laborious studies', at the expense of seeing his friends and acquaintances and perhaps in imitation of the only father figure in his life, his grandfather William Attersoll. Yet when he was in company, 'he was an excellent companion, and for the most part of a merry temper. His mirth, as he was used to say when he was far spent in his sickness, was the best cordial he had left against the consumption of his spirits.'

Culpeper's religious fervour matched the power of his intellect and he was fiercely independent of anything that tried to shackle it. 'All the religion I know, is Jesus Christ and him crucified, and the indwelling of the spirit of God in me.'[66] He opposed equally the tyranny of bishops and the enslavement of ignorant superstition that might prejudice free communication between Man and God, and saw no conflict with his acceptance of astrology, as he considered it to reveal the presence and handiwork of God. Indeed he sought to justify it from the holy scriptures, as did others of his time and tradition. An independent thinker and innovator, Culpeper, in his Puritan humility and detestation of pride, never curried favour. Rather than being patronized by the learned or the powerful, Culpeper challenged their authority and was usually found in the homes of the poor, the uneducated and the sick, whose causes he championed. Perhaps by always styling himself 'Gent.', he was making the statement that one 'born a gentleman and raised a scholar' could still opt to side with the disadvantaged and against those holding the reins of power. Such a revolutionary stance, combined with his outspoken and self-opinionated manner, inevitably encountered opposition.

Despite such opposition, new works by Culpeper continued to be published for ten years after his death and his other major works were subsequently republished many times in the remaining years of the 17th century and beyond. In addition, it was not just on these shores that his influence was felt. The last edition of his translation of the *Pharmacopoeia Londinensis*, together with the Boston edition of the *English Physitian* (1708) which matched Culpeper's work in the title and name of the author only, were the first medical books printed in the British colonies of North America.[67] It is interesting to note that it was from that continent that the revival in herbal medicine in Victorian England emanated. The part that Culpeper's writings played in this remains to be elucidated.

We learn from both Culpeper himself, writing in the November before his death,[68] and from *Mrs Culpeper's Information, Vindication and Testimony, concerning her husbands books to be Published after his death* that Culpeper had 'seventeen books completely perfected' to pass on to Peter Cole, his printer, who shared his radical views. Culpeper had probably begun writing and translating after being wounded in 1643, initially to fill his time while recovering and generally to further his own knowledge of 'physick'. Cole received and paid for these books before Culpeper died. Alice Culpeper testified that her husband also left her 'seventy nine books of his own making, or translating' which she passed on to the same printer for publication. Peter Cole issued 17 posthumous publications,[69] but it is not known what became of the other 79 books. If they truly existed, which is doubtful, it is presumed that they perished in the Great Fire of London in 1666. The works that Peter Cole did publish were mainly translations, and included works by Lazare Riviere (*The Practice of Physick* [1655] and *Four Books* [1658]), Jean Riolan (*A Sure Guide; or the Best and Nearest Way to Physick and Chirurgery* [1657]), Daniel Sennert (*Thirteen Books of Natural Philosophy* [1660], *Two Treatises* [1660], *Chymistry made Easie and Useful* [1662] and *Practical Physick* [1662–4]), Thomas Bartholin (*Anatomy* [1663]), Felix Plater (*A Golden Practice of Physick* [1662] and *Histories and Observations* [1664]) and Jean Fernel (*Two Treatises, the First of Pulses, the Second of Urines* [1662]). Two other works were completely original works by Culpeper: *Health for the Rich and Poor, by Diet, without Physick* [1656] and *Two Treatises* [1663], which explained blood-letting, cupping and scarifying.

There were, in addition, four original works issued by other printers: *Opus Astrologicum* (1654), *Culpeper's Last Legacy* (1655), *Mr Culpeper's Treatise of Aurum Potabile* (1656) and *Culpeper's School of Physick* (1659). Two other translations were credited to Culpeper but are spurious attributions. These are George Phaedro's *Physicall and Chymicall Works* [1654], translated by John Schenckius, as the title-page and preface testify, and *The Expert Doctors Dispensatory* (1657), printed for Nathaniel Brook. The latter is the work of Peter Morellus, translated by John Winand, Doctor of Physick at the University of Montpellier, who passed the book onto Culpeper for him, 'touched with an itch of fame', to put his name to the title-page. Culpeper wrote in his preface: 'Had I been before acquainted with this work, I had made it my business to have translated it.[70]

Culpeper's Last Legacy was published by Nathaniel Brook. Brook was a printer and rival of Peter Cole and a friend of Culpeper's in the early days. Indeed it was from his shop at the Angel in Cornhill that Culpeper collected the 40 shillings legacy from his grandfather, William Attersoll. Brook had published three of Culpeper's works in his lifetime, all overtly astrological: *Semeiotica*

Uranica, Catastrophe Magnatum and the *Ephemeris for the Year 1652.*
After Culpeper's death he then released *Culpeper's Last Legacy*
(1655), a disparate collection of medical writings. Whilst the
content was genuine, the preface was fictitious. This had been
written in both Nicholas's and Alice's name in order to give it the
appearance of a finished work and thus to increase its sales. Alice
Culpeper took him to task over this in her *Information, Vindication
and Testimony,* where she complained that her husband's
reputation and memory was

> blemished and eclipsed by the covetous and unjust forgeries of one,
> who, though he calls himself Nathaniel, is far from being an Israelite
> in whom there is no guile. Who was not content to publish a hodge
> podge of undigested Collection and Observations of my dear
> husband deceased, under the title of Culpeper's Last Legacy; but to
> make the deceit more taking, he steeled his forehead so far, and
> braised it so hard, as not to be ashamed to forge two epistles, one in
> mine and the other in my husband's name ... and therefore I desire
> all courteous readers of the writings of my husband, to take notice of
> this deceit, and to assure themselves that it never entered into his
> head to publish such an undigested Gallimoffery under the
> promising and solemn name of his Last Legacy.[71]

Alice's *Information, Vindication and Testimony* did not, however,
seem to deter Nathaniel Brook. He went on to release *The Expert
Doctors Dispensatory,* Culpeper's *Arts Master-piece: Or, the Beautifying
part of Physick* (1660), and *Ephemerides* for the years 1654–6 which
were also printed bearing Culpeper's name. The best that could
be said of the latter regarding their authenticity is that they were
constructed from notes remaining at his death.[72]

The jostling to capitalize on the Culpeper name continued with
other publications, *Opus Astrologicum* (1654), an unadorned
collection of rules for choosing by astrology the propitious times
for certain undertakings such as going to war), and *Culpeper's
School of Physick* (1659). *School of Physick* was yet another motley
collection of varied short pieces by Culpeper in the possession of
Nathaniel Brook.[73] Some reconciliation between the widow and
this printer must have taken place to allow the collaboration for
this book, especially as many of the friends and associates
Nicholas Culpeper had when he was alive contributed to the
book. His amanuensis William Ryves, whom Culpeper had clearly
made much use of in his lifetime, wrote a biographical sketch, *The
Life of the admired Physician and Astrologer of our times, Mr Nicholas*

Culpeper, and a preface in praise of the whole volume. John Gadbury the astrologer appended *The Nativity of Nicholas Culpeper*. Various others wrote short eulogies.

The most controversy, however, was reserved for the publication of *Mr Culpeper's Treatise of Aurum Potabile* (1656). That Culpeper was the true author of this work has remained a point of some debate since the book's first release.[74] William Ryves tells us that Culpeper was certainly involved in the selling of *Aurum Potabile*, a universal remedy. William Ryves contends that:

> It was Mr Culpeper's usual expression in the time of his health, that though he could not do for her as she deserved, that he should nevertheless leave her a competent estate, (meaning that he should enrich her with some secrets of his practice) which she hath since in the *Aurum Potabile*, and other rare secrets, found happily verified to her own expectation.

In addition Culpeper, at the very end of his life, wrote a brief statement on 'The virtues, use and varieties of operations of the true and philosophical Aurum Potabile. Now made and sold by Dr Freeman, as also by Dr Harrington and me, Nicholas Culpeper, in Spittlefields, on the East Side, next door to the Red Lyon.'[75] He states that he and Dr Freeman had perfected this universal remedy which had 'cured diverse people of that most horrid, putrid fever, which so violently seized on men's bodies (both before and after Michaelmas 1653) to the great admiration of many'. Culpeper then lists other illnesses which it cures but adds: 'but to what purpose do I go about to nominate diseases in particular when it is an Universal Remedy for all diseases, being administered as the Authors give directions? For its chief aims is exhilarating the vital spirits and heart, which supplies the microcosm as doth the Sun the macrocosm.'

Aurum Potabile, or 'drinkable gold', was reputed to be a cordial medicine containing pure gold. The value of this precious metal was supposed to be as great for the health as for the pocket. The preparation of the gold in solutions demanded both an experience of alchemical preparation and much skill and knowledge. If Culpeper's *Aurum Potabile* did actually exist it is difficult to work out exactly where Culpeper acquired the necessary knowledge in this new chemical medicine. In the third edition of *A Physical Directory*, published in 1651, in the section on 'chymical oils', Culpeper gives no reason to suppose that he

The Vertues, Use, and Variety of operations of the
true and *Phylosophical* AURUM POTABILE.
Now made and sold by Dr. Freeman, *as also by* Dr. Harrington, *and me*
Nich. Culpeper, *in Spittle-fields, on the East side,*
next door to the Red Lyon.

Courteous and Friendly Reader,

THis precious Jewel of *Aurum Potabile,* which Dr. Freeman and my self
have attained to the perfection thereof, is now only in the hands of Dr.
Freeman and my self, and Dr. Harrington, who hath long and often tried, and
known the Vertues, Use, and Manner of operation thereof, to the great comfort of many who had Diseases, which otherwise might have proved inseparable
and incurable, as sufficient witnesses can testifie : It cures all Agues, whether
Quotidian, Tertian, or Quartan ; as also it cured divers people of that most horrid, putrid Feaver, which so violently seized on mens bodies (both before and
after *Michaelmas,* 1653.) to the great admiration of many ; and when the par-
ties diseased have been both sencelesß and speechlesß, so that neither that, nor any
other Medicine or *Panacea,* though never so gentle, could safely be administred into the body ; it hath beyond all hopes by external application on the
stomach, revived them from death : It cures the Gout of all sorts so perfectly,
being administred as the Authors shall advise, that I dare undertake it shall never trouble the patient more, if the cause that first brought it, whether it be by
Diet, or otherwise, be forborn. It causeth Women subject to Abortion or
Miscarriage to go their times, and yet being administred when the time comes,
it causeth a speedy and easie delivery. But to what purpose do I go about to
nominate Diseases in particular, when it is an Universal Remedy for all Diseases, being administred as the Authors give Directions ? for its chief aim is ex-
hilerating the vital Spirits and Heart, which supplies the Microcosm as doth the
Sun the Macrocosm ; for *Joshua* knew right well that if he commanded and
made the Sun to stand still, that all the Macrocosm must : so of necessity must
Man, the Microcosm when his Heart, viz. the Microcosms Sun, is at a stand
in his operations. Thus doing, it both binds, and stops fluxes, yet purges. It
both Vomits, and staies vomiting : it causes sweat, yet cures preternatural sweating, and performs all its operations as Nature her self would have it, because
it only fortifies her in her Center, and it was never yet at any time known, but
if Nature be strengthened, and have an Enemy in the Body, but that she will to
work to expel him, or correct him.

To conclude, It's an Universal Fortification for all Complexions and Ages,
against all sorts and degrees of pestilential and contagious infection, both preventing before their possession, and extirpating of them after it. But why
Glauber (in his description of the true properties of that he pretends for true
Aurum Potabile) would not have it give any color to the hands or any thing
else, and yet it self a most pure Tincture, neither he, nor I, nor any mortal man
can tell.

I shall say no more at present, but refer you to a Treatise that shall shortly be
published on this Subject.

Jan. 1, 1653.   NICH. CULPEPER.

*Figure 3   Culpeper's advertisement for Aurum Potabile, dated just nine days
before he died.*

knows anything at all about the practicalities of alchemy:

> As to Alchemists (to whose profession the making of them belongs) I
> shall seem like Phormio the Philosopher, who never having seen
> battle, undertook to read a military lecture before Hannibal, who was
> one of the best soldiers in the world.[76]

On the other hand he was interested enough in Paracelsus's
alchemical medicine to have translated a work of the unknown
Simeon Partlitz, entitled *A New Method of Physick, or A Short View of
Paracelsus and Galen's Practice*, which attempted the construction
of a working compromise between the doctrines of each
physician, the traditional medicine and the new medicine of the
alchemist. The translational was not published until after
Culpeper's death in 1654, but the address 'To The Reader', dated
12 November 1653 informs us that it had been completed and
sold to a publisher as early as 1651:

> The ensuing discourse I finished when I was in health, which had
> been published two years since but that the Act of Parliament for
> punishing such thieves as steal away copies from those that purchase
> them did expire the nine and twentieth day of September 1651, and
> was not revived until the seventh of January 1652.

The apparent theft of Culpeper's translation, then, explained why
the text was not ready for printing until just before his death. In
1653 Culpeper had added to the physicians' list of 'chymical oils'
in the *Pharmacopoeia Londinensis* of 1653 antimony and mercury
which were the chemicals frequently used in iatrochemistry (the
medical use of chemical preparations). This only mirrored the
increasing prominence and controversy of the followers of
Paracelsus in the 1650s, some of whom advocated the
advancement of medicine only by experiment and observation
and demanded the replacement of Galenic medicines with their
new chemical preparations. As Capp records:

> Traditional medicine was itself under attack in this period from the
> disciples of Paracelsus, the sixteenth century German chemist and
> physician who (to over-simplify) replaced the four humours with the
> three 'principles' of sulphur, mercury and salt. He argued that illness
> sprang from a disorder of particular organs, to be remedied by
> specific, chemically-based medicines. This doctrine of therapy was
> part of a vaster concept of chemical transformation involving the
> regeneration of mankind and the 'divine alchemy' of the creation.[77]

Culpeper never went this far down the new road. As William Ryves put it, apparently quoting a member of the Royal College of Physicians: 'He was not only for Galen and Hippocrates but he knew how to correct and moderate the tyranny of Paracelsus.'[78] In the same year, he wrote that the nation was languishing under a disease 'now turned epidemical ... that is ignorance in physick or want of knowledge of what may do them good. The cure of this disease cannot be performed neither by Aurum Potabile, nor the philosophers' stone, but by the real endeavours of a public spirit by the fear of God, and love to poor people, by labouring to discharge a good conscience, by instructing people what belongs to their health.'[79] Furthermore, Culpeper, strangely dubbed 'Our British Paracelsus' after his death, in fact was scathing of 'our modern alchemist' who uses 'the chief enemies of gold', such as lead, antimony, sulphur and mercury, 'in making their Aurum Potabile which we shall omit in this place to speak of the evil such paltry stuff may do to the body of a man'.[80]

It would seem, then, that by 1653 Culpeper had become more informed as to the theory and practice of Paracelsian iatrochemistry and it is possible that he was now open to experimenting with a 'rare cordial and universal medicine'. Perhaps Doctors Freeman and Harrington prepared the Aurum Potabile, and once Culpeper had seen its beneficial effects (during the widespread 'putrid fever' around Michaelmas 1653, which he refers to in his notice, along with other single cures), he was ready to sell it.

It is certain, though, that Aurum Potabile was being sold in 1655 by Culpeper's widow and administered by a physician in her house near London, 'on the East side of Spittle-fields, next door to the Red Lyon'. However, the authenticity of the medicine Alice was selling was doubted. Someone was concerned enough about the matter to issue a pamphlet warning that Mrs Culpeper, 'a poor silly woman', was in league with two physicians to sell this remedy, 'a thing wholly destructive and pernicious' since it fraudulently contained 'a mixture of mercury, vinegar, sal ammoniac and tartar' and would prove a combination 'most destructive to human bodies'.[81] However, this anonymous pamphlet, entitled *Culpeper Revived from the Grave, to discover the cheats of that Grand Imposter, call'd Aurum Potabile,* could well have been penned by Nathaniel Brook, at a time when his relations with Alice Culpeper were at their worst (on account of the forged prefaces of *Culpeper's Last*

Legacy which he published at this time).[82] Yet the attack contained in *Culpeper Revived from the Grave* demonstrates some knowledge of chemistry and alchemy. It is more likely that the pamphlet was penned by a qualified medic; probably not a member of the Royal College of Physicians, but more likely one of the 'true chemists' who did not accept the medicinal benefits of such a preparation of gold and anyway suspected its impure transformation using mercury and certain acids. And he may have desired also to dissuade Culpeper's usual publisher, Peter Cole, from printing the awaited treatise which, for all he knew, would contain the method of preparation and would 'entice men under such golden pretences into their utter ruin'.[83]

In view of the controversy surrounding the sale of Aurum Potabile, Alice Culpeper went to great pains to validate the text of her husband's *Treatise of Aurum Potabile* as a genuine creation of Nicholas Culpeper, employing nine witnesses to attest to the preface she wrote, and Culpeper himself referred to a text which must be the same work. In 1654 Culpeper wrote: 'I shall say no more at present, but refer you to a treatise that shall shortly be published on this subject. It duly appeared in 1656, published by George Eversden under the title *Mr Culpeper's Treatise of Aurum Potabile. Being a Description of the Threefold World; elementary, celestial, intellectual; Containing the knowledge necessary to the Study of Hermetic Philosophy. Faithfully written by him in his Life-time, and since his death, published by his wife.* Alice wrote in her Preface:

> Neither let the name offend any man, as if there were some deceit couched herein, or as if we would have the world believe that it consists of nothing but gold, reduced to quintessential liquor. No, we are sure that it must then be sold at a far higher rate than we now afford it. Let it suffice the ingenious reader to know that it is the most precious of all Medicines (as gold is of metals) and worth its weight in gold, for the excellency thereof. And that there is in it of the substance of gold reduced into its principles, and made agreeable to man's constitution, by art, therefore it is called aurum potabile.[84]

As far as the treatise was concerned, the reader of it was not to expect 'a plain description of my husband's Aurum Potabile so that all the world reading this book might make it'. (This would have defeated the point of Nicholas leaving it to Alice as a legacy.) Rather the treatise would 'give such hints to the learned and experienced philosopher as might direct him in the search of this excellent secret'.Yet clearly the substance of the work has nothing to do with the literal making of Aurum Potabile, since nowhere in the text are there practical indications for the preparation of such a remedy. Instead, the work reflects Culpeper's interest in the less practical side and the more transcendental aspects, the 'divine alchemy' of the Paracelsian tradition as it existed in England in the 1650s. This would have accorded with his devoutly religious outlook and his long-time study of the philosophy of Hermeticism. As Harold Cook observes:

> One brand of chemistry derived from Paracelsianism and Hermeticism fitted in well with the heightened religious sensibilities of the period. An understanding of God's book of nature, proponents believed, could be aided by a knowledge of scripture; the key lay with the hands-on knowledge of chemistry.[85]

Culpeper had found himself in the currents of such developments involving the new chemistry. The search for Aurum Potabile was a common eddy to get carried along by.[86] Since his notice to sell this universal remedy from his home was effectively the last thing he wrote,[87] it was indeed his legacy left to his wife. But whether Alice Culpeper, in the absence of her husband, was selling what her husband had approved as genuine Aurum Potabile, or whether she had been duped by Dr Freeman into attaching the Culpeper name to some quack-salver's poison, we shall never know.

As well as the assault on Alice Culpeper in the anonymous pamphlet written on 'that Grand Imposter, call'd Aurum Potabile', two attacks on Nicholas Culpeper appeared in print after his death, although neither was of sufficient importance to tarnish his fame and reputation. The first came from a fellow herbalist who took exception to Culpeper's insistence over astrology. William Cole wrote in *The Art of Simpling* (1656):

> Master Culpeper (a man now dead, and therefore I shall speak of him as modestly as I can, for were he alive, I should be more plain with him) ... he, forsooth, judgeth all men unfit to be physicians who are not artists in astrology, as if he and some other figure-flingers his companions had been the only physicians in England. Whereas for ought I can gather, either by his books, or learn from the report of others, he was a man very ignorant in the form of simples.

The second attack was made in 1664 by Matthew Mackaile, an apothecary and burgess of Edinburgh. He appended to his study of a local spa '*a Character of Mr Culpeper and his writings*'.[88] This is a somewhat disjointed and free-ranging criticism of aspects of Culpeper's writings, from his 'impiety' for railing against the Church, his attacks on the Royal College of Physicians, his lack of knowledge of chemistry and the meaning of 'quintessence', to a predictable assault on astrological botany and his political predictions. The Restoration of the Monarchy, in 1660, gave Mackaile the opportunity to turn on the whole of Culpeper's astrology:

> If his astrology in medicinals be no better than it (and the astrology of others more famous than he) was in politics, in the time of the Commonwealth, (when Monarchy was said to be eternally exiled from Great Britain by all the powers in heaven), they will mis-spend their time, who will take the pains to read.

The curious thing is why these attacks should have been made a full ten years after Culpeper's death and at so great distance from London. Yet it is perhaps fitting testimony to Culpeper's continuing reputation and standing throughout the 'Three Kingdoms' of England, Scotland and Ireland.

However, it is the medical and astrological writings of Nicholas Culpeper that constitute his true legacy to readers of the English speaking nations. Culpeper was one of many English physicians notable for their use of astrology in medicine. His immediate predecessor, Robert Fludd, an eminent and successful doctor of royal patronage who served four times as a censor of the College, elucidated in his many writings a Rosicrucian philosophy with astrology at its heart. Several Fellows of the Royal College of Physicians practised astrological medicine, while others acted as patrons to notable astrologers or were sympathetic to their practice. The knowledge these men shared was all written in Latin. By writing extensively on astrology and medicine in English, Culpeper opened up the subjects for a wider audience. As a consequence, quite a number of 'students of physick and astrology' came on to the scene, inspired by Culpeper's success and fame. Among their number were Joseph Blagrave, Henry Coley, John Gadbury, William Salmon, Richard Saunders and John Tanner, who practised the art of astrological medicine, published their text-books and issued their almanacs.[89] This era of astrological medicine, which had opened with the publication of *Christian Astrology* (1647) by Culpeper's famous contemporary,

William Lilly, was elaborated during the following three decades, became less popular by the end of the 17th century but is still not closed today, thanks to the enduring reputation of Nicholas Culpeper.

Culpeper saw himself living on after his death in his writings, though he recognized that he had spent his health in this very task of teaching the common man and woman how to treat their ills. He had served the people as a soldier, during the Civil War, as a physician and as an educator trying to instil in his readership a questioning mind like his own, which always sought a reason for everything and refused to follow tradition blindly. However, Culpeper was faithful to the last to his God and to the tenets of natural philosophy and 'physick' which reflected a world of order, harmony and balance created by God. For this reason he did not accept Harvey's proof of the circulation of the blood from the heart, made in 1628, because it shattered the order and harmony of this world-view and smacked too much of the ungodly philosophy of Aristotle whom he criticized at every opportunity.[90] At a fundamental level Culpeper was solidly rooted in the concepts of traditional Western medicine, of astrology and of a unified cosmos created by the one God.

PART 2

Western Holistic Medicine

SECTION 1

The Seven Natural Things and the Constitutional Basis of Medicine

In his medical practice Nicholas Culpeper adhered largely to the medicine of Galen and Hippocrates which was known as 'physick', from the Greek *physis* meaning 'nature'. A practitioner of physick was called a physician. The body of medical knowledge gathered by these and other Greeks was elaborated and advanced by Arab physicians of the Middle Ages and this was subsequently passed on to Western Europe at a time when its learned men were coming into possession of original, 'lost' Greek texts. This influx of knowledge gave the impetus for the European *Renaissance* or rebirth of the study of Classical learning. At the beginning of the 17th century the Galenic model of health and disease was still dominant amongst the medical profession, although the fortress of its orthodoxy had already suffered some undermining in the previous century by the new thinking of Renaissance scientists such as Vesalius, the father of modern anatomy, and Paracelsus, the original and enigmatic missionary for chemical medicine. In his own lifetime Culpeper saw even greater challenges to this traditional medicine from the philosophy of Descartes, which valued reason above perception and taught that the body was like a machine, and from the call of Francis Bacon for the experimental validation of all knowledge.

This new orientation and approach, on which modern science is based, began to yield new medical knowledge by focusing on pathology, the study of disease processes, through the extensive *anatomical* dissection of dead and spiritless corpses. Such practice was quite different from that of physicians of earlier ages who were largely constrained from dissecting the bodies of the dead and who based their study of human health and disease on the living person and his interaction with his environment. Each person would be seen as unique according to the individual spirit inhabiting the physical matter that was the body. Consequently, the principles of traditional holistic medicine were based on physiology, meaning in Greek the study of the *physis* or nature of a being, rather than on anatomy, which means dissection or 'cutting up'.

Significantly, Culpeper was no stranger to the discoveries made in anatomy in his day. Indeed, he gained first-hand knowledge from autopsies and dissections. Nevertheless, this did not distract him at all from a holistic view of humankind and of the whole universe, so that his writings on the theory and practice of the medicine of Galen and Hippocrates proved to be a last defence of a particular view of the world on which was based the medical system known as Galenism.[1]

Seven subjects provided the basic principles of Western holistic medicine and a physician was required to have a complete understanding of them. These seven 'natural things', so called because they applied to the *physis* or nature of human beings, were:[2]

- The 4 elements (physics)
- The 4 temperaments (the constitution of the human body)
- The 4 humours (the primary constituents of the body)
- The similar parts (anatomy)
- The faculties of the body (physiology, psychology, nutrition and reproduction) and their associated spirits and virtues which were known as
- The spirits and innate heat (the life-giving principle)
- The 4 administering virtues or secondary physical faculties

1   The 4 elements

Nature that framed us of four elements
Warring within our breasts for regiment
Doth teach us all to have aspiring minds:
Our souls, whose faculties can comprehend
The wondrous Architecture of the world:

And measure every wand'ring planet's course
Still climbing after knowledge infinite,
And always moving as the restless Spheres
Will us to wear ourselves and never rest,
Until we reach the ripest fruit of all,
That perfect bliss and sole felicity
The Sweet fruition of an earthly crown.

Christopher Marlowe

In order to understand the manifestations and transformations in the natural world around them, Greek philosophers sought to uncover laws of nature which caused these phenomena. The continuing debate, already two centuries old, was famously resolved by Empedocles (c490–430 BC). He argued that nature consisted of 4 elements, namely *Earth, Water, Air and Fire.*[3] Each particular thing or entity in nature was composed of a combination of these 4 elements. The 4 elements were divided into two pairs of opposites, with Fire opposed to Water and Air to Earth, and the formation of anything was based on a dynamic equilibrium involving the right proportion of each element. Analogies can be made with painting or cooking. A painter with only the colour red cannot paint green grass, but with a combination of colours he or she can mix them in varying proportions to create many different colours. Similarly a cook cannot bake a cake with just flour, but given also eggs, milk and sugar a variety of different cakes can be made. Empedocles's idea became truly established in Greek physics and natural philosophy when the great philosophers Plato and Aristotle incorporated it into their theories concerning the physical universe.[4]

The elements Earth, Water, Air and Fire were not literally these things in the world but were the building blocks in the composition of everything in nature. Soil would be said to be formed of all elements but, in this case, with a preponderance of the element Earth so that it was perceived as being earthy. Likewise, Air contained Fire (heat), Water (vapour) and Earth (particles) as well as, mainly, the element Air. Elements become recognizable when the object breaks up.

Emphedocles might have watched a piece of wood burning. Something disintegrates. We hear it crackle and splutter. That is *water.* Something goes up in smoke. That is *air.* The *fire* we can see. Something also remains when the fire is extinguished. That is the ashes – or *earth.*[5]

Generally, however, the composition of such substances was known, not because the 4 elements forming any object were visible, but through the *primary qualities* of each element. Aristotle denoted the primary qualities as *hot, cold, moist* and *dry*. The human sense of touch, taste and smell were therefore able to detect the predominant qualities of any object and thus infer its elemental composition.

All matter was thought to manifest two of the primary qualities according to its predominant element. Each element was thus associated with a pair of primary qualities.

TABLE OF PRIMARY QUALITIES

The 4 elements	FIRE	AIR	WATER	EARTH
The primary qualities	hot & dry	hot & moist	cold & moist	cold & dry

By the alteration of one of these qualities to its opposite, the other remaining stable, the transformation of one element into another could occur and this was held to account for the constant changes taking place in the physical world. For instance, the transmutation of Air (hot and moist) into Water (cold and moist) would involve an alteration of its quality 'hot' into its opposite 'cold'. It is for this reason that the primary qualities were considered the first principles of nature, and, because their alteration denoted substantial change in physical bodies, they were often called 'forces of nature'.

The elements were also said to manifest *secondary qualities* which followed from their primary qualities.

TABLE OF SECONDARY QUALITIES RELATED TO THE 4 PRIMARY QUALITIES

HOT	COLD	DRY	MOIST
lightness	heaviness		
rarity (thinness)	density		
subtlety/ability to penetrate	grossness		
		hardness	softness
		dryness	slipperiness
		roughness	smoothness
		friability/easily crumbled	clamminess

Each of the 4 elements, Earth, Water, Air and Fire, manifested their primary and secondary qualities according to their proportions in the composition of a particular physical substance:

CHARACTERISTICS OF THE 4 ELEMENTS

Earth Earth was the element of absolute heaviness. It held its position in the centre of the other elements, and therefore of all existence. In its nature it was at rest and so it made any object in which it predominated stationary. When an attempt was made to move such an object, it tended to return to its original position. The element Earth was therefore thought to make objects firm, stable and lasting and to maintain its outward form. Thus the element Earth was said to fix and hold our bodies together in a compacted form. Likewise, stone which is cold and dry and therefore predominantly of the element Earth, is very stable. Indeed, many stone castles still stand in Britain, despite the ravages of time. Whilst the primary qualities of Earth were coldness and dryness, its secondary qualities included density, heaviness and hardness.

Water Water was the element of relative heaviness surrounding the element Earth, as the oceans surround the land masses of our planet. It was typically cold and moist in quality and the moisture imparted the secondary qualities of softness and the ability to change shape. In addition, the moisture protected dry objects from crumbling to a powder (friability) as the dryness prevented moisture from dispersing by fixing it. Consider the dew at night or falling rain. The water soaks into the ground and is held there, despite the effects of wind. Only when the Sun is out in the daytime is moisture drawn out of the ground by the attractive power of its heat. The evaporation imparts a moist quality to the air, so that moisture is seen to move back and forth between bodies of water and the air. On either side lies Earth and its force of gravity and Fire and its power of attraction.

Air Air was held to possess relative lightness and was judged hot and moist in quality. In turn it imparted the secondary qualities of porosity, lightness and thinness to matter and enabled objects to rise upwards.

Fire Fire was the element of heat and dryness which created the secondary quality of absolute lightness, in the sense of brightness and illumination of the stars above as well as meaning the opposite of heaviness. It was rarefied and so imparted lightness and porosity to objects. It enabled the natural ripening or development of substances by its heat and, like the alchemist's fire, counteracted the cold and heaviness of Earth and Water by transmuting them into other compounds with a different set of qualities.

The 4 qualities belonging to the elements were grouped into two pairs of active and passive qualities. Hot and cold were deemed the *active* qualities since they acted on other things. The application of heat to some object would render it dry while cold was thought to induce moisture in things. The qualities dry and moist were called *passive* in that they were said to be acted on in respect to their *form*. Moist was easily adaptable to form: it was soft, pliable and yielding and capable of 'filling something up'. It could not be confined within limits of its own and required a 'container' or a form other than itself in order to exist. Dry was hard, compacted and resistant and it could bind things together. It required no container and so was its own form. A stone is a good example, as this can easily be held up. Likewise, it is impossible to build sand-castles out of completely dry sand, but moist sand on a beach is amenable to being shaped.

It is useful to think of the elements as not literally constituting matter but rather as symbols for qualities of mass and energy.[6] In this regard the active qualities hot and cold can also be seen to denote the *dispersive* and *aggregative* aspects of energy, respectively. So, the heat of the Sun, for instance, evaporates and disperses moisture while cold will condense it into ice. Similarly the passive qualities dry and moist describe the *resistant* and *receptive* aspects of mass respectively. Consequently, dry, hard pebbles will resist being mixed with dry, hard sand, so that the two different forms will remain separate, while sand, when mixed with water, will dissolve into the liquid.

Culpeper said that 'the whole world, and everything in it, was formed of a composition of contrary elements', united into one harmonious whole. So, the human body, the 'epitome' of the world, was formed also of 4 contrary elements, with the heat and dryness of Fire contrary to the coldness and moisture of Water and the heat and moisture of Air opposed to the cold and dryness of Earth. Human health was represented by the unity of the 4 elements in harmony.

2   The 4 temperaments

The Western traditional system of medicine furnished a close relationship between the 4 elements and the medical study of the temperament or constitution of the human body as summarized in the table below.

TABLE OF ELEMENTS AND TEMPERAMENTS

The 4 elements	FIRE	AIR	WATER	EARTH
The primary qualities	hot & dry	hot & moist	cold & moist	cold & dry
The 4 temperaments	choleric	sanguine	phlegmatic	melancholic

The balance of primary qualities in any thing, acting through the elements, was termed its *temperament of complexion*. Both words come from the Latin: *temperare*, meaning 'to combine or mingle in due proportion', and *complecti*, 'to embrace, encompass or comprehend'. The determination of the complexion or temperament of a human being meant a comprehension of the basic nature of that person, their physique, the character of their personality and their physiological make-up. So to look at a person's complexion established a benchmark for the health of an individual against which to measure the degree of variation from the norm on account of seasonal changes, age and, importantly, the effects of disease. These variations were to be measured according to the primary and secondary qualities of the body.

The ideal state existed when the primary qualities were perfectly balanced with no one predominating. In other words when the opposing qualities were *quantitatively* exactly equal with exactly equal degrees of potency, so that a true mean between two extremes prevailed. This denoted the achievement of perfect health and harmony in life, indeed a physical immortality which, according to the Christian interpretation which Culpeper followed, was once Man's estate but which was lost in the Fall:

> They know that the Garden of Eden, as scripture calls it, in which Adam was created and which he was set to till, was created ... of pure elements, uncorrupted, equally and harmonically proportioned, even in the highest perfection. And that all the substance there whereupon man lived was pure, made of pure elements, not elements elementated as the rest of the world was, which the lord made for the beasts to live in. Then, if there was no corruption in the Garden, how could there be mortality? ...
>
> We conceive that the ancient philosophers studied out the cause of this change, how man being immortal came to put on mortality. Which they found to be this: after man had sinned, God drove him or put him out of the Garden to live amongst the beasts in the corruptible world, which was composed, not of pure elements, but of elements elementated, unequally proportioned in respect of heat, coldness, dryness and moisture. Being there, seeing he could not live without nourishment, he was forced to take his nourishment from corrupt food, by which those pure elements of which he was made were infected, and by degrees (though very slowly), declined from incorruption to corruption, until at last, one quality exceeding another in his body, as it did in the food which he took for sustenance. So his body became subject to corruption, after corruption to infirmity and sickness, and after sickness to death.[7]

The fall of humanity into a world of imperfectly balanced elements and a lack of harmony thus constituted, in this Christian view, a measure of spiritual decline. The striving to regain a perfect balance of elements, though it would bring excellent health and longevity would also, therefore, bring spiritual illumination or communion with God. Human eyes were to be fixed on the heavens, which were accounted free from all contrariety. Though the divergence of human temperament from such an ideal balance was small, especially when human beings were compared to animals, in which no equable temperament was thought to be able to exist and no spiritual illumination possible, it was sufficient to render human beings mortal. For the impurity of the elements of which both humans and animals were composed necessitated the fact of their growth and decay within a lifespan.

Culpeper gave the following description of a body in which the elements, qualities and humours were as balanced as possible, or, as he put it, 'the indications of a good temper of the habit of the whole body, which we state as the basis of the rest, so that you may see how much all distempers decline from it':[8]

> The indications of a moderate temperature according to the whole habit of the body are, a mixed colour in the face of red and white, as though the lily and the rose strove for superiority, the hair yellow, and moderately curling; the carnosity or fleshiness of the Body mean in respect both of quantity and quality, all the parts of the body keep the Golden Mean, and avoid excess on either hand. Excess to this are, grossness, thinness, fleshiness, leanness, fatness, hardness, softness, roughness, smoothness, all these swerve from meanness, but a man of a moderate or mean temper is such a one (according to the rule of *Polycletus*[9]) that if you feel his flesh, it is neither too hard nor too soft, too hot nor too cold; If you look upon his body, 'tis neither too gross nor too thin, too rough nor too smooth, neither hath it any excess or defect.[10]

Such a description provided by Galen needed some qualification, for there are natural variations according to race, custom and environment which had to be taken into account. Culpeper recorded the following points:

> As for the colour of hair I told you before, it is to be considered according to the country the man lives in, for although happily in *Greece* where Galen lived, good constitutions might have yellow hair, yet we find it not so in *England*, but usually brown.
>
> All distempers discolour the Skin one way or other, and from thence are indications taken, yet if the region be never so temperate, if the body be never so well in health, and of never so good a constitution, yet if he expose his naked body to the Sun in the Summer time, it will mar all the indications that can be taken from the colour, and therefore you must heed custom as well as colour, and therefore virgins which vail their faces from the Sun preserve their beauty by it.[11]

With this benchmark of a balanced temperament, and taking factors of race, climate, atmosphere and custom into account, a variation from this norm gives notice of some distemper in the body. This will be either small and remaining within the limits of health for a given person at a given age of life, or large, denoting imbalance and ill health. There are eight possible variations of the qualities which will yield differences of temperament, as numbered in the table below.

TABLE OF THE 8 VARIATIONS OF TEMPERAMENT

EXCESS OF PRIMARY QUALITY	PRIMARY QUALITIES IN BALANCE	QUALITY INDUCED	ELEMENTAL IMBALANCE	EXAMPLE
heat (1)	dryness/moisture	dryness	Fire heat & dryness (5)	a hot summer's day
cold (2)	dryness/moisture	moisture	Water cold & moisture (6)	dew accompanying nightfall
dryness (3)	hot/cold	cold	Earth cold & dryness (7)	an oil lamp run dry
moisture (4)	hot/cold	cold	Water cold & moisture (8)	getting soaked in a storm

The first 4 imbalances were termed 'simple' because only one quality stood in excess; the second 4 'compound' imbalances, because 2 qualities predominated, representing an imbalance of one of the elements. Moreover, a simple imbalance never remained so for long, but resolved into a complex imbalance, as the table shows. An imbalance of both heat and cold, or of both dryness and moisture, could not exist since in each case the qualities opposed one another and would cancel each other out. Any excess of a quality would eventually lead to cold, even an excess of heat, since it would produce dryness and in turn dryness eventually induced cold. The conclusion drawn from these alterations of simple into compound imbalances was that *heat* stood as the quality most favourable for maintaining the proper balance and general health of the body, particularly when *heat* was tempered by the correct amount and quality of *moisture* (the qualities of the element *Air*).

An excess of any primary quality was calculated by degree, from one to four. Take heat for example. The human body was reckoned naturally hot in the 1st degree. A moderate fever may render it hot in the 2nd or 3rd degree, while a burning fever pushes it to the 4th degree of heat. Likewise catching a chill is not as cold in effect as frostbite. Similarly, food could affect the temperament of the body. Sugar, for example, was reckoned to induce heat in the 1st degree and garlic and pepper heat in the 4th degree. Lettuce and cucumber, on the other hand, were considered cooling in the 2nd degree.

The transformation of primary qualities which change one element into another constituted the processes of construction (anabolism) and disintegration (catabolism). In accordance with the dictates of growth and decay, the body was altered by a transformation of its qualities over the course of a lifetime. The qualities were also affected by seasonal and other cyclical changes in the *Elementary World* as a whole, which Culpeper held to be related to the movements of the planets of the *Celestial World*.

> All time is measured out by motion, and that the original of all motion is in the heavens. For it is the motion of the Sun which causeth Day and Night, Summer, Winter, Spring and Harvest. From which conversion of times and years, all changes proceed, both heat and cold, dryness and moisture, by which four is caused life and death, generation and putrefaction, increase and decrease of elementary things.[12]

In keeping with the holistic outlook of traditional Western medicine, therefore, human life in its 4 phases of childhood, youth, middle age and old age was said to be reflected in the changing seasons of the year. In addition, the qualities associated with the ages and seasons matched those of the 4 temperaments, the sanguine, choleric, melancholic and phlegmatic.

CHARACTERISTICS OF THE 4 TEMPERAMENTS

Spring/sanguine temperament/childhood

In spring the increasing warmth frees the waters of life from the icy grip of winter and encourages growth to begin again. This bountiful combination of heat and moisture also belongs to the sanguine complexion, the most childlike of the 4 temperaments and full of the joys of Spring. Culpeper describes it thus:

> A man or woman in whose body heat and moisture abounds, is said to be Sanguine of complexion. Such are usually of a middle stature, strong composed bodies, fleshy but not fat, great veins, smooth skins,

SEASONS, ELEMENTS

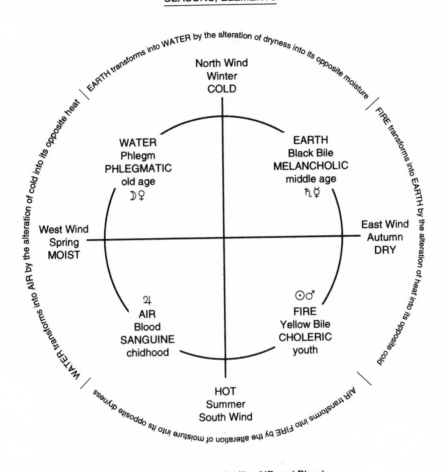

♃ Jupiter is hot and moist like AIR and Blood

☉ Sun
♂ Mars } are hot and dry like FIRE and Yellow Bile

♄ Saturn
☿ Mercury } are cold and dry like EARTH and Black Bile

☽ Moon
♀ Venus } are cold and moist like WATER and Phlegm

hot and moist in feeling. Their body is hairy, if they be men they have soon beards, if they be women it were ridiculous to expect it. There is a redness intermingled with white in their cheeks. Their hair is usually of a blackish brown, yet sometimes flaxed. Their appetite is good, their digestion quick, their urine yellowish and thick, the excrements of their bowels reddish and firm, their pulse great and full. They dream usually of red things and merry conceits.

As for their conditions [character], they are merry, cheerful creatures, bountiful, pitiful, merciful, courteous, bold, trusty, given much to the games of Venus, as though they had been an apprentice seven years to the trade. A little thing will make them weep, but so soon as 'tis over, no further grief sticks to their hearts.[13]

Culpeper's description of the sanguine temperament accords with that given in the *Regimen of Health* of the famous school of Medicine at Salerno, a Greek colony and health resort throughout the medieval period:

> Complexions cannot virtue breed or vice
> Yet may they unto both give inclination.
> The sanguine gamesome is and nothing nice [fastidious],
> Loves wine and women and all recreation,
> Likes pleasant tales and news, plays, cards and dice,
> Fit for all company and every fashion.
> Though bold, not apt to take offence, not ireful
> But bountiful and kind and looking cheerful.
> Inclining to be fat and prone to laughter,
> Loves mirth and music, cares not what comes after.[14]

Those, then, purely of the sanguine temperament appear healthy, ruddy and fresh. They enjoy the sensual pleasures of food and 'wine, women and song'. They rest easy and are untroubled in their sleep. They have but little wit and are often foolish as children or animals can seem to be. Like children they have a wavering nature, a mutable and inconstant mind and are wilful and lack maturity and discretion. By manifesting qualities attributed to certain animals, they play their part in 'the theatre of this world': the wiliness of the fox; the toying of apes; the cruelty of lions; and the extortionism of wolves.[15] Of the 4 pure temperaments theirs was considered the best state since, if it was maintained, it prolonged life and kept old age at bay.

Summer/choleric temperament/youth

The continuing and increasing heat of Summer dries out the moisture of the Spring and these qualities of heat and dryness are shared by the attributes of youth and choleric temperament. They are described by Culpeper in this way:

> We call that man choleric in whose body heat and dryness abounds or is predominate. Such persons are usually short of stature, and not fat, it may be because the heat and dryness of their bodies consumes radical moisture, their skin rough and hot in feeling, and their bodies very hairy. The hair of their heads is yellowish, red or flaxen for the most part, and curls much, the colour of their face is tawny or sunburnt. They have some beards. They have little hazel eyes. Their concoction [digestion] is very strong insomuch that they are able to digest more than they appetite. Their pulse is swift and strong, their urine yellow and thin. They are usually costive. They dream of fighting, quarrelling, fire and burning.
>
> As for Conditions [character] they are naturally quick-witted, bold, no way shame-faced, furious, hasty, quarrelsome, fraudulent, eloquent, courageous, stout-hearted creatures, not given to sleep much, but much given to jesting, mocking and lying.[16]

The *Regimen of Health* says of the choleric temperament:

> Sharp choler is a humour most pernicious,
> All violent and fierce and full of fire,
> Of quick conceit and therewithall ambitious,
> Their thoughts to greater fortunes still aspire.
> Proud, bountiful enough, yet oft malicious,
> A right bold speaker and as bold a liar.
> On little cause to anger great inclin'd,
> Much eating still, yet ever looking pin'd.
> In younger years they use to grow apace,
> In elder hairy on their breast and face.[17]

Bearing in mind that the physical description will alter from the Greek with a change of people and climate, we should add dark brown and black to the 'yellowish, red or flaxen' as possible hair colours in choleric subjects and include a range of overall colours from brown through auburn to ruddy and maybe even pale or yellowish. Their stature will not be any different, though they will have slender, lean bodies and a muscular physique, and they will be usually of medium height at most. In other words they will have a typically athletic frame and may well enjoy all sorts of sports and 'violent exercise', since this matches their inclination to be lively and to move swiftly and nimbly. They will be easily stirred to anger but it will be soon allayed and pacified. They have often been described as crafty, subtle, and deceitful and fickle of work and deed. Their eloquence and love of talking equip them to be meddlers and prattlers, 'impudently presuming to shuffle themselves into every company and place of assembly'.[18] They either achieve notable things in or for their country or else are a notable detriment to it, on account of their untractable, unruly and even villainous behaviour and their ferocity and arrogance. As Queen Elizabeth I is said to have remarked, 'Anger makes dull men witty, but it keeps them poor.' Overall they will manifest a love of action rather than enjoyment of the peaceful activities of rest and sleep.

Autumn/melancholic temperament/middle age

The vibrancy of nature during the Spring and Summer is lost in the Autumnal sadness. So, too, the middle years of life can seem like a let-down. In both cases, the previous heat now wanes and gives way to cold. Defoe wrote that 'middle age is youth without its levity, and age without decay'. Culpeper's observation was:

> The Sun causeth heat and cold, day and night, Winter and Summer. When he arrives to the house of his honour or exaltation, to wit, *Aries*, then the trees spring, living creatures are comforted, the birds sing, the whole creation rejoiceth, and sickness in the body shew themselves in their colours: Also when he arrives at his fall, to wit, *Libra*, the leaves of the trees fall, all creatures are lumpish, and mourn like the trees in *October*.[19]

The melancholic person whose temperament resonates with the Autumn is described in Culpeper's version thus:

> A melancholy person is one [in] whose body cold and dryness is predominate, and not such a one as is sad sometimes as the vulgar dream. They are usually slender and not very tall, of swarthy dusky colour, rough skin, cold and hard in feeling. They have very little hair on their bodies and are long without beards, and sometimes they are beardless with age. The hair of their heads is dusky brown usually, and sometimes dusky flaxen. Their appetite is far better than their concoction usually, by reason the appetite is caused of a sour vapor sent up by the spleen, which is the seat of melancholy, to the stomach. Their urine is pale, their dung of a clavish colour and broken, their pulse slow, they dream of frightful things, black, darkish, and terrible businesses.

They are naturally covetous, self-lovers, cowards, afraid of their own shadows, fearful, careful, solitary, lumpish, unsociable, delighting to be alone, stubborn, ambitious, envious, of a deep cogitation, obstinate in opinion, mistrustful, suspicious, spiteful, squeamish, and yet slovenly. They retain anger long, and aim at no small things.[20]

The *Regimen of Health* describes the melancholic temperament as follows:

> The melancholy from the rest do vary,
> Both sport and ease and company refusing.
> Exceeding studious, ever solitary,
> Inclining pensive still to be, and musing,
> A secret hate to others apt to carry.
> Most constant in his choice, tho' long a-choosing,
> Extreme in love sometime, yet seldom lustful,
> Suspicious in his nature and mistrustful.
> A wary wit, a hand much given to sparing,
> A heavy look, a spirit little daring.[21]

This temperament was thus held in the least esteem, as is apparent from these descriptions. Yet there was an understanding in the Renaissance period that melancholy held a key to a greater knowledge of the world, a knowledge derived not just from experience and experiment but also from a quiet contemplation of profound matters, a heightened sensibility of what it is to be alive. The intellectual has replaced the physical as the dominant activity. Cicero praised 'that old age which has its foundations well laid in youth' and exhorted his audience:

> to resist old age; to compensate for its defects by a watchful care; to fight against it as we would fight against disease; to adopt a regimen of health; to practise moderate exercise; and to take just enough of food and drink to restore our strength and not to overburden it. Nor, indeed, are we to give our attention solely to the body; much greater care is due to the mind and soul; for they, too, like lamps, grow dim with time, unless we keep them supplied with oil. Moreover, exercise causes the body to become heavy with fatigue, but intellectual activity gives buoyancy to the mind.[22]

Winter/phlegmatic temperament/old age

In the Winter months the coldness of the season induces dampness or moisture. All activity is frozen and congealed beneath the surface. The pure phlegmatic temperament or complexion is associated with the qualities of the Winter season and similarly demonstrates in a younger body some of the tendencies associated with the aged. Culpeper records the following physical description and condition:

> Such people in whom coldness with moisture abounds are called phlegmatick, yet are usually not very tall, but very fat. Some you shall find almost as thick as they are long, their veins and arteries are small, their bodies without hair, and they have but little beards. Their hair is usually flaxen or light brown, their face white and pale, their skin smooth, cold and moist in touching. Both appetite and digestion is very weak in them, their pulse little and low, their urine pale and thick, but the excrements of their bowels usually thin. They dream of great rains, water and drowning.
>
> As for Conditions [character], they are very dull, heavy and slothful, like the scholar that was a great while a-learning a lesson, but when *once* he had it – he had quickly forgotten it. They are drowsy, sleepy, cowardly, forgetful creatures, as swift in motion as a snail, they travail (and that's but seldom) as though they intended to go 15 miles in 14 days. Yet they are shamefaced and sober.

The *Regimen of Health* has this to say:

> The phlegmatic are most of no great growth,
> Inclining to be rather fat and square.
> Given much unto their ease, to rest and sloth,
> Content in knowledge to take little share,
> To put themselves to any pain most loath.
> So dead their spirits, so dull their senses are,
> Still neither fitting, like to folk that dream,
> Or else still spitting, to avoid the phlegm.
> One quality Doth yet these harms repair
> That for the most part Phlegmatics are fair.[24]

Phlegmatic types are stable and seemingly indifferent people with a poor memory and a conspicuous lack of guile or quick-wittedness. They indeed may suffer repeated head colds or chronic catarrh and may be prone to noises in the ears (tinnitus) and hardness of hearing, for their head is like a house which cannot keep out the wind and rain. Their hair is likely to turn grey or white long before they might ever become bald. They tend to be slow and lazy and have a dislike for exercise of any kind. Yet for all that they are gentle and quiet, lovers of ease who are neither irascible, fraudulent nor lustful.[25]

The salient feature of each of the primary qualities and of the 4 temperaments are therefore as shown below:

TABLE OF CERTAIN PHYSICAL SIGNS ASSOCIATED WITH EACH OF THE PRIMARY QUALITIES

	HOT	COLD	DRY	MOIST
Feel of skin	hot & rough	cold & smooth	dry & hard	soft & smooth
quantity of hair	plentiful	sparse or balding		
form of hair	curly	straight	curly	straight
colour of hair	red or black	brown		
build of body	lean	fat	slender	fat

TABLE OF PHYSICAL SIGNS ASSOCIATED WITH EACH OF THE 4 TEMPERAMENTS

	SANGUINE	CHOLERIC	MELANCHOLIC	PHLEGMATIC
Temperature of skin	hot & moist	hot & dry	cold & dry	cold & moist
Feel of skin	smooth & soft	rough	rough & hard	smooth
Stature	middle	short	middle	short
Build	fleshy	lean	slender	fat
Quantity of hair	hairy	very hairy, curly	hairless	hairless
Hair colours	dark brown/ flaxen	red, yellow	brown	light brown/ flaxen
Pulse	great & full	swift & strong	slow	little & low
Appetite & digestion	good, quick	strong digestion	appetite greater	both weak
Urine	thick & yellow	thin & yellow	pale	pale & thick
Faeces	reddish & firm	costive	pale & broken	thin
Dreams	merry/ colour red	fire, quarrelling	darkness, frights	water/ drowning
Associated emotion	joy	anger	fear/worry/grief	indifference

Compound Temperaments

Usually, however, a person consisted of more than one temperament displaying characteristics of two, or occasionally three, although one was likely to dominate the overall picture. This was called the principal temperament. The whole matter of assessing the temperamental balance in an individual was further complicated by their sex and age, for the temperament was not completely made manifest, Culpeper thought, until the person had reached full maturity, that is, around age 30. A basic melancholic nature (cold and dry), for instance, might be less apparent in childhood because of the prevailing qualities of that period of life (hot and moist) but become very accentuated in middle age (cold and dry). In addition the balance was also believed to be affected by consideration of the sex in that males were seen to be relatively hot and dry and females relatively cold and moist. The acme of the choleric temperament would therefore be seen in a young man of that complexion.

Culpeper listed 8 possible compound temperaments, taken from Galen:[26] sanguine-melancholic (the first – in this case sanguine – being the principal temperament), melancholic-sanguine, sanguine-phlegmatic, phlegmatic-sanguine, choleric-melancholic, melancholic-choleric, choleric-phlegmatic and phlegmatic-choleric. Culpeper ruled out the combinations where an active quality was twice in evidence, ie sanguine-choleric (hot and moist, hot and dry) and melancholic-phlegmatic (cold and dry, cold and moist), on the grounds that, since heat would induce dryness and cold attract moisture, the former combination would resolve into a choleric temperament and the latter into a phlegmatic. The combinations of 'opposite' temperaments, ie. sanguine-melancholic and choleric-phlegmatic, were quite in keeping with the notion of a world held in a dynamic equilibrium of opposing elementary qualities. Culpeper's descriptions of the 8 compound temperaments are summarized in the tables below:

COMPOUND TEMPERA-MENT	SANGUINE-MELANCHOLIC	MELANCHOLIC-SANGUINE	SANGUINE-PHLEGMATIC	PHLEGMATIC-SANGUINE
Skin temperature	warm	slightly warm		somewhat cold
Feel of skin	smooth	slightly soft		smooth & soft
Other skin features	dusky red cheeks; big veins/arteries	dark red colouring of face	face paler than in sanguines	white colouring
Stature	middling	tall	taller than sanguine	middling
Build	strong, well compact, fleshy	big, fleshy, firm, strong	strong, well-set, not very fat	rather fat

COMPOUND TEMPERA-MENT	SANGUINE-MELANCHOLIC	MELANCHOLIC-SANGUINE	SANGUINE-PHLEGMATIC	PHLEGMATIC-SANGUINE
Quantity of hair		somewhat hairy	less hairy than sanguine	little hair
Hair colours	dark brown, black			brown, flaxen, straight
Pulse	great & full		moderate	small & low
Appetite/digestion		good	digestion poorer than appetite	digestion poorer than appetite
Urine	yellow, not thick or thin	light saffron, not thick or thin	subcitrine, not thick or thin	pale & thick
Faeces	reddish, thin	reddish, soft	red with white	
Dreams	deep pits & wells, flying	pleasant, prophetic	flying in the air, rain & water	falling from high places into water
Character	like sanguine but not so merry or liberal	more liberal, bold & merry than melancholics and less pensive, solitary & fearful	less bold, liberal or 'addicted to the sports of Venus' than sanguines	a mean between phlegmatic & sanguine; fearful rather than valiant

COMPOUND TEMPERA-MENT	CHOLERIC-MELANCHOLIC	MELANCHOLIC-CHOLERIC	CHOLERIC-PHLEGMATIC	PHLEGMATIC-CHOLERIC
Skin temperature	slightly warm	cold	slightly warm	
Feel of skin	rough & hard	rough, dry, hard	slightly moist	
Other skin features	swarthy colour	face darkish but pale	face of tawny yellow colour	tawny red face, full of freckles
Stature	taller than cholerics	tall	middling height, stout, lusty, strong	tall
Build	little & lean	slender	well-set, neither fat nor lean	less big and fat than phlegmatics
Quantity of hair		little hair	hairy	moderately hairy

COMPOUND TEMPERA-MENT	CHOLERIC-MELANCHOLIC	MELANCHOLIC-CHOLERIC	CHOLERIC-PHLEGMATIC	PHLEGMATIC-CHOLERIC
Hair colours	chestnut or light brown	dark brown	yellowish or sandy	chestnut, neither curly nor soft
Pulse	strong, slightly slow	slow	swift	moderate and fairly full
Appetite/ digestion	moderately strong	both weak	good	indifferent, since well met
Urine	pale yellow & thin	subcitrine & thin	saffron & thin	subcitrine, neither thick nor thin
Faeces	yellow & hard	sallow & thin	yellow & hard	pale yellow, thick
Dreams	falling, robberies, murders, injuries from fire & anger	falling from high places; vain, idle and fearful things	fighting, lightning & rain; hot baths and waters	swimming in water, snow and rain
Character	quick-witted, studious, solitary, quarrelsome, less scornful, more suspicious, retaining anger	very gentle, sober, studious, solitary, bashful, constant, true & willing to do good	similar to cholerics but with moderated passions and less vicious	less drowsy and lazy than phlegmatics; nimbler, bolder, kinder, merrier and more quick-witted

Temperaments of organs

Just as a person was seen to manifest a certain temperament, so too were each of the organs and parts of the body. In the same way, therefore, a divergence of an organ or part of the body from the normal temperament denoted disease of that part or organ. The skin was said to possess the ideal balance of temperaments and was thus especially sensitive to any imbalances such as differences in heat, cold, dryness and moisture.

The temperaments of other parts and organs of the body diverged from this mean towards heat, cold, dryness and moisture, as shown in the table below. For instance, the heart was regarded as extremely hot but tending neither to dryness nor moisture, while the liver was less hot but moist. The third principal organ, the brain, was classified as particularly moist and a little cold. We may note in passing that the lungs were considered not naturally moist but were made so by accumulated moisture from the gaseous products of the whole body which are exchanged there, and from 'phlegmatic distillations' or catarrh from the head. Similarly, the stomach was held to manage the first main 'concoction' or digestion of food, not by virtue of its own heat but because it is adjacent to the heart above, to the liver, another hot organ, on the right, and to the omentum in front, whose fatty substance appeared to retain heat easily and to reflect it onto the stomach.

TABLE OF THE TEMPERAMENTS OF ORGANS

```
                          COLD
   phlegm                                hair & nails
                                              bones
                                           cartilage
                                          ligaments
                                            tendons


                                   membranes
M                                  nerves
         brain
O                                                        D
     fat
I                                                        R
          lungs            SKIN
S                                                        Y
        breasts                  veins
T
     testicles & ovaries         arteries
            kidneys
          spleen
                           muscles
                             flesh
          liver
   blood
                      heart & vital force
                          HOT
```

3 The 4 humours

> Four humours reign within our bodies wholly
> And these compared to four elements,
> The sanguine, choler, phlegm and melancholy.
> The latter two are heavy, dull of sense.
> The other two are more Jovial, quick and jolly
> And may be likened without offence
> Like Air both warm and moist is sanguine clear,
> Like Fire doth choler hot and dry appear.
> Like Water cold and moist is Phlegmatic,
> The melancholy cold, dry Earth is like.
>
> *The Regimen of Health*

The 4 temperaments of the body, then, were said to arise from the interaction of the 4 elements and their primary qualities. This four-fold variation in the human body was matched specifically by the predominance of one of the 4 humours or body fluids. Indeed, the humours, elements, qualities and temperaments were all related.

TABLE OF RELATIONSHIPS

THE 4 ELEMENTS	FIRE	AIR	WATER	EARTH
The primary qualities	hot & dry	hot & moist	cold & moist	cold & dry
The temperaments	choleric	sanguine	phlegmatic	melancholic
The humours	yellow bile	blood	phlegm	black bile

Thus an excess of blood, correlating with the element Air and qualities of hot and moist, denoted a sanguine temperament (the Latin *sanguis* actually means 'blood'). A relative preponderance of yellow bile, of the nature of Fire and qualities of hot and dry, produced the choleric temperament (the Greek *chole* means 'bile'). The presence of more than a little black bile represented a disproportion of the element Earth with the qualities of cold and dry and resulted in a melancholic temperament (*melas* and *chole* in Greek mean 'black bile'). And excessive phlegm, pertaining to the element water and to the qualities of cold and moist, gave a phlegmatic temperament.

In the same way in which the elements were not literally those things in the world, so too the humours were not simply reducible to body fluids. The phlegmatic humour, for instance, was not constituted simply of phlegm, lymph or serous fluid and neither was it simply all three. Urine, through a body fluid, was not regarded as a humour. Instead, the 4 humours were thought of as 'essences' or 'radical humours', quasi-material in nature and therefore more than the actual body fluids with which they were associated.[27]

The 4 humours, therefore, stood as components of the smaller world or microcosm that was the human body, in reflection of the 4 elements constituting the larger world or macrocosm.

> Nature was constituted by the four elements, the human body by the four humours, and elements and humours had their elementary qualities in common. They formed the bridge between the microcosm and macrocosm.[28]

Observation and reasoning on the 4 humours of the body came from the Hippocratic school of medicine. They fitted comfortably with the physics of elements and qualities taught by Aristotle and were easily assimilated into Galen's theory of medicine.

Greek physicians believed that they had found actual evidence of the existence of four humours in the contents of an emptied blood vessel. It was noted that when blood coagulates, an upper, light red layer (oxygenated red corpuscles), which was reckoned to be the blood humour itself, separates from the dark red coagulum (poorly oxygenated red corpuscles), called the black bile humour, below. Further contraction of this coagulum releases a clear yellow liquid (blood serum), corresponding to the yellow bile humour. If the blood was whisked before coagulation, a fourth humour, phlegm, was seen as a yellowish-white, fibrous mass (fibrin), sticking to the whisk.[29]

The stickiness of the phlegm humour, tending towards solid form, was interpreted as a likely cause of dangerous and unhealthy obstructions in blood vessels and an explanation for the arising of many diseases. When coagulated blood from sick patients was studied, it was found that, in cases of inflammation, eg in pneumonia, a distinctly deeper layer of a pale coagulum without any red corpuscles was present on its surface. This increased quantity of phlegm in the blood was interpreted as the cause of the disease present. Doctors today still test for this state of the blood as a general indication of inflammation, their attention specifically focused on the speed of sedimentation of the red blood corpuscles (the erythrocyte sedimentation rate or ESR), by which the layer of phlegm was revealed to Greek physicians.[30]

The basic concept of the body's organization was, in Galen's theory, that each organ has an attractive power, a transforming or assimilative power and an expulsive power to rid itself of unwanted residues. Galen believed that each organ works for itself and contributes to the whole. For example, the stomach attracts food from the mouth and is nurtured by it. The wholesome part of food, that which can be turned into actual flesh, is separated out from the dross by a 'first concoction' or 'cooking' in the stomach. The liver then draws to itself the resulting milky, semi-fluid mass, which is called 'chyle' via the mesenteric and portal veins. In the liver a second concoction takes place by which the chyle is turned into blood, yellow bile, black bile and phlegm.[31] These 4 humours in correct proportions are then transformed into the various tissues of the body while the gall-bladder holds the excess of yellow bile or choler and uses it to cleanse the bowels of the dross, the faeces, separated out in the stomach.[32] The spleen then attracts the superfluous black bile or melancholy which is used to stimulate the appetite for the next meal.[33]

Thirst will cause a person to drink more than the strictly required amount of fluid in order to render the blood in the liver more watery. This is to facilitate the passage of chyle through the narrowest channels of the liver. Once the blood then leaves the liver it is too watery for further needs so the superfluous fluid, along with the waste products of the second concoction, are siphoned out in the kidneys and stored in the bladder for subsequent excretion from the body as urine. Faeces and urine, the waste products of the first two concoctions, were termed 'excrementitious' fluids or 'superfluities' and had to be expelled from the body because they could not be transformed into actual bodily substance.

A third concoction, subsequent to the creation of the 4 humours in the liver, occurs in the distributed blood now coursing through the veins of the body. This is the intermediate stage before the subsequent fourth concoction in which the blood is transformed into tissue. The fluid, at first like dew sprinkling over the tissues, becomes 'glutinous' – the fluid begins to condense and finally becomes 'cambial' – in other words it transforms itself into the tissue substance itself. The waste-products of the third and fourth concoctions are eliminated from the body in various ways: by sweat and insensible transpiration, in the hair and nails, and by secretions from the ears and nose. Faultiness of the third concoction allows various deposits to remain in tissues and blood vessels with damaging effects.

CONCOCTIONS AND EXCRETIONS

3rd Concoction

Blood first passes from the liver to the most 'noble' organs, the heart and brain, where vital and then animal spirits are elaborated. Waste products from these processes are removed via the lungs, as exhaled air, and via the nose, as mucus, respectively. Blood is otherwise altered in the veins in preparation for the 4th concoction, the waste products removed via the kidneys or skin as sweat or insensible transpiration.

4th Concoction

Blood is transformed into tissues, and other substances such as breast milk and spermatic fluids. Waste is excreted via the kidneys or skin as sweat or insensible transpiration.

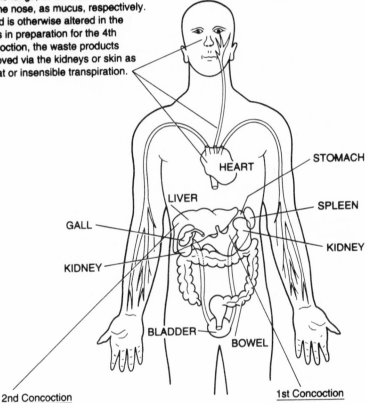

HEART

STOMACH

LIVER

SPLEEN

GALL

KIDNEY

KIDNEY

BLADDER

BOWEL

2nd Concoction

Chyle is cooked and differentiated in the liver into the 4 tumors, which are distributed in proportion via the veins. Excess of black bile is held in the spleen, yellow bile in the gall bladder. The waste of the 2nd concoction passes to the kidneys, then to the bladder for excretion as urine.

1st Concoction

Ingested food is cooked in the stomach. The nutriment (chyle) is separated out and passes by the mesenteric and portal vein to the liver. The waste passes down the digestive tract to be excreted as faeces.

Heat and cold were understood to have an effect on the production of all 4 humours in the body. When the heat within the body is temperate, blood is formed; when it is excessive, choler and a melancholic residue are produced; when in great excess, so as to burn the substance black, a toxic melancholy is the result. When the cold is temperate, normal phlegm is formed; but when in excess, the innate heat is compromised and the digestive powers weakened. Less blood and more melancholic humours are formed, causing congestion, obstruction to the flow of the spirits and a sluggish habit of the body. The importance of maintaining a balance of heat in order to produce a healthy proportion of humours is therefore vital since any excess of heat or cold helps to produce disease-causing humours.

The relative quantities of each of the 4 humours in the body were also determined by the degree of heat and moisture in the stomach and liver. All 4 humours would be produced by concoction in the liver according to the person's temperament but the different types of foods, seasons and other environmental or lifestyle factors could alter the balance. Where the digestion was excellent, all foods in a moderate diet would be turned into blood, together with the other humours in their correct and healthy proportions. However, the eating of a lot of hot and dry foods, such as garlic and onion, or a preponderance of fats, oils and sugar, foods that were reckoned easily combustible, could produce more choler, as could the strength of heat in the body of a young adult. Likewise, cold and moist food would produce more phlegm, especially in old age. Cold and dry melancholy would then be produced out of sour, tough or overcooked foods, and more easily in middle age, in autumn or in a state of continued anxiety. As an imbalance in the humours could thus cause ill-effects or even disease, so the temperament of the body could be affected in favour of a better balance of humours through the effects of foods, seasons and other factors. In the following descriptions the quotations are from Culpeper's *Astrologo-Physical Discourse*.

CHARACTERISTICS OF THE 4 HUMOURS

Blood

'*Blood* is made of Meat perfectly concocted, in quality hot and moist, governed by *Jupiter*. It is by a third concoction transmuted into Flesh, the superfluity of it into seed, and its receptacle is the veins, by which it is dispersed throughout the body.'

NORMAL

- *Normal blood* was described as red in colour with a sweet taste and no unpleasant odour. The Blood Humour included blood itself, its constituents (eg red and white cells and platelets) as well as the system of blood vessels and lymphatic channels in the body.

ABNORMAL

- *Abnormal blood* was basically of two types: when it was mixed with abnormal choler, phlegm or melancholy, or when its moisture increased so as to diminish its heat. This second form was very prone to putrefaction or bacterial infection, resulting in fevers and inflammatory diseases.

Phlegm

'*Flegm* is made of meat not perfectly digested; it so fortifies the vertue expulsive, as makes the Body slippery, fit for ejection; it fortifies the Brain by its consimilitude with it; yet it spoils Apprehension by its Antipathy to it. It qualifies Choler, cools and moistens the heart, thereby sustaining it, and the whole Body, from the fiery effects, which continual motion would produce: its receptacle is the Lungs, and is governed by *Venus*, some say by the *Moon*, perhaps it may be governed by them both.'

NORMAL

- The phlegmatic humour, sometimes called the serous humour, was classified as moderately cold and moist in quality and, *in its normal form*, was very sweet. It was regarded as imperfectly matured blood, the product of the less choice part of assimilated food, but it could subsequently undergo full conversion into blood. Otherwise it formed the lymphatic fluid and was thought to mix with blood in a certain proportion to nourish cold and moist organs and tissues of the body, particularly the brain. In this regard, there is a correlation to be made between healthy phlegm and carbohydrates. Since it was also said to help to keep the joints and other parts of the body moist its presence was necessary in the body. The classification also included nasal mucus, saliva and the mucus of the digestive tract.
- Several sorts of *abnormal phlegm* were identified. Since phlegm could harden when affected by either extreme heat or cold, it ranked as the main cause of obstruction

A
B
N
O
R
M
A
L

to the flow of blood and spirits in the body. The action of heat on phlegm could thin a part of it, producing a serous or watery discharge, while what remained would be very thick, dense and obstructive. The most hardened forms of abnormal phlegm were likened to glass, the 'vitreous' form to which old people were particularly subject, and the 'tophi' or deposits seen in the joints of those afflicted by gout, to chalk.

Choler

'*Choler* is made of Meat more than perfectly concocted; it is the spume and froth of blood: clarifies all the Humours, heats the Body, nourisheth the Apprehension, as Blood doth the Judgement. It ... fortifieth the attractive faculty, as Blood doth the digestive; moves man to activity and valour: its receptacle is the Gall, and it is under the influence of *Mars*.'

N
O
R
M
A
L

- Choler, also known as yellow bile or the bilious humour, was considered *in its normal state* to be hot and dry in quality and bitter to the taste. It was call the 'froth' of blood, to use the simile of wine (as melancholy is the 'lees' or sediment) and described as clear, light, pungent and of a yellow colour. As a fluid, it is the bile found in the gall-bladder. It was said to serve two purposes in the bloodstream: very small amounts thin the blood so as to facilitate the passage of the blood through the smallest channels of the body and also to nourish those organs and tissues which require choler, eg the lungs. A larger quantity of choler, which is extra to these needs, is then held in the gall-bladder to stop it polluting other parts of the body and for secretion into the bowels. This secretion cleanses the walls of the bowels of food residues and thick phlegm, and stimulates the muscles of the lower digestive tract for defecation

A
B
N
O
R
M
A
L

- *Abnormal choler* was formed when the digestive process was impaired due to an excess of heat, the chyle being burned by degrees. These types of combusted choler were considered toxic, varying in colour according to the degree of their abnormal heat, from the vitelline bile, likened in colour to an egg yolk, through leekgreen, verdigris and red to black. The leekgreen bile in particular was thought to be produced by the heat from certain types of food such as garlic, leeks, onions and watercress. The darker the abnormal choler, the less moisture it contained and the more toxic and inflammatory it was. It was said to be produced in the stomachs of very overheated bodies. When choler was charred black, like wood in a fire, it was termed adust choler.

Melancholy

'*Melancholy* is the sediment of blood ... fortifying the Retentive Faculty, and Memory; makes them sober, solid and staid, fit for study, stayes the unbridled toyes and fooleries of lustful thoughts, and reduceth them home to the Centre: it is like a grave Counsellor to the whole body: its receptacle is the Spleen, and it is governed by *Saturn*.'

N
O
R
M
A
L

- Melancholy, also called black bile, the atrobilious humour or sauda, was cold and dry in quality. *In its normal form*, it had a taste between sweetness and astringency. The melancholic humour was said to be stored in the spleen because, on dissection, that organ appears to contain a thick black matter made of decomposed red blood cells like that seen when blood separates out into its constituents. The spleen was nourished by melancholy in the same way that the gall-bladder derived sustenance from the choler it drew into itself, whilst traces of melancholy remained in the blood to give it strength, stamina, density and consistency as well as to supply a balanced nutriment to organs requiring it such as the bones, hair and nails. A small amount of black bile was also believed to be regularly attracted into the stomach with the purpose of stimulating the appetite by its sour bitterness and to strengthen the ability of the stomach to retain the food eaten until it was fully digested. Moreover, this humour was thought to help in the process of dissolving the food because of its likeness in taste and acrid nature to vinegar.
- *Abnormal melancholy* was regarded as an ash or residue resulting from the combustion of the denser portions of food material, or indeed any fluid in the body, by

A
B
N
O
R
M
A
L

unnatural heat. Thus this abnormal black bile is yellow bile or choler, phlegm or blood burned black. Being hotter and lighter than the natural form, it was thought to manifest a strong penetrative power of moving from the upper parts to the lower and also to have a destructive, corrosive and ulcerating action. The 4 basic kinds of abnormal melancholy are:

1 Residue from complete combustion of choler (verdigris-green and other colours of bile), bitter in taste and extremely toxic.

2 Residue from the combustion of phlegm, which may taste salty if the phlegm is watery, acid or astringent if otherwise. Less morbid.

3 Residue from the combustion of blood, tasting salty and faintly sweet. Less morbid.

4 Residue from the combustion of melancholy, which if thin, will be very acrid, like vinegar, or, if denser, will be astringent and slightly bitter. This was considered a slow-acting poison unless it was burned black, in which case it was more toxic.

Abnormal melancholy was said to be increased in the body as a result of

a excessive heat in the liver, causing the cooking to be burned

b weakness or inefficiency of the spleen to contain the humour

c excess cold in the body which congeals and solidifies excretions

d prolonged stagnation, from the same cause, and

e chronic diseases which burn the humoral matter.

The excess of melancholy was thought to lodge between the liver and stomach, interfering with assimilation of food and the production of blood so as to produce results such as anaemia.

The Unity of the Humours

Colour was an important indication of the nature of the morbid humours. Blood red stood for the normal sanguine humour; a darker red, together with yellow and green, for an abnormal choler; black for adust choler and abnormal melancholy; and white for phlegm. The tissue in a cancerous tumour is black due to necrosis and so was labelled a disease of the extremely toxic form of melancholy. The black faeces of melaena, due to the presence of altered blood, and haemorrhoids were reckoned to be other manifestations of this humour. In contrast, the tissue destruction (the whitish caseating necrosis), of the appearance and crumbliness of cheese, which is caused by the tubercle bacillus (tuberculosis), was thought to be a form of abnormal phlegm. And the fluid contained in cysts (literally 'bladders') was regarded as an accumulation of yellow bile or choler, or, where the fluid was clear, it was simply deemed a watery humour.

Although an impure or 'corrupted' humour would indicate the nature and process of disease present and had to be evacuated from the body, the unity of the humours in a living being was ultimately more important than the condition of any of the humours taken separately. In this the holistic nature of traditional Western medicine is reflected. The ability of the organism to function well as a whole was conducive to its health. The more it was torn by conflict, the sicker it would become. The Greeks defined a healthy temperament as a *eucrasia* or 'good mix' of elements composing the body, even though there might be a divergence from a perfect balance by dint of one element being slightly in excess. Furthermore it was not thought that everyone sharing a temperament, or the equivalent balance of humours, would be exactly alike. For the *physis* or nature of a person in their unity was considered unique, and was therefore ranked by Hippocrates as of higher importance than any of the individual humours or elements. Moreover, the exact blending of the 4 humours into the individual person was regarded as something mysterious and impossible to elucidate, defying further analysis without the risk of losing sight of that unity. Such a concept prevented the considerations of health and sickness from becoming a simple reduction of the person to a matter of the quantity of humours present in the body. These had to be evaluated with reference to the totality of being.[34]

Yet, as life is a constant interplay between the *physis*, or nature, and the environment, it was thought useful to have some rationale for interpreting the effects of the one upon the other. This interaction is a two-way affair, for while the environment affects the organism, so the organism shapes and changes the environment for its own benefit, and grows and develops at its expense. For Hippocrates, the study of the 4 humours of the body gave an explanatory theory, but not a binding doctrine, for the effects of the interplay. Since the internal humours were added to by the external food eaten, the processes of digestion (*pepsis*) or indigestion (*dyspepsia*) seemed a pertinent analogy for success or failure in interacting wholly and successfully with the environment.[35] Such an analogy is brought out in descriptions like 'he could not stomach it' or 'she could not swallow it'. Thus any kind of dyspepsia which is producing discomfort on a physical level could have its origin on any of the physical, mental, emotional or spiritual planes which constitute the *physis* or nature of the human being in its unique and mysterious unity.

4   The Parts

Aristotle decreed that all perceptible objects, both living and non-living, are composites, that is, they are made up of smaller *parts*.[36] If we take the human body as an example, we can divide the whole into major subdivisions: the head, the chest (thorax), the abdomen (pelvis) and the limbs (extremities). Further subdivisions can be made: for example the leg has a part called the foot and the foot a part called the toe. Finally we arrive at the similar parts, the parts which constitute other parts. These are *skin, bone* together with *cartilage,* and *ligament, vein, artery, nerve, tendon* and *fat,* collectively called *flesh*.[37] Each of these was considered homogenous: for instance if bone is broken up into smaller fragments, each separate fragment appears like the others, differing only in size but not in basic nature. This basic nature of such similar parts was, like everything, analyzed in terms of elements. Bone, for example, was said to be composed of all the 4 elements but with a preponderance of the element Earth which gave it the qualities of coldness and dryness ('bone dry').

In the human body the similar parts are found together in whole units, such as the knee, the lower leg or the foot; units which on dissection are found to be quite different from each other. These dissimilar parts were termed organs, along with other composite tissues which we refer to today as organs, such as the liver, heart and stomach, so that, in Culpeper's day, the term 'organical' was synonymous with 'dissimilar'. The whole of the human body, therefore, was seen as a composition of various organs, made up of an aggregate of similar parts which could be reduced to the 4 elements. But the body is material: it is composed of matter, has spatial extension in the world and manifests certain qualities so that we can perceive it with our senses. The body also has *form*, which determines that the object in question is specifically one thing and not another thing. For example, a chimpanzee is a living being composed of organs which are constructed out of the same group of similar parts as a human being is but it is not human because it possesses a different form.

Three characteristic properties of form were noted.[38] First, it is indivisible, existing entire and whole in the smallest or the greatest mass. For example, the same appropriate form exists whether it be in the fennel seed or in the fully grown plant. Secondly, form fills all matter which embodies it. Thus, form is not absent from any part of the fennel plant as it grows and develops. Thirdly, form is capable of multiplication, as is the fennel plant.

There was understood to be a hierarchy of forms both in the natural world and within any composite body. In nature those forms dealing with more complex motions or activities were seen as the more 'noble'. Thus the nutrition, growth and reproduction which plants demonstrated set them above non-living matter. More noble and higher were the animals, by virtue of their more complex physiology incorporating sensation and motion, while at the apex of this hierarchy sat Man, whose perfection was measured by the myriad activities he performed, in thought and deed. The same system of rank was then applied to the human body. The similar parts and lesser organs were concerned with the disposition of their own material and its functioning and the 'nobler' principal organs, the brain, heart, liver and sex organs, which had the first share of newly formed blood, regulated the various functions of the whole body via their own networks of other organs and similar parts.

5 The Faculties of the Body

In Galenic medicine there was a fundamental concern with the dynamic aspects of reality; with function and activity. It was felt that what a thing was, its essential nature, was related to what it did. The explanation of the powers of an object to function in a certain way and to produce particular effects was therefore thought to reveal the basic nature of that object. These powers, also called Virtues or Faculties by Culpeper, were derived from the primary qualities inherent in the object. For instance, the power of oak bark to tan leather resides in its strong drying or astringent quality. The faculties and qualities of any thing were also closely connected with its form, that is to say, with the active principle which dictated its formation and determined its structure and characteristic appearance. Indeed it was believed to be through the qualities of an object that its form was made functional.[39]

The function and activity of an object thus related to its primary qualities which were detectable by the human senses. Yet physicians also noticed that certain objects produced efforts which were not explained by their manifest qualities of heat, dryness, cold or moisture: the force within a magnet which attracts iron, for example, also the properties of purgative plants, the force that lurks within the saliva of a mad dog (rabies) and the poison of a scorpion. These were thought to possess some other quality to account for such effects and these qualities were termed *occult* or *hidden* qualities. It was felt that they were present by virtue of their form and 'from the whole substance' of them but they could not be perceived directly by the senses, only understood indirectly from their effects. These then also provided a basis for the Faculties.[40]

Thus the principal organs of the body, the heart, brain and liver, and the gonads were thought to possess qualities emanating from their complete form and in these cases the qualities were hidden qualities. The *faculty* of the liver, for instance, would not be discovered by dissection of that organ. Nor was it apparent in the manifest feel or taste of a liver. Like the *physis* or nature of a person, or the 4 humours said to be present within the body, the faculties of the body's principal organs had an existence beyond the merely physical. They were to be understood as metaphysical entities displaying actual activities. The whole was to be understood in effect as greater than the sum of its integrated parts.

Galen identified three faculties of the body and associated three 'spirits' with them. These spirits were thought to be hot and vaporous 'breaths' emanating from the principal organs. Culpeper described them as 'airy, subtle and quick.'[41] The vital spirit radiated from the heart, passing along the arteries throughout the body and so effecting the vital faculty, the principal faculty to which every part of every living thing owed its existence. In turn this spirit vivified the other two, the natural spirit in the liver and the animal spirit in the brain. No part of the body could perform its activities and processes without first being vivified by the vital spirit.[42]

The Vital Spirit, the Radical Moisture and the Innate Heat

The spirits with the body were also called *pneuma* meaning 'wind', 'air', 'breath' and also 'spirit' (the breath of life). Pneuma is traditional Western medicine's equivalent to *prana* in Indian Ayurvedic medicine and the *chi* in traditional Chinese medicine.

Life-giving air was said to be drawn into the lungs during inhalation and sucked into the heart by its own expansion and contraction via the pulmonary vein. Here it mixed with the 'light and vapoury' portions of the blood flowing to the heart to form the principal pneuma, the vital spirit, which then radiated throughout the body.

The heart was sometimes likened to a brazier's bellows which suck in air from one direction and blow it out in another. In another sense it was a great furnace. The air taken into the body through the lungs served a double purpose of not only replenishing and refreshing the vital spirit but also helping to cool the heart, thus tempering the heat of the organ and of the innate heat. The sooty exhalations of this fiery process (carbon dioxide) were believed to be conveyed back to the lungs via the pulmonary vein to be exhaled from the body.

Pneuma as it was conceived cannot be regarded simply as the equivalent of oxygen which animals and humans have to breathe in order to live. Nor is it to be thought of as a force like electricity or heat, that can be investigated physically or chemically. It is not even what is meant by 'soul'. Instead it should be regarded as a sort of aura or life-giving principle which takes over the whole of the being.

It was apparent from the pulse felt in the arteries of the body that the pneuma or breath of life, like the natural rhythm of breathing in and out, ebbed and flowed in a regular manner. This alteration from one state to another found correspondences in nature, such as day and night, activity and rest, masculine and feminine, the cyclical changes in the seasons and their qualities (from hot to cold and from dry to moist and back again), and finally in the generation and corruption of all life forms. The beating of the heart is the pulse of all life.

Culpeper argued another alteration in the state of pneuma, from a divine form to an earthly one. In his words, Man

> had an immortal spirit breathed into him, according to that in Gen.2.7. 'God spirited into his nostrils the spirit of life, and he became a living soul,' which spirit cannot be corrupted because it is not nourished by food, and experience teaches us that even in our own bodies it still maintains a continual enmity and combat against the vices of the flesh.[43]

This spirit or 'breath of God' had a mundane counterpart which, being of the elemental world, could be tainted. The spirit was derived from the Sun, the source of motion in the world, and the maintainer of the vital spirit in humans and animals who breathed it. Culpeper added:

> According as this spirit is retent or remiss, vehement or not, according to the administration of other planets, so are the qualities and appetites of things below, either acute or dull, vehement or moderate.[44]

We can thus identify the spirit or breath of God in the first quotation as sustenance for the higher mind or 'rational soul', as it was called. This rational soul had the potential to become aware of realms of reality higher than that of the senses and to follow the spiritual path in life. The second earthly pneuma maintained a spirit which co-ordinated the faculties and functions of the body and operated at the lower level of the mind as a self-directing force.

It is clear, then, that Culpeper, as a devout Christian, agreed

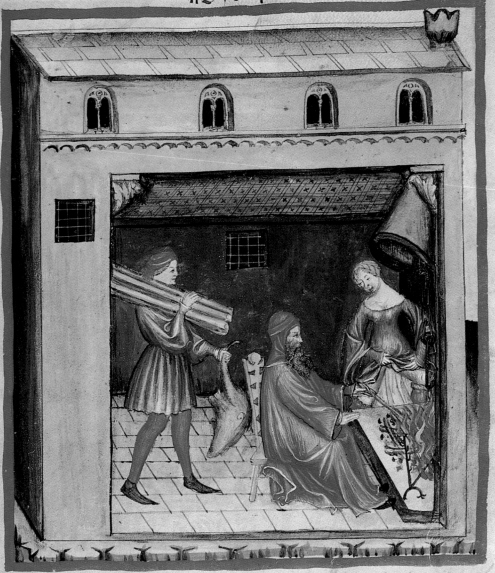

hyemps · 2plo · fri · iiz · hu · iii · malie se hiis. Aceto finis ei · uiuiiiituiii egtudiiiib; olicis et ꝯfoztit digōnez. nocuii · nocet egtudiiiib; flaticis Ꝉ auget ſtā. Remō noeti eiiigiie Ꝉ ueſtiiiiis Coiueit · ca · Ꝉ · siccis · iuueiiib; niidiaiiis Ꝉ maritiiiiis regioiiib; ·

PLATE 1

The text reads: 'Winter. complexion: cold in the third degree, moist in the second, of a bad quality.
Better at its end. Helpful for rank illnesses and strengthens the digestion. Harmful for phlegmatic
illnesses and increases phlegm. Removal of harm to the disposition with fire and clothing.
Agreeable to hot and dry youths and to southerly and maritime regions.'
From the **Tacuinum Sanitatis in medicina.**

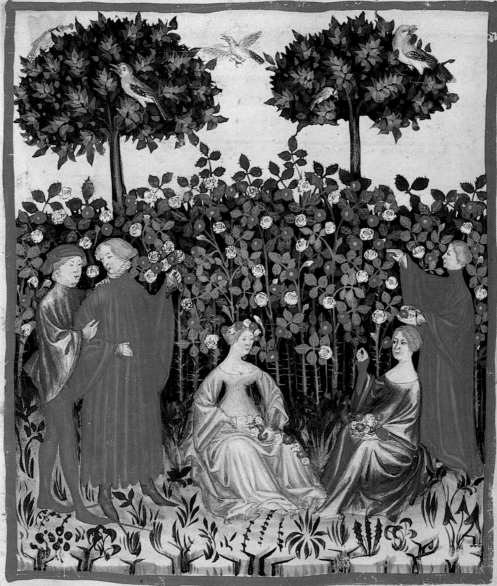

Uer. cplo. ca. tpate. hui. mi. Acct medui. ci. uuani. cfcit ulr aialibz 7 tir nafccitbz. nocii.
nocet cozbz ihumidis. qz facit i eis putredine. Remo nocti mundificando cozc. Genatur
i co humoz bonus 7 sanguis multus puenit fri a. sic 7 tpatis uuenibz 7 alus tpatis regio
mbz. 7 fere omnibz.

PLATE 2

The text reads: 'Spring. complexion: temperately warm, moist in the second degree. Better in the
middle of it. Agreeable to animals in general and especially to those born of the land. Harmful to
humid bodies as it causes putrefaction in them. Removal of harm by purging the body. It generates
in the body a good humour and much blood. Agreeable to cold and dry temperaments,
to temperate youths and to other temperate regions and to almost everything.'
From the **Tacuinum Sanitatis in medicina.**

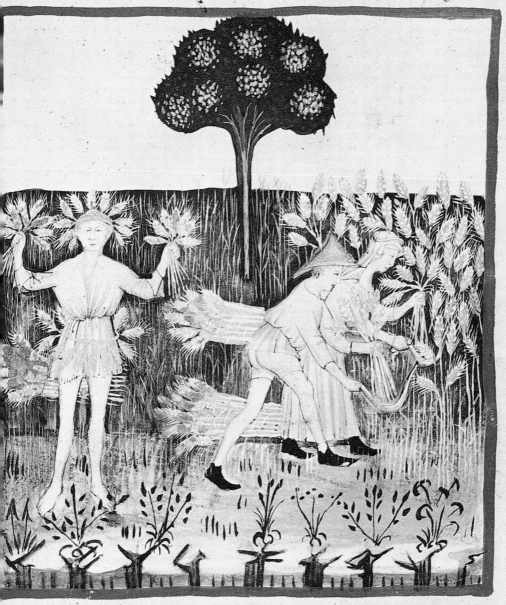

Eftas. ꝯplo. ca. iuʒ. ⁊ fic inᵉ. Electio iᵖſ ꝑꝑuiu. melⁱ é coꝛpoꝛibʒ. iuuini. diſoluit ſup
fluitates. ⁊ egritudies fir. nocuui. miuuit digōnes. ⁊ auget. colam Rem̄ nocti ei regi-
mē i ſtitate ꝟuido. Qᵤⁱd auget humoꝛes colicos. ⁊ ſicᶜ ꝺuenit. frⁱ⁊buʒ ſcibʒ. ⁊ ſeptᵉtᵒalib·

PLATE 3

The text reads: *'Summer. complexion: hot in the third degree and dry in the second. Better for the body
at its beginning. Helpful in resolving superfluities and cold illnesses. Harmful in impairing digestion and
augmenting choler because it increases choleric and dry humours. A regime of cold and moist things
removes its harm. Agreeable to the cold and the moist elderly and to northerly places.'*
From the **Tacuinum Sanitatis in medicina.**

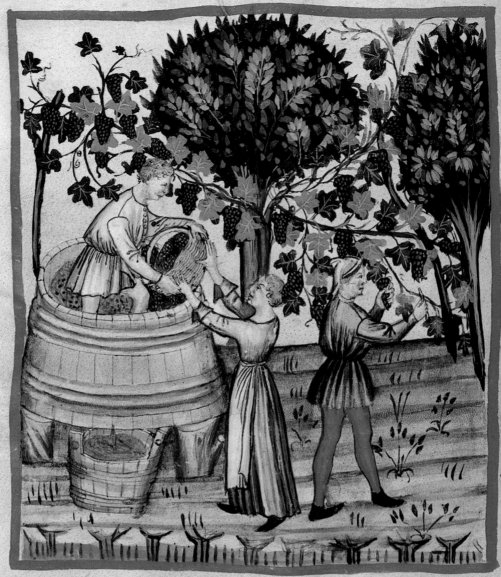

Autumpn̄. ꝯplo. fri̇. t̄p̄ate m̄t̄. Electo medui ı̇p̄i̇. uı̇uam̄i̇. q̄datum. pꝯb; aꝺ ꝺꝛıa. ut aꝺ caliꝺu
т̄.bu͛ſnocuum. nocet т̄patıs ꝯplꝓnıb; ⁊ dıſpo͛ⁿ aꝺ pᷓſız̄; Remı̇o noctı̇ cu̇ hu̇cet̄mtıb; ⁊ balneo .O:
augẹt huoꝛes mel̃ecolıcoꝛ; hueıt. ca.т̄.hū.uı̇uentıb; ſı̇ue aꝺolesectıb;. ca.⁊.hū. regıoıb; al̄̄т̄p̄atıs .

PLATE 4

The text reads: *Autumn. complexion: temperately cold in the second degree. Better in the middle of it. Helpful in proceeding by degrees to its opposite as far as a hot and moist state. Harmful to temperate complexions and dispositions to bad coughs because it increases melancholic humours. Removal of harm with moistening things and with bathing. Agreeable to hot and moist youths or adolescents and to hot and moist and other temperate regions.*'
From the **Tacuinum Sanitatis in medicina.**

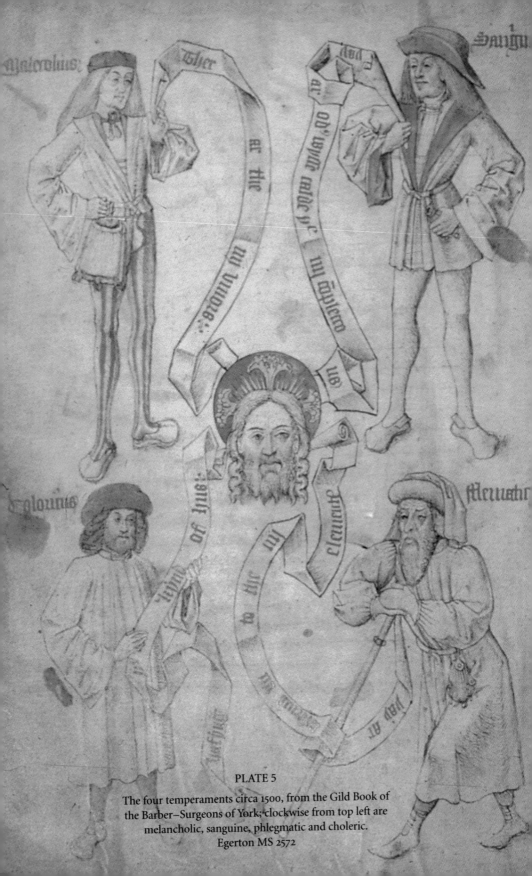

PLATE 5

The four temperaments circa 1500, from the Gild Book of
the Barber–Surgeons of York; clockwise from top left are
melancholic, sanguine, phlegmatic and choleric.
Egerton MS 2572

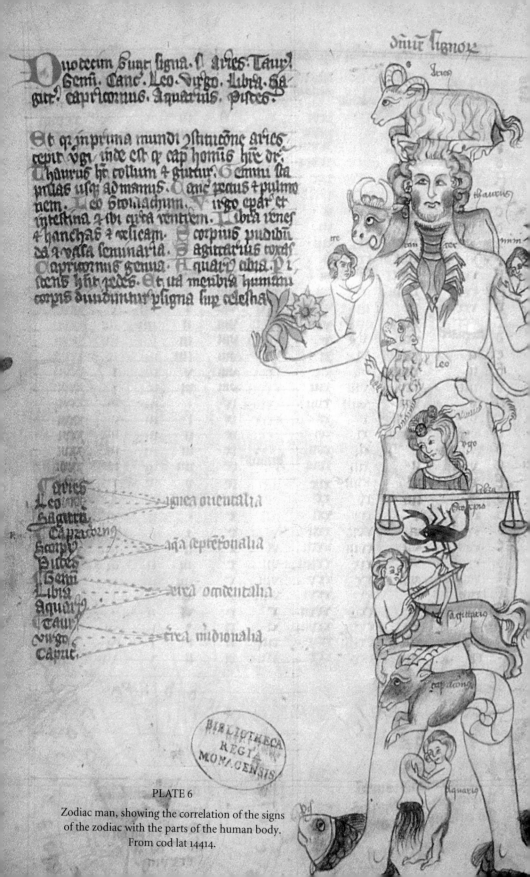

PLATE 6

Zodiac man, showing the correlation of the signs
of the zodiac with the parts of the human body.
From cod lat 14414.

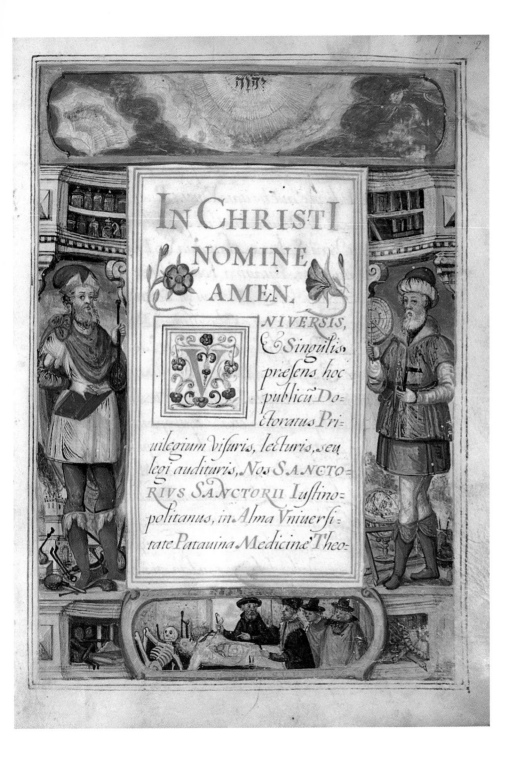

PLATE 7

A doctoral diploma in medicine from Padua, 1618, bearing the coat of arms of J Rave, a German
Physician. Note the medical instruments on the left and astronomical instruments on the right.
Santorio Santorio, a friend of Galileo, taught medicine at Padua between 1615 and 1624.

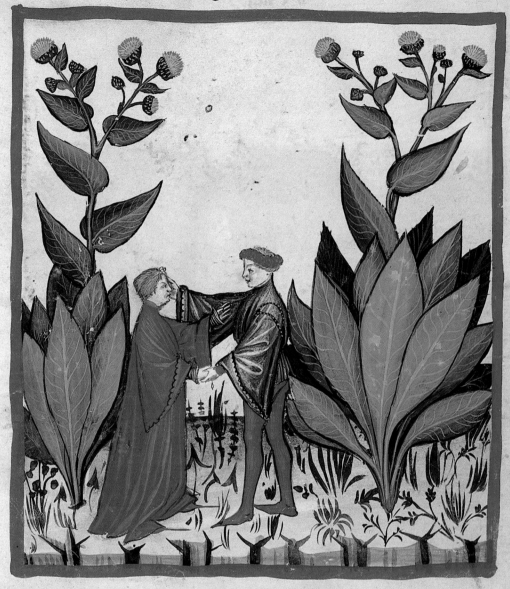

Gnula. ꝯpl'o. cala. inȝ. humia.in ȝ. al'. fic. inȝ. Gcecto melior ē ortulana domeſtica. uua
nitum. apit opilatices. ꝯfert cordi. mundificat pect ab humorib; groſſis noeunitur.
cit ſodam ꞇ minuit ſanguine·Remoto noeuniti eu ȝuch. oleo amigdola ꞇ aceto ꞇ ſale.
Qo gñat ſanguine calȝ. no bonuȝ ꝗue nit. fris. ꞇ ſic. ſcib; ꞇ decrepitis. hyeme. ꞇ ſepte
trionalib;·

PLATE 8

ELECAMPANE (*Enula*).

The text reads: '*Elecampane. complexion: hot in the third degree, moist in
the second, others are dry in the second. Better from a domestic garden. Helpful in opening obstructions,
comforting the heart and purging the breast of thick humours. Harmful in causing a migraine and
diminishing the blood because it gives rise to hot and not good blood. Take with sugar, sweet
almond oil, vinegar and salt to remove its harm. Agreeable to the cold and dry elderly and
to those made decrepit in winter and in northerly regions.*'
From the ***Tacuinum Sanitatis in medicina.***

with Plato in regarding the soul as immortal, immaterial and separated from the body, unlike Aristotle or Galen, who did not believe in a soul existing apart from the body. Many times Culpeper found fault with Aristotle's concepts or he criticized him for 'marring Plato's philosophy'.[45] He obviously rejected Aristotle's view that the 'inbred' pneuma each person was born with was supported by the nutritive faculty, and instead found himself sharing the view of many philosophers and physicians, Galen included, that the inbred pneuma was preserved, nourished and cherished in the living being through the inspiration of air which was said to contain 'accidental' pneuma (ie it did not belong naturally to the body but entered it from outside). In Galenic teaching, this point was qualified inasmuch as the three faculties and their spirits, considered as powers of the soul through which the body functioned in life-as-action, were partly derived from the individual temperament of the body and therefore varied in their powers from person to person.

Aristotle himself argued that pneuma possessed soul, which he called *psyche*, and which he said correlated with the form and organization of the living being. His teaching on reproduction had it that only male semen contained the formative pneuma. He likened pneuma to *aether*, the material from which he said the stars were made since both were generative, the one of stars and planets, the other of human beings. Moreover, both mediated motion: aether transmitted the motor effect of the 'Prime Mover' or *Primum Mobile*, the source of all movement and the maintainer of the eternal motion of the universe, while pneuma communicated the motor effect of the soul to the menstrual blood in the creation and animation of new life.[46] Thus, in Aristotle's view, pneuma was unlike anything else: being very hot in quality, it provided the original innate heat of the body from conception to death, as the Sun continually provides warmth, light and life to planet Earth. This 'natural heat' innate in humans is simply the manifestation of the pneuma-containing vital spirit which gives life and motion and, when free to emanate unobstructed, provides a wholeness and unity of the being which maintains it in full health and vitality. In Culpeper's words, 'The Celestial Sun gives a vital seed and stirs up all to motion and action. It dries, cherishes, quickens, defends and preserves what it has quickened.'[47]

EXPLANATION OF RADICAL MOISTURE

Pneuma, then, represents the spark of life at conception and, in the air which we breathe, the maintainer of life after birth. Menstrual blood provided the moist pabulum for the hot pneuma at conception so as to meet the requirements of heat and moisture which nature needs and receives each Spring in order to produce new life. A special moisture came to be regarded as essential for maintaining the innate heat of the body throughout life and a concept of a *radical moisture* was developed, particularly among Arab physicians.[48]

Radical moisture was likened to a humid, fat or oily substance and was said to be found in all tissues. As the 'inbred' pneuma was nourished by the 'accidental' pneuma entering the body during breathing, so the radical moisture was added to as well, albeit imperfectly, at the fourth concoction. During this some of the blood, which was at the glutinous stage before its complete integration into tissue substance, was held back. It was this fluid that became radical moisture. The relationship of radical moisture to innate heat was explained by the metaphor of the lamp.

THE METAPHOR OF THE LAMP

In traditional Western medicine the oil lamp came to be used as a metaphor for individual life.[49] While the flame burns there is light and life and while there is oil in the lamp, the flame is fed. When the lamp is first lit the flame burns brightly, but when the quantity of oil in the lamp becomes diminished, the flame starts to weaken and dim. Eventually when the oil has been consumed, the flame starts to splutter and is then extinguished: no more light, no more life.

In this metaphor, the flame was thought to represent the innate heat in the body and the traditional belief decreed that it was furnished by the pneuma originating from the father's semen. This traditional belief then stated that the pneuma, the spark of life, animated and shaped the menstrual blood of the mother (the oil or moisture which feeds the spark and makes it a flame) creating a new life in the womb. The parts that the male and female fluids played were likened by Aristotle to a carpenter's effect on wood, the material being provided by the female, which is shaped or operated on by the male.[50]

Culpeper, however, rejected the traditional notion that only male sperm formed and energized new life. For him, the seed of both the mother and father came together equally to form a new life as the Sun and Moon equally influence procreation. Similarly, he held radical moisture to be an active force existing throughout the body in parallel with and as a complement to innate heat, cherishing and maintaining the flame while ensuring that its Fire conserves rather than destroys the body. He wrote:

> The *Sun*, as is well known to every one, gives heat to the world; and if so, then also to the body of man, because our life consists chiefly by heat which animates the moisture, so the *Sun* must needs be the Author of life, and father of all living creatures, and therefore must of necessity be first formed in the Seed of both Sexes, being mixed in respect of order, if not in respect of time. He is formed in the very midst of the Seed, from whence he quickens, inspires and moves every part to its particular action. Indeed what *Aristotle* attributed to the heart in the generation of man, is very true, if he had spoken it of the *Microcosmical Sun*, and therefore some real Philosophers (scarce dare reckon *Aristotle* in the number of them) having imagined that the seat of the *Microcosmical Sun* in the body of man was the heart. Yet I can scarce be of that opinion, that the *Microcosmical Sun and Moon*, which reign like King and Queen in the body, should be confined to any particular place. However, the office of the *Microcosmical Sun* both in and after Conception is to give vital Spirit, and stir up all things to motion and action.
>
> As the water moistens the Earth, that so it might not be burnt up by the scorching heat of the *Celestial Sun*, so the *Microcosmical Moon* adds moisture to the conception from the very beginning of the *embrion*, even to the utmost term of life. And this is what they call *radical moisture*, a term familiar enough amongst all *Physitians*, yet understood by very few.[51]

The oil in the lamp and the radical moisture of the body were thought to be of a limited quantity, which varied from person to person, according to how much each was endowed with at birth. The lifespan of an individual thus depended on this initial quantity, but then also on how fast the radical moisture was consumed in the course of his or her life. At the start of life the lamp was brimming with oil and this quality of moisture was much required for the foetus to grow, to be shaped into the form of the species and to be made into an individual with characteristics inherited from the two parents. Once born, a child would continue to grow and develop quickly, thanks to the great abundance of oil still in the lamp. The growing strength, vigour and capability of the child was mirrored in the increasing strength of the flame and the greater consumption of oil in the lamp as childhood progressed.

In youth or young adulthood, the period of life characterized by heat and dryness, the lamp's flame was at its maximum intensity and perhaps brighter than during childhood,[52] as a fire would be when the damp wood is fully dried out or tinder-dry. Dryness meant a diminution of moisture; some of the oil in the lamp had been consumed in the course of growing up, so that there was no longer sufficient to sustain the growing process but enough to maintain the flame in its full vigour. Then, in middle age, there was a diminution in the flame as yet more of the precious radical moisture had been consumed in maintaining the flame and the flame had begun to dim in the continuing state of relative dryness. The diminution of the flame – and the innate heat – rendered the digestive process less efficient, increased the production of a cold moisture, and the formation of phlegmatic humour instead of blood. This, in turn, further diminished the innate heat and the powers of digestion by diluting the radical moisture – or oil – in the lamp with the cold moisture so that the voracity of the lamp's flame was reduced still more. In this way an unavoidable spiral of decline was set up, leading in old age towards coldness, loss of radical moisture and death. This pattern of diminution continued until death when the oil or radical moisture was exhausted and the flame, with nothing to feed on, was snuffed out.

The combination of innate heat and radical moisture was therefore deemed crucial to the preservation of health. The balance of such a heat, with its potential to dry out the body, and a moisture that, if excessive, could dampen down the flame of life had to be carefully maintained. The moisture was also said to cherish and nurture the heat as well as to protect the body from its effects. The heat attracted moisture to it and consumed it at the same time for its own maintenance. Physicians thus became focused on preserving life and on halting the ageing process in two ways: by stopping the heart in particular, and the body in general, from drying out to such an extent that it ceased to function (heart failure); and by maintaining the innate heat for optimum digestion so as to avoid the production of crude

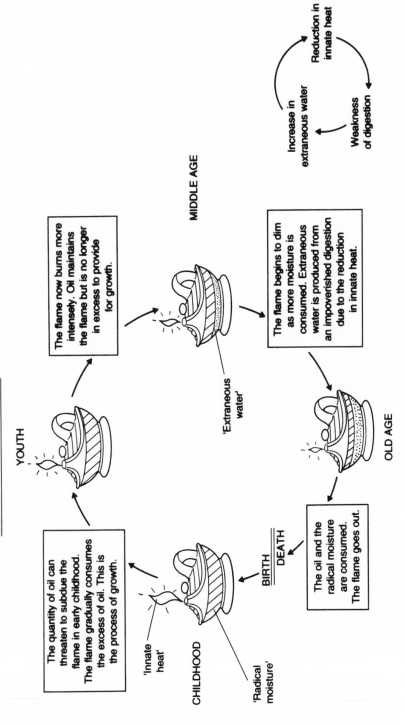

THE METAPHOR OF THE LAMP

YOUTH

The flame now burns more intensely. Oil maintains the flame but is no longer in excess to provide for growth.

MIDDLE AGE

'Extraneous water'

The flame begins to dim as more moisture is consumed. Extraneous water is produced from an impoverished digestion due to the reduction in innate heat.

Increase in extraneous water

Reduction in innate heat

Weakness of digestion

OLD AGE

The oil and the radical moisture are consumed. The flame goes out.

BIRTH
DEATH

CHILDHOOD

'Innate heat'

'Radical moisture'

The quantity of oil can threaten to subdue the flame in early childhood. The flame gradually consumes the excess of oil. This is the process of growth.

humours created in the body by faulty concoction. The key to both was thus to protect the radical moisture from being consumed faster than it needed to be.

PUTREFACTION

Putrefaction occurred when excess moisture in the body dampened the innate heat and allowed the body to be governed by an *extrinsic* or *foreign heat*. While the innate heat was strong, the natural faculties could work successfully, effecting the digestion and maturation of the humours of the body and thereby maintaining them within the range of the healthy state. If the innate heat was weak, however, the natural faculties could be hindered in their operation by foreign heat. Aristotle stated that any body had intrinsic or natural heat capable of drawing its own moisture to itself but that extrinsic or foreign heat could overcome the body's own heat and then draw natural moisture out of the body.[53] Gruner comments:

> *If the innate heat is feeble*, the natural faculties are harassed in the regulation of the humours. For the instrument – the intermediary between the natural faculties and the humours – is enfeebled. Stagnation sets in and foreign heat now finds the humours no longer opposed to its action. It overcomes them. It utilizes them in its own way, and imparts a foreign movement to them; and the result is what is known as 'putrefaction'.[54]

Putrefaction (meaning in Latin 'making rotten') was a hot state because of the fever produced. Whilst fevers were classed as diseases in their own right, Hippocrates had interpreted fever as an attempt of the body to throw off an underlying disease by concocting the crude humours which were the cause of it and bringing them into a form in which they could be more easily voided from the body. One effect of a fever, particularly if it was chronic, was to induce a dryness of the body through a destruction and dispersal of moisture, which was apparent in the sweating of a feverish body.

Putrefaction was largely seen to come about through what we now call bacterial infection, although the term then was also applied to the effects of poison. It was regarded as the effect of an external heat, which overcame an enfeebled innate heat and corrupted the humours of the body, causing the heat of fever and the destruction and dispersal of the radical moisture, notably through sweating. Putrefaction could be life-threatening. Serious cases of infection with a high fever could easily end in death, and chronic fevers could reduce the body to a state of complex *marasmus* (complete wasting) which, being hot and dry in quality, could consume the radical moisture and thus bring the life of the sufferer to a speedier end. In less serious cases of putrefaction, some increased loss of radical moisture might occur but if the innate heat could be speedily restored by a complete recovery, then life would continue much as before.

Avoidance of putrefaction was therefore necessary for the purposes of preserving health and for living out the full span of years, since this was commensurate with the quantity of innate heat and radical moisture within a person. This meant that the integrity or 'wholeness' of the person, both body and soul, had to be preserved. Moreover sanguine types had to be careful since the abundance of moist blood in their bodies could easily dampen their innate heat, making them prone to diseases of putrefaction.

Culpeper knew that a calm mind and an appropriate and moderate diet was the way to ensure that the innate heat and radical moisture were preserved. He warned his readers

> to beware of care, grief, pensiveness, anger, of surfeits [excesses of food and drink] and venery [too much sexual intercourse]; to keep good hours, not to break the usual custom of their sleeps in the night; not to perplex themselves with too much worldly business, which brings on age and death.[55]

Perturbations of the mind were thus considered detrimental to the health of the body since they might affect the heart, situated at the centre of the body and regarded as the seat of the emotions.[56] The English language is full of examples of how we locate emotions in the heart. There are 'heartaches', 'heart-warming' moments and 'heart-rending' events. It has been said of some people that 'they died of a broken heart' and the expression 'a heaviness of the heart' denotes a depression of spirits. We instinctively understand the meaning of the symbolism employed: that a heart so compressed by heaviness is a heart whose vital force is contracted and whose faculty is depressed. To 'take heart' is then to be encouraged. Feelings of all sorts, when sincere and not feigned, come 'straight from the heart' and are described as 'heartfelt', while a frank and honest conversation may be described as a 'heart-to-heart'. If others toy with our affections, they are playing with our 'heart-strings'.[57] Thus we speak of the heart as the seat of our emotions and our true desires, the source of genuine, earnest and enthusiastic expression and spontaneous activity, often tempered by kindness and pity (unless we are 'hard-hearted'). A person may display these sincere, inner feelings quite openly when she wears her heart on her sleeve.

The opinion was that if the mind was tranquil and the feelings contented, as in hope, for example, or moderate joy, love, mirth, trust, mildness or in the act of singing, there would be a gentle and gradual expansion of the spirits and blood outwards throughout the body, which comforted and strengthened the person. When anger or hatred was involved, however, this movement became sudden and forceful, so that the spirits were rapidly dispersed and the pulse quickened. If these emotions were very strong, it was thought that they could overcome the rational mind temporarily.

Fear and terror, on the other hand, were said to confine the spirit inwards, as do other feelings of discontent, such as sorrow, grief and care. In the case of fear, the confinement or drawing of the spirits to the centre of the body would choke and constrict the heart. The extremities wax pale and cold, with trembling, chattering teeth, interrupted speech and loss of strength. There could be a 'loosening of the belly' or an involuntary urination and, when severe, it could cause fainting or even death ('scared to death') by extinguishing the vital faculty.

Gloom or mental depression was reckoned to maintain a prolonged and gradual contraction of the heart. With the spirits drawn inwards, the now concentrated innate heat they carried would begin to dry up the radical moisture and produce a pale, lean body with a weak pulse, cold and full of woe. Despondency was thus considered a drying state which, if unmitigated, could hasten old age. The vital spirits were rendered thick by the cold, increasing melancholy in the body, and the depression compromised the powers of digestion and diminished the resistance of the body to disease.[58]

Intense emotions altered the temperament and the altered temperament would then make those emotions habitual. Anger was associated with the choleric, joy and desire with the sanguine, and fear, terror, worry, despair or sadness with the melancholic.

The phlegmatic could be more stable and indifferent. If the heart was then inclined to a certain passion or the mind fixed in a predominant feeling, permanent changes to the body could ensue. Wasting and weakness were the concomitants of long-standing passions, as is reflected, for example, in the view today that continually raised blood pressure relates to contained or unexpressed aggression.

Sudden extreme passion of whatever kind, including excessive joy, could even cause the heart to break by violently contracting or expanding it, thus bringing about death. As Shakespeare wrote of King Lear:

> His flaw'd heart –
> Alack! too weak the conflict to support;
> Twixt two extremes of passion, joy and grief,
> Burst smilingly.

The Animal or Nervous Faculty

The animal faculty was believed to be created in the ventricles of the brain and its animal spirit therefore was supposed to govern mental activity and motor and sensory function. The difference between this and the vital spirit was that whilst the vital spirit energized every part of the being to perform its function and thus, in a general sense, enabled organs to receive sensory and motor activity (via the sympathetic nervous system, as we now know it, which innervates the internal organs),[59] the animal spirit actually caused the being to be animated – to effect specific voluntary motion and to relay back sensory information from outside the body. For example, a limb may be paralyzed and flaccid due to an obstruction for a variety of reasons of the animal faculty, but the limb does not decompose since the vital faculty is still maintaining it. However, when the passage for the vital spirit and the blood to a limb is obstructed, that limb will turn gangrenous and will mortify (die) from loss of the vital faculty.

A second distinction was made between the brain as the seat of reason and the heart as the seat of the emotions. The qualities of the brain from which the animal faculty was believed to originate were cold and moist, like the phlegmatic humour. The phlegmatic discharge voided from the nose or lungs by sneezing

Culpeper's Astrologo-phys. Discourse of the Human Virtues in the Body of Man

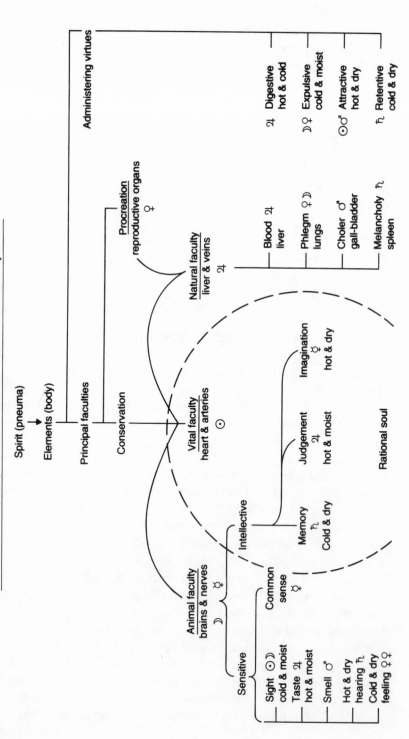

or coughing was therefore thought to be the waste produced by the creation of animal spirit in the brain.

There were differing opinions on whether phlegm had a receptacle or organ to which it belonged. Galen affirmed that there was no organ to excrete phlegm so that an excess of the humour was retained by the body.[60] Others named the pituitary gland lying at the base of the brain as its organ because it was thought to serve as the excretory pathway for the phlegmatic discharge from the brain into the nose.[61] To account for phlegm in the lungs, it was conjectured that it first *flowed down* from the brain and this is the meaning of *catarrh*, to flow down. The teaching that head and lung problems were caused by 'distillations from the brain' was being challenged in Culpeper's day, however, since physicians could not prove that the phlegm did always flow down from the brain to the lungs. Culpeper, presumably, also could not, which would explain why he suggested the lungs themselves as the receptacle for excess phlegm.[62]

Culpeper followed tradition in dividing the functions of the animal faculty into sensitive and intellective. The sensitive function was then further separated in two more parts, particular and common. The particular side of sensitive function dealt with perception through the 5 organs of sense, the eyes, ears, nose, tongue and hands, which provide sight, hearing, smell, taste and touch. Each sense was said to possess qualities; the power of sight was cold and moist, the faculty of hearing was cold and dry, that of smell was hot and dry, and the sense of taste was hot and moist. Of touch however he says:

> The *feeling* is deputed to no particular Organ, but is spread over the whole body; is of all qualities hot, cold, dry and moist, and is the Index of all tangible things; for if it were only hot alone, it could not feel a quality contrary, viz. cold; and so might be spoken of other qualities.[63]

The common part of the sensitive function (or 'common sense') was, Culpeper says, an imaginary term for that which united and preserved harmony between and among the five senses. Common sense received all forms and images perceived by the senses and combined them into one common mental picture.

Culpeper then goes on to divide the intellective function into imagination, judgement and memory:

Imagination is seated in the forepart[64] of the brain; it is hot and dry in quality, quick, active, always working; it receives vapours from the heart, and coins them into thoughts; it never sleeps, but always is working, both when the man is sleeping and waking; only when judgement is awake, it regulates the imagination, which runs at random when judgement is asleep, and forms any thought according to the nature of the vapour sent up to it. *Mercury* is out of question the disposer [regulator] of it ...

The imagination thus preserves what has been perceived by the senses and is able to recall and reproduce these mental images. In so doing, an emotion may be re-experienced and the faculty of invention given something to work on.

The imagination is constantly active, forming thoughts in the vapours of vital spirits which rise to the brain and generate the animal spirit. However, imagination, also called 'fancy', can be a dangerous thing too. If it provokes 'tempests in the mind', these uncontrolled thoughts will be transmitted to the heart, where they will stir up the passions and make the spirits of the body impure so as to drive man or beast to act in any way conceivable, for good or evil.

The second aspect of the intellective function, judgement, could, in fact, control the tempests in the mind. As Culpeper says:

Judgement is seated in the midst of the brain, to shew that it ought to bear rule over all the other faculties; it is the judge of the little world, to approve of what is good, and reject what is bad: It is the seat of reason, and the guide of actions, so that all failings are committed through its infirmity, in not rightly judging between a real and an apparent good. It is hot and moist in quality, and under the influence of *Jupiter*.

Judgement then includes the discursive processes of reason, whereby an intellectual analysis and synthesis of sensory information takes place. Understanding leads to decision-making based on what is concluded to be most advantageous, expedient or proper. The notion of judgement has been put in the following way:

Reason possesses the power of judgement, which permits it to understand universals, grasp innate ideas, and reflect upon one's own thoughts and actions ... Reason also possesses the power of will, which allows it to command the senses so that the potent drama of imagination conforms to judgement's script and thus to control human passion and behaviour. The imagination imperils insanity when its illusory powers are not plotted and directed by reason.[65]

The liver and judgement share the qualities of hot and moist. In the unity of body and mind, therefore, the influence of one upon the other goes either way. Just as passions of the mind can manifest physically in a disruption of the vital spirit, for example, so the temperament of the body and the qualities of the food it digests were thought to affect the mind. In addition, hot vapours from an overheated stomach, spleen, liver or womb were held to affect the mental function as well.

Lastly there is memory. Of its operations Culpeper writes:

> Memory is seated in the hinder cell of the Brain, it is the great Register to the little world; and its office is to record things either done and past, or to be done. It is in quality cold and dry, and melancholick, and therefore generally melancholick men have the best memories, and most tenacious every way. It is under the dominion of *Saturn*, and is fortified by his influence, but purged by the luminaries.

Memory therefore preserves the ideas discovered by judgement.

The three aspects of the intellective faculty – imagination, judgement and memory – thus had the power to affect the state of mind of a person.

> ... Judgement always sleeps when men do; imagination never sleeps. Memory sometimes sleeps when men sleep, and sometimes it doth not. So then where memory is awake, and the man asleep, then memory remembers what apprehension coins, and that is a dream: The thoughts would have been the same if memory had not been awake to remember it.

Furthermore:

> These thoughts are commonly (I mean in sleep when they are purely natural) framed according to the nature of the Humour, called Complexion, which is predominate in the body; and if the humour be peccant, it is always so. So that it is one of the surest rules to know a man's complexion, by his dreams ...

Thus dream interpretation was a part of holistic diagnosis. The quality of dream was supposed to reflect the qualities of the prevailing temperament. However if the mind was distracted by study or concern, or food was still being digested in the stomach during sleep, the quality of the dream could be altered. In

Culpeper's opinion there was then one more exception in that 'false dreams may happen by the illusion of evil spirits, true dreams may be caused by the revelation of good angels'.[66] Generally, though, it was believed that if the mind was not distracted and, to use Milton's phrase, 'his sleep was aery light, from pure digestion bred', the quality of dreams provided a useful indication of the prevailing state of being.

By way of example, Culpeper quotes some verses by his friend, the Republican poet Thomas May,[67] for each of the four temperaments:

Sanguine Complexion

There all together flye in Companies
Of different colours, shapes and qualities
Bright Sanguine Dreams, that seem to cheer the night
With beauteous shapes, and rosie wings as bright,
As in the morning, or those flowers that grace
In midst of Spring, the painted Flora's face:
Within the Temple merrily do sport,
To whom the little Cupids oft resort:
The little Cupids from fair Venus Grove,
Stealing by night, do thither come and love,
With those bright Sanguine dreams to pass away
The hours of night, in sport and amorous play.

Cholerick Complexion

There dreams of choler in a flame-like hue,
Through th'air, like little fiery meteors flew
With swift and angry motion to and fro,
As if they sought within that place, a foe,
Sometimes up to the Temples roof, on high,
They soar, as if they meant to scale the Sky:
Or some impossible achievement sought
T'allay the thirst of an aspiring thought.

Melancholick Complexion

But down below, with sad and heavy cheer,
On dead mens tombs, and every sepulcher
The dusky dreams of melancholy dight,
With sable wings, like bats, or birds of night,
Fluttering in darkest corners here and there,
But all alone, and still each other fear:

Courting dead skulls, and seeming to invite
The dismal Ghosts, for company by night.

Flegmatick Complexion

There all along the temples whited wall,
Flegmatick lazy dreams, not wing'd at all
But slow like slimy snails, about do crawl,
And evermore, and thence afraid to fall,
And so be drown'd, for on the floor below
They do suppose great pools of water flow.

The vital and animal faculties (along with their respective spirits) can therefore be viewed in one sense as aspects of energy, concerned with or operating through the psyche (spirit, soul, mind) while the natural faculty was associated with the soma (body).

The Natural Faculty

The natural faculty governs nutrition and the material composition of living things. It was said to reside in the liver and to be conveyed in the blood by the natural spirit. This faculty maintained the life of the individual. In addition, the natural faculty supplied blood to the sex organs and the potential for procreation depended on a proper supply of good blood beyond the quantity necessary for the nutrition of the individual human being. Thus the natural faculty maintained both individual human life and that of the race or species.

The procreative aspect of the natural faculty was said to be manifested in the sexual drive as well as the processes of reproduction and development. In addition, Galen believed that since the testes were organs of great force and power, the natural spirit within them could produce such distant effects as the growth of hair on the chin and a deepening voice by some occult or hidden quality. A comparison was made between the penetration of the Sun's rays in the macrocosm of the world and distribution of this power of the testes throughout the body,[68] so that it was argued:

Not only do the testes produce semen, in Galen's view; they also are a fountain of strength and augment the activity of the heart in supplying the whole body copiously with heat. The heart is a source merely of life; the testes, of the good life.[69]

Galen, after all, had to account for the dramatic physical changes seen in animals and men as a result of castration or removal of the testicles. Endrocrinology, the science of the body's internal secretions, particularly the hormones, was only born in the last few years of Culpeper's life.[70]

Culpeper, however, rejected the traditional view formulated by Aristotle that it was only the male sperm that formed and energized new life. For him, the seed of both the mother and father came together equally to form a new life. He wrote:

> The use of the stones in women is the same that it is in men, viz to concoct seed; and of this judgement was *Hippocrates* in ancient days, and yet *Aristotle* had the face to deny that women had any seed at all, though against both reason and experience. Also *Jovian Pontanus* in his Coelestial Observations, goes about to prove the very same thing in the *Moon*, which *Aristotle* quotes in women; he affirms, that the *Moon* only supplies matter for the *Sun* to work upon in the generation of things here below, even as the female doth to the male in the generation of man; and that he learned of *Aristotle*, and so confesses; but those that have studied *Hermetical Philosophy* know well enough that the moisture which the *Moon* bestows upon the Earth, hath an active principle in it, yea such an active principle, that the world cannot stand without it, nor Philosophers operate without it.[71]

In asserting that the woman's role in the conception of new life was as active as that of the man's, Culpeper showed just how forward-thinking and liberated he could be. He did not, as some have suggested,[72] anticipate the discovery of the eggs released by the female ovary by the use of the microscope which was invented some years after his death. Instead, he used his knowledge and logic to reject the traditional view and put forward his own.

TABLE SUMMARISING THE FACULTIES AND SPIRITS OF THE HUMAN BODY

	SITUATED IN	QUALITIES	ACTIVITY
Vital faculty & spirit	the heart	hot & dry	vitality & emotional life
Animal faculty & spirit	the brain	cold & moist	sensory, motor & mental
Natural faculty & spirit	the liver the sex organs	hot & moist	nutrition & reproduction

The 4 Administering Virtues
or Secondary Physical Faculties

The four administering virtues were the attractive, retentive, digestive and expulsive virtues. Shah[73] calls these secondary physical faculties, and their central process is digestion whilst 'the others like hand-maids attend it'.[74] For there would be nothing to digest if there was nothing to eat or drink in the first place. Secondly the process of digestion would be hindered if food was not retained in the stomach long enough for concoction to take place. Then, once digestion was under way, the superfluous or bad portion of the food and drink consumed had to be expelled from the body.

The attractive virtue operated through hunger and appetite to draw or attract food and drink into the body. A deliberate move to enter a restaurant at lunchtime, for example, would suffice. Culpeper writes:

> The *Attractive* virtue is hot and dry; hot by hot quality, active or principal: and that appears, because the fountain of all heat is attractive, viz the Sun; dry by a quality passive, or an effect of its heat; its office is to remain in the body, and call for what nature wants.

Thus the Sun is the symbol of the attractive virtue. We see it literally after a shower of rain, when the Sun comes out again and draws the moisture up towards itself by evaporation. Metaphorically it is apparent in the way a fire draws the attention of the bystander to gaze, sometimes almost spellbound, at the changing patterns in the flames. Imagination, too, coining thoughts from the vaporous vital spirit which rises to the brain, is a form of attraction of mental images called apprehension. We may, for example, envisage the meal which would satisfy our appetite and then act to obtain it; or we can be apprehensive of an imminent event, one which has not yet happened in fact, but which we anticipate and move towards with joy or fear in our thoughts. In every case the emphasis is on movement, in the same way that the hot and dry quality of the vital spirit energizes the organism and endows it with movement.

Of the retentive virtue Culpeper says:

> The *Retentive* virtue is in quality cold and dry; cold, because the nature of cold is to compress, witness the ice; dry because the nature of dryness, is to keep and hold what is compressed. It is under the

influence of *Saturn*, and that is the reason why usually saturnine men are so covetous and tenacious.

Cold was said usually to inactivate and anaesthetize every function but in this case the coldness and dryness held the food in the stomach through a constriction of the fibres,[75] a sort of 'gripping' action. Likewise the memory, when functioning optimally, maintained a tight grip on every experience and thought and stored them all away in the rear part of the brain, in compressed form, for future recall.

The digestive virtue had the qualities opposite to those of retention, namely heat and moisture. Heat was required for the concoction of food and for its differentiation into the various humours, and moisture was needed for its liquefying action which allowed the chyle to be more easily assimilated through the narrow channels of the intestines and liver during the second concoction and to prepare the nutriment for subsequent transformation into differently-shaped organs and parts. This is similar to the way that the procreative aspect of the natural faculty is hot and moist, since the process of reproduction involves the formation of the whole body from the elemental building blocks derived from food and these are garnered by means of the 'plastic' principle of moisture under the guidance of the formational principle of heat (pneuma). So too was the faculty of judgement of these qualities. Through judgement we can sort out the various thoughts and imaginations in the brain and sift the good from the bad. We can elevate and transform a particular idea into one of universal application or bend our minds to reflect on our own thought processes.

Finally, Culpeper describes the expulsive virtue:

> The *Expulsive* virtue casteth out, and expelleth what is superfluous by digestion ... The *Expulsive* faculty is cold and moist; cold, because that compresseth the superfluities; moist because that makes the body slippery and fit for ejection, and disposeth it to it.

When the expulsive faculty was weak, there was difficulty in the processes of excretion of waste products from the body. Excessive heat in the body, for example, could cause a secondary dryness and this might manifest as constipation by opposing the quality of moisture of the expulsive virtue. Coldness assisted expulsion both by condensing faecal material in the bowel and thereby lessening its decomposition and the production of gas or wind, and also by contracting the longitudinal fibres of the digestive tract so that the faeces were moved down and excreted.

Each administering virtue could be strong or weak in a given person at a certain time. When weak, each could be corrected and strengthened by medicinal agents and correct diet according to that person's temperament and humoral balance.

Section 2

The Preservation of Health and the Prevention of Disease: The Six Non-natural Things

If health is to be preserved, there has to be clear understanding of what exactly is meant by health. It was certainly not defined simply as an absence of disease, not only because this is a negative statement more applicable to a machine than to the complexity of a human being, but also because it suggests that there are only two states of being, that is, in health and in sickness. In traditional Western medicine three states were considered to exist, the third being a neutral state which was neither health nor sickness but a decline from health towards sickness.

For Culpeper, health is a condition in which the seven natural things are 'in good decorum', while St Thomas Aquinas stated that 'health is a harmony of the humours'.[1] The words of Aquinas emphasize a concept, that of a dynamic equilibrium, which stretches back to the earliest Greek philosophers.

> In a well-known passage of Plato's *Phaedra* (86b) we are told by Simmias that the Pythagoreans held the body to be strung like an instrument to a certain pitch, hot and cold, wet and dry taking the place of high and low in music. According to this view, health is just being in tune, and disease arises from undue tension or relaxation of the strings. We still speak of 'tonics' in medicine as well as in music ... Health in fact was an 'attunement' (Gk *harmonia*) depending on a due blend of opposites, and the same account was given of many other things with which the physician is concerned, notably of diet and climate. The word 'blend' (*crasis*) itself was used both of bodily *temperament*, as we still call it, and of the *temperature* which distinguished one climate from another. When we speak of 'temperance' in eating and drinking, we are equally on Pythagorean ground.[2]

Thus when Culpeper speaks of the seven naturals being in good decorum, he means that a condition of harmony exists between them so that the whole being is in tune and able to operate efficiently and happily. The person feels at ease with himself and has a sense of contentment with his life, there being nothing to trouble the body, mind or spirit. A balance is being maintained between conflicting aspects of the being. Any discord arising is coped with and taken in the stride, so that health is also the ability to adapt successfully to changing circumstances.

> In Heraclitus' own view, everything is at all times pulled simultaneously in opposite directions (like the bow and the bowstring), yet this very tension of opposites is the *sine qua non* [essential requirement] of the harmony, the integrity, of physical objects. Harmony entails an adjustment or balance, but by no means an abolition, of the strife that is everywhere present.[3]

As to sickness, this is normally apparent to the sufferer by the sense of something wrong, of feeling out of balance and dis-eased. It was defined as the exact opposite of the state of health, with a disturbance of normal function due to a disorder of temperament or structure of the body and mind. It is significant that both health and disease were considered to be states that people come to be in, rather than something which someone catches or which is imposed on them so that emphasis was put on the person rather than the disease.

What of the neutral state, between full health and sickness? This has been clarified to mean that although the person feels ill, there are no definite lesions and so, as yet, no definite diagnosis of disease.[4] Physicians routinely accounted the very young, the old and the convalescent in this state. It was also applied to those who were ill in one season and well in another. Culpeper says the neutral state exists where, for instance, one organ of the body works well while another is intemperate or where healthy concoction does not take place but there is not yet an unhealthy production of crude, undigested humours in the body, so that overall there is no manifest disease but a sense of unease as if the person knows that he or she is heading for sickness.[5] Thus the range of states from health to disease comprise:

- perfect health
- normal health
- unhealthy without any specific disease
- uncomplicated convalescence

- slight ill-health or disease
- fully developed disease

Culpeper lists the following signs, as they arise with some regularity, as indicators of a neutral state heading towards sickness:

- increased or decreased appetite, or irregular meals or unusual foods being eaten
- weight gain or loss
- altered excretions (assessed by colour, consistency, frequency)
- too frequent sexual intercourse, or long abstention from it
- absence of, or heavy periods (amenorrhoea/menorrhagia)
- excessive sweating
- haemorrhoids
- troubled sleep
- deafness or dullness of sight; dullness of mind and forgetfulness
- change of body colour
- sneezing, belching or breaking wind.[6]

Culpeper provides another list of symptoms which, he says, are not yet diseases or impediments to daily life but are not natural either:

- a gnawing sensation in the stomach
- pain
- vomiting
- headache and heaviness of the head
- excessive sleep or wakefulness
- salty or bitter taste in the mouth
- ringing in the ears, odd smells or spots in the vision (floaters)
- numbness or soreness.[7]

Culpeper writes that 'the body of man is always subject to alteration, corruption and change'.[8] Consequently, the preservation of health lies in the maintenance of harmony within the body. This cannot help the person to avoid death or escape external afflictions but harmony and balance in life encourage longevity and contentment.

Despite being able to identify general symptoms, physicians did not believe that what is good for one person is necessarily good for all. Each of the 4 temperaments which characterize individuals has its own blend of humours within which they remain healthy. This is their *eucrasia* (Greek for 'good mixture'). Illness arises as a *dyscrasia*, an unhealthy disproportion and state of these humours.[9]

In order to concoct healthy humours in the right proportion, proper regulation of the innate heat and the three spirits within the body was necessary. This would ensure the vitality of the body and its resistance to disease. Through the spirits the proper functioning of the vital, animal and natural faculties were performed. Levine Lemnie lists the following as 'things which dull, quench and damnify inward spirits':

- impure, gross and offensive air
- excessive sex
- excessive wakefulness
- excessive heat
- chasing and labour
- long fasting
- heaviness of the mind and sadness.[10]

To breathe good air is essential for the spirits of the body because it contains the accidental pneuma by which they are sustained. Polluted air harms them. All the other factors affect the spirits, either by reducing directly the innate heat carried in the spirits and the blood or by consuming the radical moisture which nurtures it. So the body is rendered drier by excessive heat, notably through too much activity and motion, or when the person has not had sufficient sleep to refresh the body (by 'cherishing' innate heat with moisture as the evening dew refreshes the earth made dry in the heat of the day). If not enough food is consumed the requisite amount of blood for the maintenance of the spirits will not be produced. The relative lack of the moisture or oil (from the blood) will thus result in a failure to temper the innate heat which, in turn, will allow the flame to burn excessively and to consume more rapidly what moisture there is in the body. This state along with various other deficiency diseases was called *anaemia* (from Greek, meaning 'no blood'). This could produce what Galen called a simple *marasmus* (wasting of the body) which he likened to the withering of fruit.[11] It was termed simple because only one quality, dryness, was in excess; heat and cold were still balanced. To counteract dryness of this state, a regimen of fatty meats, pulses, almonds and bread was proposed, together with increased sleep and the arousal of the subject to mental excitement. As for sadness and other perturbations of the mind:

> A merry heart maketh a lusty age, but a sorrowful spirit dryeth up the bones. Heaviness bringeth old age before the time and carefulness weareth away a man's days.[12]

Thus the spirits have to be comforted, by quiet and seasonable sleep, good-quality wine, merry company, moderate exercise and by sweet smells and fragrant savours.[13]

The innate heat then is intimately connected with the spirits since it is conveyed by them through the body. In the vital spirit the innate heat maintains the wholeness and integrity of the body and protects the humours from putrefaction and disease. In the natural spirits, it properly concocts food so that only healthy humours are produced. This will then prevent hot vapours rising from overheated organs or from obstructed vital spirits as the organs in the lower part of the body will be in an optimum state. The innate heat will thus be protected.

At the other extreme to anaemia, a diet in excess of either the needs of the body or its ability to digest it will produce an imbalance of humours. In the first case, any excess of food is turned into blood, so creating the danger of its moisture subduing the innate heat and increasing the likelihood of putrefaction (infection) and fever.[14] The sanguine temperament can be predisposed to this. This state is termed *plethora* (Greek for 'fullness' or 'satiety'). Plethora can also be caused by the retention of waste matters that should have been evacuated from the body, including those in the lymphatic channels (most apparent as lymphoedema) or anything which produces a state of excessive moisture in the body, such as a phlegmatic temperament; a failure to exercise and the too frequent taking of baths, especially after meals, may contribute to a plethoric state. Even high blood pressure would have been regarded as an example of this. In the second case, if the diet is incorrect for the person not all the food can be properly concocted so the remainder will enter the body as crude, undigested humours. The filling of the body with such humours simply diminishes further the digestive power of the innate heat and encourages the continued generation of unconcocted humours. These products of incomplete or faulty digestion were called 'crudities' by Culpeper and were considered the root cause of most diseases and that which predisposes the person to ill-health. For an abundance of such humours can cause congestion of the blood and the obstruction or 'choking' of the spirits, while if the humours are strong in quality, according to the nature of the food eaten from which they derive, they give rise to an imbalance of temperament or dyscrasia of the same nature. Culpeper said:

> Excellent and true was that speech of Galen: 'plures Gula periere quam Gladio', the throat destroys more than the sword doth. Excess in either meat or drink causeth crudities; crudities sickness, and sickness death, and this is the absolute and indeed undeniable reason, (unless to such as will carp at every thing) why so many are taken away in the prime of their youth, viz. because they keep not a temperate diet.[15]

Treatment of these two cases differed. If plethora occurs, the production of blood has to be decreased by reducing food intake and basing the diet on fruit and vegetables, in other words bulky foods which do not add to the quantity of humours. Where undigested humours abound in the body, moderation in food is still required but in addition the congestion of the liver needs treating and evacuation of the crude humours encouraged. The latter would be done with medicines to induce sweating and by purging, usually with laxative agents. In cases of obesity herbs to thin the humours (attenuating medicines), strong diuretics, pepper and anise were recommended, together with regular baths before but not immediately before meals, avoidance of excessive sleeping and active exercise followed by massage with oils inducing a sweat.[16]

Another way in which the humours of the body are continually affected is through the ambient qualities of the changing cycle of the seasons.[17] In Spring the cold and moist humours which Winter brought forth are stirred up and can be hardened into obstructions by the increasing heat. Chronic diseases, especially of melancholy, are thus reactivated, while those of a phlegmatic temperament would show a tendency to arthritis, paralysis and stroke. Those who have overeaten and exercised little over the winter are more liable to Springtime diseases, the most common of which are coughs, bronchitis, pneumonia, flu, inflammations, angina, abscesses and aggravation of varicose veins. In order to avoid or lessen such diseases the person would have to fast or restrict the diet, avoiding very hot and moistening foods, to drink more fluids but abstain from alcohol and take moderate exercise whilst purging excess humours with diuretic and sweat-inducing herbs. Despite these diseases, Spring was generally considered a healthy season, especially for adolescents, because of its temperance.

In Summer the humours are easily dispersed by the ambient temperature, rendering some more healthy and lessening the impact of some diseases. However, because the innate heat is also dispersed, phlegm is increased in the body. Those already weakened by disease can therefore grow weaker and die. A wet summer in particular produces thick, clammy humours which will prolong diseases. Fevers, diarrhoea (the movement of humours downwards), eye problems and boils are typical Summertime problems. The diet should be spare and cooling in quality, with drinks and exercise moderated. Old people do well in this season and during the first part of Autumn.

Autumn was reckoned a bad season for diseases. The innate heat is still weak from the Summer heat, and hot days and cold nights make keeping a balance even more difficult. Choler, which increased over the Summer due to the heat and dryness, is still strong, partly due to a relatively smaller amount of blood in the body. The body is also full of the phlegmatic humours from the Summer, which may be added to by the overeating of the moist fruits available. The phlegmatic humours would then be subject to combustion by the increased choler, thus producing melancholy. Otherwise, they would be concocted by the heat of fevers, brought by the 'pestilential' or infection-laden air of late Summer and early Autumn, and purged from the body in sweat or urine. Other diseases of this season include impetigo, scabies, pustules, worsening chest problems, back and hip pains, diarrhoea, throat problems and mental disaffections. General advice is to protect oneself from the variations in temperature, to increase the variety and quantity of the diet while avoiding all drying foods, excessive cold water drinks and sleeping on a full stomach and in a cold place.

Diseases in Winter are usually phlegmatic in origin, due to the qualities of the season of cold and wet. The innate heat is once again strong, in order to keep the body warm, but the cold and wet mean that colds, inflammations such as sinusitis and sore throats, and, less commonly, chest problems such as pleurisy are more prevalent. Eating liberally in this season is recommended, because the innate heat is strong, but cooling foods are to be avoided. Exercise must be increased. The middle-aged fare best in this season.

The Doctrine of the Six Non-Naturals

The external factors affecting the health of a person were called the *non-naturals* because they affect the body from outside.[18] They were said to incur inevitable effects on the individual, for good or ill, and intemperance in any or all of them were judged to be a necessary cause of disease because they cannot be avoided.[19] However, a proper ordering of the non-naturals could prevent or by itself remedy many cases of plethora and dyscrasia. They are six in number:

- air
- diet
- exercise and rest
- sleep and wakefulness
- retention and evacuation of waste matter
- perturbations of the mind

For health to be maintained, all six *non-naturals* need regulation and their consideration comes under the heading of *hygiene* in its widest sense. In this regard, the physician, in order to understand and assess the patients correctly and to exercise good judgement over their care, also has to apply rules of hygiene to his or her own life. For, as Galen says, 'the physician will hardly be thought very careful of the health of others who neglects his own'.[20]

Air

Robert Burton stated: 'If the air be impure and foggy, it dejects the spirits, and causeth diseases by infection of the heart ... Such is the air, such be our spirits; and as our spirits, such are our humours. It offends commonly, if it be too hot and dry, thick, fuliginous, cloudy, blustering, or a tempestuous air.'[21] We require clean, healthy air to breathe. This should be neither contaminated by industrial pollutants, sewers, swamps or car exhausts, nor rendered stale by confinement in caves, high walls and mountains and closed houses, where winds have difficulty entering to cleanse the air.

A key work in the Western medical tradition which explores the question of air quality in various locations is the Hippocratic text *Airs, Waters, Places,* an essay on the influence of climate, winds, water supply and situation on health.[22] Written in a country and at a time when most physicians were itinerant practitioners, the text affords an evaluation of the effects of seasonal temperatures and types of local water supply on the nutrition and vigour of the human body and gives lists of expected diseases in a population inhabiting a particular place and exposed to winds from a certain quarter.

Culpeper's writing on the subject is much more brief and rooted in Galenic systematization but sufficiently to his purpose of providing some basic notions on the topic for his audience, the people of England.[23] He states that air is the author of life, diseases and death to people. Thus the quality of air must rank, in Culpeper's mind, as equal to the consideration of quantity and quality of diet in the preservation of health.[24] He defines air as basically cold (one of its effects is to cool the heart) and moist, since it carries vapour, but it can become hot and moist in sunshine. Exposure to winds prevailing from each of the four compass points, Culpeper says, affects the various operations of the body. The East wind is hot, dry and blasting and thus strengthens the attractive virtue (of the four Administering Virtues). Hot air disperses the pneuma, relaxes the body, loosens the joints, weakens digestion and promotes thirst. So if the heat is excessive it will weaken the body and dry it out. In places continually exposed to hot winds the length of life will thereby be shortened. Winds from the West are cold and moist. The coldness strengthens digestion by driving and aggregating heat inside the body. It closes the pores of the skin and reduces insensible transpiration, its binding effect on the body in some cases extending to constipation, although there is an increase in the amount of urine passed. If the cold is intense, it causes head catarrhs (for cold in particular was reckoned very hurtful to the brain). The South wind is hot and moist and encourages putrefaction and the spread of infections. A very moist air softens and moistens the body and clears the skin, the pores remaining open. Yet it makes the body slow and heavy, increasing its excrements and dulling the brain. The North wind is cold and dry and augments the retentive virtue; as a dry wind it has a hardening effect on the body. The best air to be recommended is that which is temperate both for heat and cold so that it neither freezes with continual frost in winter nor evaporates too much in summer. A location with hills on some sides is good but living on top of a hill and subject to all wind and weather is not thought healthy.

Air which is gross, thick or cloudy, perhaps in a still, damp and misty mountain valley by a lake, produces fat bodies, Culpeper says, by disturbing the humours. It can also dull the wits by depressing the mind. Pure and clear air makes for nimble bodies and quick wits. Any sudden change of air is bad, since Nature abhors all sudden changes. Each of the temperaments benefits from air which opposes its qualities or effects and yields an equable state. So moist airs are good for hot types and warm air, good fires and draughtproof homes benefit cold types. Dry bodies also benefit from moist air as moist bodies do from a dry atmosphere.

As for the lie of the land, Culpeper says that stony ground, perhaps in more rocky or mountainous terrain, denotes a cold and dry environment. Sandy ground shows a hot and dry quality. Damp ground such as fenland gives a more cold and moist atmosphere whilst woody and 'fat' land is of a hot and moist quality. Once again, the physical state of the land can be matched with a person's temperament so that balance and harmony prevail. Overall, the qualities of wind, aspect of a town and its local terrain provide a useful context in which to consider the accidents of ill-health in an individual living there or the benefits and drawbacks of relocating. The same applies, in larger relief, to the climate of a country and its inhabitants. For example the British Isles are damp or moist but neither particularly hot nor cold. Countries in which great seasonal changes take place expose their inhabitants to all the effects of heat, cold, dryness and moisture.

Culpeper's considerations of the quality of air and local terrain for the health of the inhabitants was simply an addition to what was a complex but very developed subject for study by physicians. Hippocrates's work *Airs, Waters, Places* has been greatly added to by the contribution of other observers over the centuries, although specific detailing of environmental causes of disease came rather late on. Paracelsus had drawn a connection between fibrosis of the lung and the environment in which miners worked, notably the dust-filled air. Then in 1700 Professor Bernardino Ramazzini published the first book to be written on diseases of occupation in which he described 'the lung diseases of miners and stonemasons, the eye diseases of blacksmiths, gilders and "cleansers of the jakes" [toilets and cess-pits], the lead poisoning of printers and potters, mercurial poisoning of surgeons who treat patients by inunctions, and the diseases of midwives, bearers of corpses, vintners, tanners, tobacconists, fishermen, washerwomen, and even learned men.[25] However, the usefulness of the study of the geography of diseases was called into question in the late 19th century with the discovery of bacterial infection and the existence of pathogenic micro-organisms, which in the opinion of Henry Sigerist, the famous historian of medicine, 'overshadowed all other factors that might have been considered and led to a somewhat oversimplified view'.[26] Today, however, environmental factors of all sorts, from pollutants in the air to processed foods, are being implicated in the development of diseases. For those living in inner city areas, for instance, the quality of the air which they breathe is entering very much into their health equation, as testified, for instance, by the dramatic rise in the incidence of asthma in recent years.

Diet

The importance of diet to health has been maintained since earliest times. The effects of malnourishment or food-poisoning have been experienced in every age. Food and drink of the right quality, taken in an adequate quantity from a local supply grown in the natural environment, were required to sustain life and it was believed that people were naturally drawn to that which they needed. Henry Sigerist wrote:

It can only be attributed to instinctive behaviour that man all over the world, under the most different geographic conditions, invariably found a *balanced* diet, one best adapted to the climate ... And just as man in health sought and instinctively found the animal parts, plants and minerals that his organism required for sustenance, so man in illness craved and instinctively found other plants, animal parts, or minerals that his body needed to overcome illness, or he ate foodstuffs in different combination or quantity. There is no sharp borderline between food and drug.[27]

In the same way that an overdose of a potent drug will do more harm than good, so habitual excess of regular food and drink can occasion sickness by virtue of its frequency. Hippocrates recognized that overeating causes just as much sickness as excessive fasting.[28] Correct diet for the preservation of health or the healing of disease was central to Hippocratic medicine, and so to Western holistic medicine. To preserve the body in health, the diet had to vary in quality and quantity according to the degree of health or disease being present, to temperament, physique, age, season of the year, locality and habit. Culpeper says 'a good nature appetites no more than it concocts', meaning that a desire for food should be commensurate with the ability to digest it properly. This makes for a life in harmony with nature, which primitive peoples practised and would continue to do, according to Sigerist, if they were allowed.

Under the most different climates primitives devised a balanced diet. If they had not, they would soon have died out. The great deal of malnutrition among them today is the result of prevailing social and economic conditions, the consequence of colonial exploitation.[29]

What of the situation in Culpeper's day? Life expectancy at birth may have been less than 35 years, compared with 40–45 years for country people in the mid-16th century, and with the three score years and ten spoken of in the Bible which we have re-attained today.[30] The doubling of grain yields in the period 1500–1600 was matched with a doubling of the population and the failure of one harvest in six meant unavailability of food, high prices for what did exist, and malnourishment and sickness for those who could only afford a little food of poor quality. As Keith Thomas wrote:

The dietary deficiencies of the lower classes, by contrast, reflected not so much ignorance as simple poverty. Not until the nineteenth century did labourers get enough meat and butter. In the seventeenth century they may have escaped gout and stone which plagued their betters, and may even have had better teeth from eating more vegetables. But they were chronically under-nourished and vulnerable to tuberculosis and gastric upsets ('griping in the guts') caused by bad food.[31]

The rich created their own problems through an intemperate diet, by eating too much meat and by disdaining the consumption of fresh vegetables and milk. This resulted in vitamin deficiency, notably chlorosis or 'the green sickness', and rickets. All classes, however, fell victim to infections brought on by a lack of hygiene, the absence of effective sanitation and ignorance of antisepsis. In London there were periodic epidemics of influenza, typhus, dysentery and smallpox, whilst bubonic plague was endemic until the late 17th century, with severe outbreaks in 1603, 1625, 1636 and 1665.[32] The failure of society to deal adequately with such overwhelming health problems cannot, however, rest on the simple attribution of ignorance of the causes of infection but is more complex. For instance:

> Ancient Egypt, Greece and Rome had admirable systems of public hygiene and the Old Testament has ample evidence of the excellent code of the Hebrews. The fall from grace in this respect in the Middle Ages, and even up to the nineteenth century, may have something to do with the Christian attitude towards the body as the merely temporary dwelling place of the soul and the acceptance of suffering and disease, even on a vast scale, as inflicted by God.[33]

Culpeper, despite his Christian faith, was not one to readily assign disease to the Will of God as a punishment for sin. Rather he attributed sickness to natural causes aided by ignorance and folly. His whole endeavour was to teach his fellow countrymen how to look after their own health, by correct use of physick when ill and by observance of a sober life when well.

> By a sober life, I intend such an exact quantity of meat and drink, as the constitution of the body allows of, in reference to the services of the mind ... This exact proportion being found out both according to quantity and quality is to be kept in a constant measure ... Although the matter of this sober life or diet be mainly conversant about meat and drink; yet it forbids excess in all other things called 'not Natural'.[34]

By the services of the mind, Culpeper means that the studious should not eat as much as the more physically laborious, since the whole power of the spirits is called up to serve the brain and understanding so that insufficient would remain for good concoction of too large a meal. In such a case 'fuliginous, sooty' vapours would arise from the stomach, liver and spleen to trouble the brain 'with cloudiness and dizziness' and this was taken as a sign, along with other symptoms of dyspepsia, that the due measure of food and drink had been exceeded. Generally, overeating would make the body dull, heavy and weary instead of refreshed, since the 'abundance of ill humours' from faulty digestion would stop up the passages through which the spirits passed in their proper ordering of the body. This in turn prepared the ground for diseases. It was not considered helpful to try to work off the effects of an excess with some strenuous exercise ('burning up the calories') since this only 'confusedly stirs the body, and that many times with much perturbation of the humours, with much heat and hazard of sickness, with much pain and grief'. A general avoidance of excess was promoted as the better way. On a practical note of how to avoid overeating, Culpeper urges:

> Keep as much as may be from the view of dainty feasts and banquets. The difficulty of keeping a just measure in diet proceeds from appetite, and appetite proceeds from apprehension of the fancy, which conceives meats to be delightful and pleasant. Which fancy is stirred up by their sight and smell. The presence of every object doth move the fancy to what pertaineth to itself; so vain a thing is man. It is far more difficult to restrain the appetite from good cheer when it is present, than from the desire of it when it is away.[35]

Such 'curiosily and daintily dressed' food was thought to prolong the appetite beyond the satisfaction of hunger and thirst into excess. However, Culpeper did not equate the pleasure of eating and drinking with the sin of gluttony. In his practice, he was 'never too rigid in prescribing of his diet for the sick' and he himself feared that his own declining health was due to some intemperance.[36] He advocated that people 'now and then eat a little of any meats they desire' and if they sometimes exceed the due proportion at one meal, they may correct this by missing the next – 'What a piece of matter is it, when one hath eaten too much at dinner, to forbear eating any supper?'[37] Hippocrates himself said that of two foods the one preferred by the patient should be prescribed even it if is slightly harmful,[38] on the basis, perhaps, that appetising food would be easily digested. The 'sober life' however was still the rule.

In accordance with the teachings of Hippocrates,[39] the due measure of food and drink must be altered according to various factors, and this must be done by degrees, not suddenly. The seasons, for example, demanded certain variations. As to quantity, 'Winter requires a larger quantity of meat than Summer' since the bodily spirits are less dispersed in the cold season and the natural faculty is stronger. The *Regimen for Health* puts it thus:

> In Spring your dinner must not much exceed
> In Summer's heat but little meat shall need.
> In Autumn ware you eat not too much fruit,
> With Winter's cold full meats do fittest suit.[40]

In keeping with the Hippocratic axiom that the diet should be opposite in character to the prevailing climate of the season, so as to ensure a balance, Culpeper advised in the Winter the eating of food of a hot and dry quality and, for the Summer, cold and moist food. This is consistent with our present habit of eating cooling foods such as lettuce, cucumber and soft fruits in the Summer and usually preferring cooked foods such as nourishing soups in the Winter.

A diet was recommended for each individual to match his or her temperament and age as well as the season of the year. Certain foods, such as bread, chicken, mutton, the flesh of young goats and veal, were held to be good and wholesome in general because they avoided excesses of being too hard or too soft, too cloying or too insubstantial, too heavy or too light, and created few excrements. Physicians regarded other foods, such as bran, beef, goat's meat, pulses, hard cheeses and cabbage, to be 'of evil juice', thick, heavy and hard to digest. They recommended that a person with a strong digestion could eat more of the foods that were hard to digest because their stomachs were able to cope with them and because easily digestible foods might be 'overcooked' and so putrefy in the stomach. Those with weak stomachs, however, were advised to consume the easily digestible foods such as lamb, veal, soft boiled eggs and fresh fish.

As to age, children were to be given plenty of food because they were growing but this had to be young, moist and easily digestible flesh, eg lamb, together with some cooling foods, such as barley, vinegar, lettuce, cucumbers and Summer fruits, to temper the heat of their growth, unless their stomachs were weak. Cooling and moistening foods were certainly recommended to young adults to balance their heat and dryness, although the quantity was to be less than for young children. Wine, although it was thought detrimental to the young, was always recommended in moderate quantity for the old because of its heating quality and its effect of thinning the humours and cleansing them from the body via the urine. Typically, the diet of those of greater years had to be hot and moist, especially moist in order to preserve what remained of the radical moisture, but low in quantity because of the weakness of their digestion. This 'moistening regimen' put emphasis on soft foods like milk, peeled barley, wheat, honey and wine.

The diet was similarly tailored to suit the prevailing temperament of an individual. The primary qualities of foods – hot, cold, dry and moist – along with the secondary qualities such as lightness or heaviness, hardness or softness, were evaluated in order to decide which foods represented the best nourishment for an individual. Wine, pepper and other spices, vegetables of the onion family, parsley, mint and salty foods were considered to be among the heating foods.

Herbs and spices, salt and pepper should be used only in small quantities, depending on the person, to add heat and flavour to the various components of the diet and to aid their good digestion, but the choice of foods eaten should reflect the same concern. For heat is generally more conducive to health than cold, and warming foods increase metabolism with minimal residue while cooling foods diminish metabolism and tend to increase crude humours in the body.

Culpeper made the following observations on the qualities of common dietary items.[41]

Drink

Of the various sorts of drink, wine is heating and, if moderately drunk, comforts the heart and quickens the wit. Good wine breeds good humours and so should be taken with meals. Ale, a natural drink for Englishmen, gives strength but encourages thick humours, while beer is a cold drink which 'inflates the belly'. Cider also is cold and thus hinders digestion except in those who 'are constantly used to it'. Mead, made of honey and water, was recommended, being gently warming by virtue of the honey. In addition, honey has a cleansing faculty and it nourishes and preserves life. Water (as long as it is pure and fresh) is also a good drink if taken in moderation with or after meals, with more needed in the Summer. It is also good when mixed with wine as wine tempers its coldness.

Bread

Grains can be hard to digest. Of those used to make bread, leavened wheat bread is the most easily digested as long as it does not have too much bran in it and is thoroughly cooked. It should be eaten one-day old and not after five-days old, for stale bread dries up the natural moisture of the body. Excessive consumption of bread is harmful, because it has a glutinous quality which can clog up the digestive tract and cause obstructions there. Oats are also warming and wholesome but breads made from rye and barley are not so, because of their coldness. The *Regimen of Health* advises:

> Eat not your bread too stale, nor eat it hot,
> Not fresh of purest grain that can be got.
> The crust breeds choler both of brown and white,
> Yet let it be well baked or eat it not,
> Howe'er your taste therein may take delight.

Dairy produce

The yolks of hens' eggs are temperately hot and are a cordial (reviving and stimulating) but the white of an egg is viscous and cold, slow to be digested and does not create good blood. Culpeper recommends pheasant eggs and partridge eggs but not duck or goose eggs. Butter is hot and moist in quality, nourishing and softening. However, since it is easily combustible, like all oils and fats, it is not good to take when feverish or for choleric temperaments. Cheese is of various qualities depending on its form. New cheese, eg cottage cheese, is cold and moist. Soft cheese is the most easily digested, being hot and moist. Hard cheese, however, is hot and dry and therefore hard to digest. The overeating of cheese, warns Culpeper, is wont to produce thick humours and render the eater constipated. Goat's cheese is the least favoured because of its sharpness. Milk, however, whether from a cow, goat or sheep, is moistening and nutritive and good for the melancholic, the old and children. It is not good though for sanguine types nor for any illnesses except a hot and dry state of consumption. Very fresh cream, the top of the milk is preferred to clotted and prepared creams which, because they are not as fresh, 'are eaten more for the sensual appetite than for any good nourishment'.

Fish

Sea fish are recommended above freshwater fish, and fish caught in the flowing waters of rivers, streams and brooks are better than those found in ponds and lakes. Fish provide cold and moist food and yield phlegmatic humours in the body, so that persons of such a temperament should restrict fish in their diet. Those deemed the best nourishment are plaice, flounder, sole, gudgeon, whiting, skate, salmon and trout. However, little is gained by eating anchovy, cod, turbot and mullet, according to Culpeper, while the oily fish herring and mackerel he thought positively harmful to health because of their 'thick, clammy and suffocating substance'.

Shellfish, such as oysters, shrimps, cockles, lobsters and crabs are very nourishing food, hot and moist in quality. They restore flesh and are aphrodisiacs. Mussels, however, he deems bad for the health. Eels too are unwholesome since they live in the mud, but sea or conger eels afford good nourishment for hot stomachs in the Summer.

Fish may be cooked in whatever manner but in regard to this Culpeper reminds his reader that 'one good old fashion is not yet left off, viz to boil fennel with fish, for it consumes that phlegmatic humour which fish most plentifully afford and annoy the body by'.[42] Thus since fennel is a herb, and hot and dry in the third degree, it is able to temper the coldness and moisture of the fish and produce a cooked product more equable in quality. All dishes can be prepared with similar regard, so that a truly 'balanced' meal may be enjoyed.

Meat

Animal flesh is generally accounted hot and moist. The meat of young animals is softer and more moist (but makes more excrements) than that of old animals, which can be dry and tough. So, also, the flesh of domesticated animals is more moist than that of wild ones.

Generally, moist meats should be roasted and dry meats boiled, for ease of digestion. Fried and baked meats are harder to digest and less recommended, except in small quantities for the phlegmatic, since they breed choler and melancholy. Chicken is more digestible than duck or goose, and more nourishing. Of wild fowl, the partridge, pheasant, woodcock and moorhen are the best to eat. Small birds are good and light to digest whereas most water fowl are hard to digest. Pigeons are good for choleric and melancholic persons. Veal is excellent, but beef from an older animal produces thick, melancholy humours. Mutton, notes Culpeper, was recommended by Arab physicians but not by Galen. A well-nourished sheep will breed good blood if eaten by a sickly person. 'Lamb is moist and phlegmatic; it is not good for old persons, except of a melancholy complexion, nor for phlegmatic men to feed, except very moderately'. Pork, although from the unclean pig, is nutritive if from a young animal, otherwise not. Bacon is not good for those suffering from kidney or bladder stones because of the salty astringency of the meat.

The flesh most recommended is that of a young goat or a rabbit. The hare, like the pig, is an unclean beast according to Scripture, and its flesh is drying and conducive to melancholy.

Vegetables

In Culpeper's day, those plants eaten as vegetables were called 'pot-herbs'. Some were what we call vegetables and others were herbs, and both types were used medicinally. For instance, Culpeper recommends the roots of borage to engender good blood, while parsley root is diuretic. Fennel bulbs are good for the lungs and sight, while turnips increase fertility if eaten with meat. Parsnips and carrots are nutritive. Radishes, unless they are sweet, cause unpleasant belching and spoil the goodness of other foods. Onions encourage good appetite, sleep and sexual arousal, while leeks create bad blood. Garlic 'opens the breast and it doth kill worms in the belly ... heats the body and dissolves gross winds'. Culpeper advises in his herbal, too, that garlic is very hot and dry (in the maximum fourth degree) 'and all vehement hot things send up but ill-savoured vapours to the brain. In choleric men 'twill add fuel to the fire. In men oppressed by melancholy, 'twill attenuate the humour and send up strange fancies and as many strange visions to the head. Therefore let it be taken inwardly with great moderation.'

Cabbage (although only hot in the first degree and dry in the second) and watercress are likewise 'of bad juice' and only moderately wholesome. Instead Culpeper highly recommends potatoes and asparagus as nourishing foods. Artichokes are also good to eat as well as being aphrodisiac. Lettuce, on the other hand, works against the sexual urge and, furthermore, cools the brain towards sleep, remedies a hot stomach and causes good blood to be made. Cucumbers also restrain sexual desire and 'as they are cold and moist, corrupt the stomach, and if they are not well ordered and moderately eaten, engender thick and gross humours and are within few degrees of poison to persons of a weak digestion'. Sorrel too is cooling for the digestion and opens the bowels, like the bitter succory and endive. They correct a tendency to choler. Spinach is cold and moist and generates watery humours if not corrected with spices.

Fruit
Both pears and apples can cause wind and pain, because they are cold fruits and therefore less easily digestible. Pears create watery blood so they should be cooked. Apples are best when fresh off the tree after a frost, or when old, red and mellow. If eaten raw, fennel or aniseed (hot foods) should accompany them, and, like any cold fruit, should be taken at the beginning of a meal. Baked apples, however, 'comfort the stomach and cause good digestion' because their coldness has been tempered by cooking. Grapes are sweet and wholesome, and figs and large raisins are counted some of the best fruits. In particular, stewed figs cleanse the lungs and open obstructions of the liver and spleen. Being hot and moist, they increase fertility and are aphrodisiac. Raisins help digestion, if eaten before meals. Gooseberries and pomegranates are nourishing. Dates and currants, however, if eaten to excess, tend to obstruct the workings of the liver and spleen, melons and gourds breed bad humours, and apricots do both. Peaches and cherries are cold and moist and 'mollify [soften] the belly', so, like raspberries, are not good for cold stomachs. Strawberries are the best berries, since they temper the heat of the liver and breed good blood. Lemons are cold and dry in the third degree and are often used for fevers. The juice taken on its own will cause griping but the whole fruit is more tempered and is a cordial. Quinces help digestion and protect from drunkenness, while cold and moist prunes and damsons are purging. Olives and capers provoke the appetite.

Nuts, spices, salt and sugar

Nuts should be eaten fresh or new when they are nutritive and increase fatness. However, when old they are too choleric, too heating and drying. Peas, beans and pulses are nourishing and stimulate sexual desire but very windy foods are hard to digest. Ginger heats the stomach and helps digestion. Pepper of all kinds heats the body, helps digestion, dissolves phlegm and wind as well as being a diuretic. Cloves are restorative and ease pains in the joints. Mace is a cordial. Saffron also comforts the heart and stomach, while nutmeg is good for the brain. Cinnamon is another cordial with astringent properties to counteract looseness of the bowels. Since all these spices have a pungent heat which will rise in the body to the brain, they all help digestion by their heat and are comforters of the heart and brain by virtue of their fine aromas. Of salt Culpeper writes:

> Salt moderately used is very wholesome. Taken excessively, it engenders choler, dries up the natural moisture and inflames the blood, stops the veins, hardens the stone and gathers together viscous humours, causing sharpness of urine, consuming the flesh and fat of the body. Those who are cold, watery and phlegmatic may feed more plentifully of salt and of salt meats, but choleric and melancholic persons must eat it moderately, and sanguine persons must take no more of it than lightly to relish their meat.

Salt helps to hinder putrefaction, and so is used to preserve or 'cure' meat. It is astringent and dries up superfluous humours. Sugar is temperate in heat and nourishing, pleasing to the stomach, liver and blood and good for the lungs. It was thought not as hurtful to choleric temperaments as honey. It was used for syrups, lozenges, conserves, cordials and other medicinal preparations as well as part of the diet. Culpeper was of the opinion that refined sugar was the purest and best form of cane sugar, 'melting as salt doth speedily in any liquor'.

DIET AND TEMPERAMENT

Those of a sanguine temperament 'need not be very scrupulous in the quality of their diet, provided they exceed not in quantity, because the digestive virtue is so strong'.[43] However, drinking too much mild beer or ale may cause cholic and pains in the back, while inordinate quantities of strong beer, ale and wine cause fevers

TABLE OF THE QUALITIES OF SOME COMMON ARTICLES OF DIET

HEATING FOODS	COOLING FOODS	MOISTENING FOODS	DRYING FOODS
wine & mead	beer, cider & water		
fresh bread		fresh bread	old bread
oats	barley		
egg yolk	egg white		
		butter	
	cottage cheese	cottage cheese	
soft cheese		soft cheese	
hard cheese			hard cheese
		milk	
	fish	fish	
shellfish		shellfish	
chicken		chicken	
veal		veal	
lamb		lamb	
	beef		beefmutton
mutton			
garlic, onions, leeks			garlic, onions, leeks
artichokes			artichokes
cabbage			cabbage
fennel			
asparagus		asparagus	
	spinach	spinach	
turnip		turnip	
carrot			carrot
chickpeas & beans		chickpeas & beans	
	lentils		lentils
parsnip			parsnip
	lettuce	lettuce	
	cucumber	cucumber	
	oranges & lemons		oranges & lemons
olive oil		olive oil	
	pears & apples	pears & apples	
figs, raisins, dates		figs, raisins, dates	
	other summer fruits	other summer fruits	
	quinces		quinces
nuts		nuts	

and inflammations of the skin, lungs or head. Choleric types, whose stomach 'fire' is too strong, can easily digest any kind of food but are more often harmed by fasting as by excessive alcohol, both of which add dryness and heat to their bodies. Spices and any other heating foods are also to be avoided. A moderate amount of cooling beer, however, is reckoned good. The melancholic person, while wary of all excess in food and drink, should also seek to avoid foods that are hard to digest, such as hard cheese, heavy breads and roasted, fried and salted meats, 'especially such as are students or lead a sedentary life'. Easily digested foods, such as eggs, with plenty of fluid to drink at meal times, like milk or a little white wine, is recommended instead. Excesses of food or drink cause crude humours to be formed in such people which create chest and digestive problems, headaches and other symptoms. But the provoking of appetite in the stomach by an abundance of melancholy in the spleen can result in an insatiable hunger for food and drink with deleterious consequences.

Of all the temperaments, the phlegmatic benefits most from fasting, since this allows an opportunity for the body to be cleansed of the thick and unconcocted humours that the weakness of Fire engenders in these types. Otherwise the diet should be light, and include cooked rather than raw foods. Wine and strong beer taken here and there is wholesome for such people because of their heating effect. Garlic, onions, pepper and ginger are recommended on the same grounds. An excess of food or drink in these people causes indigestion, wind and catarrhal problems.

Regarding the compound temperaments, the choleric-melancholic should 'observe great moderation in meat and drink, for meat hard of digestion engenders tough phlegm in such bodies and will bring their bodies to an asthma ere they are aware of it'. More particularly, they should avoid excess in drinking, for light ale and beer create phlegm and strong beer and wine cause the 'breaking out of heat about the body'. Great moderation applies even more to the melancholic-choleric type. 'Let their care be to suffice nature and not to stuff their guts with meat, nor make a hog-wash-tub or their bellies with drink', otherwise the tough and congealed humours produced will provoke lung and digestive problems. Instead, a glass of wine or strong beer here and there after meals will help digestion.

The melancholic-sanguine and sanguine-melancholic types have a reasonably good digestion and can be a little more liberal in their diet, but 'much fasting fills their bodies full of wind and much strong beer and wine inflames the blood'. Those of a sanguine-phlegmatic temperament have only an averagely strong digestion. Therefore they must eat only a moderate amount of foods which must be easy to digest and they may be helped by the use of some heating wine or strong beer. The same applies to the phlegmatic-sanguine type, in whom an excess of food and drink creates plentiful humours and sour phlegm.

Of the phlegmatic-choleric temperament Culpeper says that 'although they may be a little bolder with their food than the phlegmatic may, yet is digestion in them none of the strongest, and excess in meat fills their bodies with choler and punishes their carcasses with choleric diseases'. Furthermore an excess of drink 'spoils their digestion and weakens nature'. Where choler predominates over phlegm, the warning against frequent fasting for simple choleric types holds true in the compound temperament, the harmful effects being of the same quality if less so in degree. Too much wine and strong beer inflame the blood and putrefaction is the sequel to this inflammation.

Exercise and Rest

Moderate exercise, Culpeper says, stirs up the natural heat by which digestion is improved, and equally distributes the spirits of the body.[44] It opens the pores to let the waste products of the third concoction escape, an important, cleansing transpiration through the skin, and helps rid the body of other waste through the lungs. Exercise generally strengthens the physique and comforts the body, senses and spirits. It is 'a principal means for preserving health, above all other things except temperance'. Hippocrates said that the way to preserve health is not to glut the stomach with food and to be laborious in exercise. Aristotle explained the reason why this is so, that 'the superfluity of humours causeth diseases, which show themselves chiefly when either a man exceeds in diet or is wanting in exercise'. Galen even suggested that, provided a person exercises regularly, the occasional excess in diet will do no harm.[45]

Excessive exercise, on the other hand, hurts by its drying and wearying effect on the body and spirits, and can disturb normal functioning. In the same way rest, as a necessary corollary to exercise, also strengthens the body and maintains good health, but excessive rest, or idleness, is bad for the body. For rest activates the phlegmatic humour, as exercise sets in motion the blood and the choleric and melancholic humours. Excessive resting brings the effects of excessive phlegm in the body: a dullness of the mind and senses and the production of crude humours in the body through diminished digestive power. The result will be cold diseases, continual sickness and a hastening of old age.

The amount of exercise and rest that should be taken as a part of healthy living varies according to the temperament and age of a person as well as his or her physical capabilities. A child should exercise moderately and an elderly person should exercise lightly. The sick and convalescent may benefit from certain specific, gentle movements depending on their condition. Young adults are those most suited to the most vigorous forms of exercise, the more so if they are robust. Yet the degree of vigorous exercise falls well short of the 'No pain, no gain' theory. Exercise should stop when the body becomes weary, breaks out in a sweat or becomes reddened or swollen.

Exercise should be taken before meals when the activity helps to remove waste products from the body before more food is taken in. Moderate walking is cited as a most commodious and often used form of exercise. A gentle walk may be taken after a meal, but nothing more vigorous, else the motion will cause humours to be taken into the blood, which will obstruct the liver, trouble the brain and cause various diseases such as itchy or scabby skin.

The sanguine or choleric person should avoid violent exercise because it inflames the blood and may provoke fevers. Yet the active choleric type is probably the one most likely to exercise to excess. Hot exercise is very good for the cold temperaments, the melancholic and phlegmatic types, since it will help digestion and the distribution of vital spirits through the body, as well as clearing the skin and the mind. Exercise is good for a compound temperament of choler and melancholy, especially where the latter is predominant since the innate heat is weak in such people. Such moderate activity is also good for the combination of sanguine and melancholic since it purifies the blood, clears the skin and strengthens the body. If the sanguine predominates, however, vigorous exercise must be avoided. Where the sanguine and phlegmatic temperaments are mixed, on the other hand, 'the more they accustom their bodies to exercise, the better 'tis for them', since it will consume the undigested humours of their bodies. Moderate exercise is also required for the combination of choleric and phlegmatic temperaments.

Sleep and Wakefulness

Sleep, says Culpeper,[46] is caused by a sweet vapour rising to the brain which is condensed by the coldness of that organ into a humour which blocks the nerves and puts a temporary end to movement and stimulation of the senses. However, this sweet vapour may be affected by other vapours such as those rising from the organs of digestion, if a meal has not yet been fully concocted, or from other overheated organs. Thus food, temperament or the distemper of an organ could affect the quality of sleep.

Sleep was judged to affect the body in several ways. It helped digestion by stopping the dispersion of the innate heat and this, in turn, encouraged the immature humours in the body to be fully matured. Thus complete digestion by the end of the day was considered a very important requirement for good sleep. Good sleep would then bring the sensitive faculties into repose and renew and restore them. It remedied the weakness due to dispersal of the innate heat by bodily fatigue, sex, anger and emotional disturbance and the like, and so restored strength. Overall, sleep brought about an equilibrium in the quantity and quality of humours by good digestion and the removal of excrements, and instigated a warming and moistening action to refresh the mind and cheer the spirits. This was considered particularly beneficial to the cold and dry elderly, for whom good sleep was very important. The waking state created opposite effects to this, as day is opposite to night.

Generally the best time for sleeping was at night, in harmony with the period of passivity in the macrocosm. Moreover, the humidity and drowsy stillness of night was thought to contribute to perfect digestion. Sleeping in the day was bad, on the other hand, because it overmoistened the body at an inappropriate time and filled the head with catarrhs, unless the sleep was short enough to prevent this from happening. However, if it was short, it could not particularly benefit the digestive process and might cause heaviness in the stomach, acidity, wind and gurgling noises from the bowels, once the person was again awake. Only the weak and sickly, those who have laboured hard in the morning and those who did not sleep the night before were thought to benefit from sleeping for any length of time in the day. An exception was made, however, in those countries where, due to the fierce heat of Summer, the 'siesta' was customarily observed. The *Regimen for Health* of the School of Salerno summarized the matter as follows:

> If R be in the month, their judgements err that think that sleep in the afternoon is good.
> If R be not therein some men there are that think a little nap breeds no ill blood.
> But if you shall herein exceed too far, it hurts your health, it cannot be withstood.
> Long sleep at afternoons by stirring fumes breeds sloth and agues, acking heads and rheums.
> The moisture bred in breast, in jaws and nose are called catarrhs or tysique or the pose.[47]

It was thought bad to go to sleep with the stomach still full of food since this would disorganize and diminish the digestive faculty, and good, deep sleep would be impossible because of the resulting tossing and turning of the sleeper. Thus a gentle walk after a meal and before sleep, a 'constitutional', was recommended. Equally, sleeping on a quite empty stomach, that had not received food for some time, was held to be weakening. All this shows that there was a clear notion of when to eat in relation to sleep. The quantity of sleep in relation to wakefulness was important too. Seven to eight hours was the amount usually required. In correct balance, sleep would have the same effect as rest, whilst wakefulness influenced the body in a similar way to exercise. For movement of any sort, like exercise, causes the innate heat and the humours to be stirred up.

Excessive sleep, like idleness, was believed to be harmful in several ways. It dulled the senses by overmoistening the brain. The excess of moisture then dampened the innate heat, closed the pores of the skin and slowed transpiration. Furthermore, since the only natural evacuation for the body during sleep is by transpiration, the effect of this is prolonged retention of waste products, which could lead to harm. The brain in particular would be full of superfluities. On the other hand, those of a phlegmatic temperament whose digestion is slow or those who have overeaten needed to sleep longer than others in order for their digestion to be completed.

Excessive wakefulness, such as a state of insomnia, was said to consume and dissipate the spirits, to dry the body and the brain, making the latter 'giddy' and weakening its reasoning power. Catarrhs or 'rheums' from the brain consequently troubled the body and spirits, and the digestion could be hindered. Putrefactive changes and hot diseases due to excess choler might ensue, leading to the formation of abscesses. Sometimes diseases of cold followed a relative lack of sleep if the innate heat was sufficiently dissipated.

Retention and Evacuation of Waste Matter

Retention and evacuation refer to the excrements of the body, namely faeces, urine, sweat and transpiration through the skin, menstrual blood and semen.[48] The over-long retention of these substances in the body was judged a cause of diseases. Such a situation could come about because of a weak expulsive virtue or an unduly strong retentive virtue. The expulsive virtue might not be strong enough to deal with an excess of waste matter. In such a situation the waste matters could be reabsorbed to set up a disease process in another part of the body. On the other hand, the retentive virtue might hold food and waste in the body for a long time because the digestive power was weak and the concoctions worked slowly. Otherwise, channels in the body might be narrow or obstructed by coarse and glutinous matter. For whatever reason, the continuance of waste products in the body, a condition of plethora, can only harm. Constipation will hinder digestion, cause nausea and adversely affect the appetite. The fermentation of the unevacuated excrements will irritate the stomach and cause colic due to the trapped gas. These 'putrid vapours' will rise higher in the body to cause giddiness and headache. Other effects may include atony or laxity of the bowels, inflammations and septic conditions such as boils, obstructions and ruptures (hernias). In addition, obstruction of normal transpiration through the skin, because of pores closing due to external cold or bad humours within, can cause serious diseases such as pleurisies, pneumonias and other fevers.

Perturbations of the Mind

As previously discussed, the unity of psyche and soma in the human being implies that thoughts and emotions will have just as much impact on the health as other, more physical aspects of living. Proper ordering and equilibrium of the thoughts and feelings is achieved by the regulation and balance of the breath or pneuma, which in turn can be upset by the mind and the passions it can transmit to the heart, the seat of the emotions. All aspects of being, the physical, mental, emotional and spiritual, are thus mutually dependent within the whole and attention must be paid to each of these factors in the preservation of health.

SEX

The Hippocratic school taught that the moisture of semen was derived from a phlegmatic humour in the brain and was passed down the spinal chord and by some channel through to the sexual organs.[49] Levine Lemnie recommended the Hippocratic idea of moderate 'spending of seed' as a means to rid the body of excess phlegm and warned against both excessive intercourse and abstinence from sex which was considered just as harmful.[50] The 'spending of seed' by a man was considered a direct drain on the vital spirit and innate heat since semen contains pneuma. Excessive sex therefore was reckoned to cool and dry the body and to weaken the brain, eyes, nerves and senses. The ensuing cold would diminish the natural faculty to allow less than optimum digestion and result in the production of crude humours in the body.

> In immoderate intercourse the testes place inordinate demand on their blood vessels for the juice out of which they make semen. As these vessels are exhausted they communicate the demand to other vessels until the whole body is depleted not only of the spermatic ingredients but of pneuma; the consequence is debilitation.[51]

Lemnie specified gout and joint inflammations (gonococcal arthritis?) amongst diseases caused by excessive sexual intercourse, whilst an absence of sex brought troubled sleep and cardiac problems by heat and fumes rising from the womb to annoy the hearts of 'old maids' (the connection formerly made between 'hysteria' and *hysteros*, the Greek for 'womb').

Culpeper expressed a Puritan view on the subject and his objection to excessive sexual intercourse was as much on the grounds of sin as of health. His opinion was that sex was for procreation or it was the sin of *concupiscence*. He gave a remedy for such desire in a chapter entitled 'A sober Diet allayeth the heat of Lust',[52] where he reminded the reader that the sin of lust was deleterious, not only for the soul but for the body also:

> It is in vain to object to me what lustful thoughts either to this or any other sin, the Devil may cast into the heart, for if there be no corruption in the body answerable to this temptation, he had as good be quiet and keep his breath to cool his pottage.

He had earlier specified this corruption:

> People extremely addicted to lust, are seldom long-lived, because nothing so exhausteth the spirits, and best juice of the body, as lust doth, nor more weakens and overthrows nature.[53]

Culpeper seemed to regard excessive intercourse as just as harmful to women – although tradition had it that excessive 'venery' (pursuit of sexual desire) was more harmful to men than to women[54] – because the fact that 'there is an essential, vital spirit in the seeds of both sexes, is without all question':[55] and that 'in the act of copulation, the woman spends her seed as well as the man'.[56] Both Lemnie and Culpeper agreed that healthy sex should take place after digestion and not immediately after a meal, nor on an empty stomach. Riviere said that the morning was the best time of day for sexual intercourse, and Winter and Spring the best seasons. Sex was thought hurtful to those who were too young or too old for it. For the purpose of conception, Culpeper advised against drunkenness in either partner during intercourse as he felt that such an unhealthy state would affect the quality of pneuma.[57]

Central to the preservation of health is therefore the correct maintenance of the innate heat and the conservation of radical moisture in the body. Their functioning is affected by the normal human activities of breathing, eating and drinking, sleeping, bodily evacuations, movement and sex. The climate, changing seasons and ageing will exert their effects also. All the while, a balance must be maintained whereby the spirits of the body and the blood, which carry the innate heat, flow free without impediment. Each of the above factors which have an impact on this balance are measured in terms of the primary qualities they bring to bear on the human organism. Armed with this knowledge, every person can strive to maintain the balance within their own unique being, according to their temperament, by countering a superimposed quality with its opposite. Thus, for example, in Summer the ambient temperature heats the body and this is corrected by the taking of cooling foods and drinks. The causes of the production of heat, cold, dryness and moisture are summed up below.

TABLE OF CAUSES

Causes of Heat (Galen's 5)
- outward heat, eg Summer, moderately hot baths, heating external applications
- movement, eg moderate exercise, light massage, moderate friction, hot foods, drinks and medicines; nourishment generally
- emotions, eg anger, mild worry, moderate joy; also moderate wakefulness and sleep
- putrefaction

(also tightening or shrinkage of skin, reducing perspiration and so increasing internal heat)

Causes of Cold (Galen's 5)
- excessive exercise or repose
- external refrigerants, including cooling foods, drinks and medicines
- excessive heat, eg very hot air, thermal waters, hot fomentations, which disperse the innate heat by relaxing the body [the prolonged application of moderate heat eg staying in the bath too long, will have the same effect]
- insufficient food
- extreme aggregation of humours within the body which strangles the innate heat

(also excessive rarefaction which relaxes the body and disperses the innate heat, excessive retention of excretions, an abundance of crude humours and undue evacuations all refrigerate the body) (also emotions: excessive worry, fear, joy or pleasure)

Causes of Moisture
- baths, especially after meals
- moistening food and medicines; food taken to excess
- retention of matter ordinarily eliminated from the body
- evacuation of a desiccant or dry humour
- rest and sleep
- moderate joy
- things which cool the body, thus causing humours to be retained
- applications which, being mildly warm, liquefy the secretions

Causes of Dryness
- external cold, which congeals humours, constricts channels in the body and obstructs moistening nutrient materials
- excessive heat, which disperses moisture
- diet: drying foods and medicines, insufficient food
- exercise
- wakefulness
- frequent emotional disturbance
- violent evacuations, including sexual intercourse

PART 3

As Above, So Below:
Astrology, Medicine and Hermetic Philosophy

The application of astrology to medicine to which Culpeper was heir arose from a co-operation of Greek and Egyptian scientific minds in Hellenistic Egypt after the time of Alexander the Great. It is true that astrological lore had been transmitted from its birthplace in ancient Babylon to Greece around the end of the 5th century BC, for 'Berosus was said to have settled on the island of Cos, the home of Hippocratic medicine, and astrology early found its way into the Hippocratic corpus of medical writings.'[1] But the full development of astrological medicine took place in Egypt. It was called *Iatromathematica* by the Greeks.

Many early works form a compendium of this astrological medicine, supposedly written by a priest named Petosiris for a fictitious King Nechepso[2] with divine guidance from Asclepios, the Greek god of medicine[3]. In reverence for the greatness and antiquity of Egyptian medicine, Asclepios was identified with the Egyptian pharaoh-priest Imhotep of the 4th millennium BC.[4] However, the principal text in antiquity on the subject of astrological medicine was attributed to that other divine source of revelation, the Egyptian Hermes Trismegistos or 'thrice-greatest' Hermes. He, an all-wise Egyptian priest, philosopher and law-giver (the three aspects of his greatness[5]), was also the Egyptian god Thoth (the god of mental disciplines) in another guise. The text bearing his name was the *Iatromathematica of Hermes Trismegistos to Ammon the Egyptian* of the 2nd century BC.[6] The fact that a version of this short text was included in the second edition of Culpeper's *Astrological Judgement of Diseases* in 1655, and that Lilly published a version of his own in his *Christian Astrology* eight years before this, indicates the close and unbroken connection between 17th-century medical astrology and the first development of iatromathematica.

The Greeks believed that the Babylonians worshipped the Sun, Moon and planets, and took from them the notion that the movements of the heavenly bodies bore a relation to human existence. They adopted, conceptualized and rationalized the art of astrology and incorporated it into their science and philosophy. This was especially true of the Stoics who believed that the course of human existence followed and was determined by the movements of the heavenly bodies in the cosmos. In Hellenistic Egypt in the first centuries AD, when disaffection with rational Greek philosophy became apparent, and when mystery cults of all sorts, including Christian gnosticism, began to flourish in the Roman Empire, a new philosophy started to emerge, a consensus of Greek strands of thought but with a religious aspect. Plato's philosophy had taught that the human being possessed an immortal soul within the physical body and that the mundane world this body inhabited was but a shadow of the real nature of the cosmos found in the metaphysical realm of images and ideas of which the soul had knowledge. This transcendent reality, coupled to late Stoic philosophy with its emphasis on the relationship between human life and the stars, and in Egypt to the indigenous religious and magical beliefs, thus produced there a doctrine supposedly drawn from the ancient teachings and wisdom of Hermes Trismegistos.

Hermetic philosophy, as Culpeper explained it,[7] posited three connected worlds, the elementary, celestial and intellectual, within the unity of the cosmos. The elementary world is that of mundane existence, occupied by objects and life forms which are composed of the four elements in their varying proportions. This is the 'sublunary' world comprising everything on Earth beneath the orbit of the Moon. Above the elementary world lies the celestial world of the Sun, Moon, planets and stars. This realm was said to rule over the lower elementary realm, its planetary bodies representing active and ever-changing forces operating on passive matter to form, shape and alter it. Culpeper explains it thus:

> Consider that all time is measured out by motion and that the original of all motion is in the heavens, for it is the motion of the Sun which causeth day and night, Summer, Winter, Spring and Harvest. From which conversation of times and years all changes proceed, both heat and cold, dryness and moisture. By which four is caused life

and death, generation and putrefaction, increase and decrease of
elementary things ... The Sun gives a vital seed and stirs up all to
motion and action, quickens and defends what it hath quickened.
The Moon subministers moisture to preserve what the Sun hath
generated from the scorching heat which is caused by motion. Both
Sun and Moon make use of the other five planets [even as the Heart
and Brain make use of the liver, spleen, gall &c in the Body of Man]
for the effecting and varying things below, and tempering them
diverse ways according to their several motions, else all the things
generated in the elementary world would be of one nature and
quality and then the world could not subsist. For Man, having all
qualities in him, cannot subsist without any one of them.[8]

The celestial bodies, existing externally because they are formed
not from the four elements but from a fifth element, which
Aristotle called Aether, alter by their constant movement and
interaction in the heavens the elementary bodies below, like 'a
carpenter, when he hews a timber log, the timber log must needs
change form according as 'tis hewed, but the carpenter himself
changeth not'.[9] This close affinity of the elementary and celestial
worlds furnishes what Culpeper called the 'excellent and true'
motto of Hermes Trismegistos, namely 'as above, so below',[10] and
constitutes the cosmic sympathy between human beings and the
stars which the art of astrology makes known.

The third realm, the intellectual world, contains the higher
truths and knowledge of the oneness of all creation. It is the
realm of Plato's Ideas and Images and of the Christian God. The
rational human soul has an inkling of this world but the faculty
must be developed. As Culpeper says in his Christian
interpretation, Man is

> capable of the intellectual world, as having an epitomy of that in
> himself, whereby he knows that there is a God and that God made this
> world and governeth it now he hath made it; that there are angels,
> and that he hath an immortal spirit in himself, which causeth him to
> hope and expect immortality.[11]

As the celestial world is a cause of effects in the elementary world
over which it rules, so the intellectual world governs the celestial
by having its higher truths mirrored in the 'harmony of the
spheres'. Consequently the human rational soul, not by necessity
subject to the same celestial effects as the elements which
compose the human body, is free to act with or resist them when

it has crossed from ignorance to wisdom for 'the influence of the stars reacheth not to the mind or rational part of man, because it is an epitome of the intellectual world which is superior to them'.[12] Thus it is said that wise persons rule their stars (because they are aware of higher truths) while the fool (who is unenlightened and remains in ignorance) obeys them. In this sense, the right use of astrology is dependent on the spiritual awareness of the practitioner and a knowledge of the intellectual world is something a human must aspire to and work diligently towards over the years, and 'happy, yea, thrice happy, is he that attains it'. In pursuit of this aspiration, the spiritual purpose of right living, in order to extend the lifespan, is to gain a true understanding of the intellectual world and to 'attain the divine mysteries in philosophy'. Moreover, the attainment of wisdom by contemplation would necessarily be bound together with 'a quiet, serene body in respect of health'. On the other hand, says Culpeper:

> intemperancy not only causeth both a short and sickly life here, but also by crudities chokes the intellectual and angelical part of man, whereby his brains are made so muddy, that he is pro tempore made incapable of the understanding of what Great things God ... hath left for him to know and study after.[13]

The three worlds of Hermetic philosophy thus form one undivided whole. Culpeper speaks of a 'trinity in the deity' (the Father, Son and Holy Spirit) and of a 'unity in the godhead' in his works, meaning a unity of the three worlds 'and a dependency between them, and not that God made the Creation to hang together like ropes of sand'. He felt that God, as the first cause of things, set in motion the planets to act as natural second causes of things below in the elementary world. 'The most high Creator of all things has given commission to Nature to be princess both over the celestial and terrestrial worlds.'[14] He sees the number 3 as 'a most powerful number, a number of perfection' and states that everything in the vegetable and mineral world consists of 3 principles, namely sulphur, mercury and salt. A similar trinity is found in the 3 essences of body, soul and spirit which compose the human being.[15]

The human body is thus composed of the four elements, it contains a microcosmic Sun, Moon and planets which respond to their celestial counterparts, and it houses a rational soul that is nurtured by contemplation of the intellectual world. The human being is thus the epitome in miniature (or microcosm) of a fully alive cosmos (or macrocosm).

Reference to astrological medicine was made in the most famous astrological textbook of the classical period, Claudius Ptolemy's *Tetrabiblos* or 'four books' on astrology, written in the 2nd century AD. In discussing the extent of knowledge attainable through astrology and its usefulness, Ptolemy cites as his example the Greek-

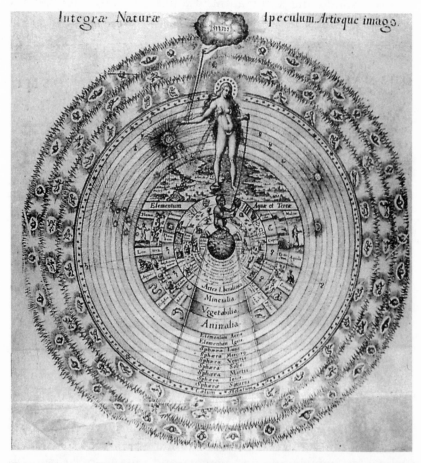

Figure 8 In this illustration, entitled The Mirror of the Whole of Nature and the Image of Art, from Robert Fludd's History of the Macrocosm and the Microcosm *(Utriusque Cosmi ... Historia, 1617), the three worlds described in Hermetic philosophy are clearly depicted. In the centre is the elemental world of Water and Earth surround by the circles of Air and Fire. Around these are the seven circles of the planets, the 'eighth' circle of the fixed stars and, beyond this, the realm of God and his angels. Nature, shown as a beautiful virgin, straddles all three worlds and is connected by a chain to God above and to the Ape of Nature, or human art, below.*

Egyptian iatromathematicians who have 'completely bound medicine to astronomical prognostic'.[16] These Egyptians, he said, recognize that the predictive power of astrology, like the power of preventive medicine, was not infallible but nevertheless valuable. However, in the *Tetrabiblos* this iatromathematical practice remained a reference only, because Ptolemy had a problem with the kind of horoscopes these astrologer-physicians were using. They would cast a horoscope for the time when a sick person either took to his or her bed or first consulted them. Such a horoscope is called a *decumbiture* (from the Latin *decumbere* meaning 'to lie down').

The point of Ptolemy's work, on the other hand, was to establish a scientific base for astrology along Aristotelian lines, in other words, according to the moments of conception and birth. These were put forward as the only valid moments for the astrological effect. According to Ptolemy's 'hypothesis of seeds', the moment of conception is an instant when the Sun, Moon and stars can impress the qualities of the heavens onto the seed that is to develop into a human being. The moment of birth is the other instant of importance, that of true human existence, when the developing being emerges into the world, like the first leaves from a seed bursting forth from the ground. For Ptolemy the more readily knowable moment of birth was more fully impressive of the complete living being and so he used this to provide the scientific data and starting point for the assessment of the nature (temperament) and fate (including the length of life) of its subject.

These two separate practices, which each validated a different orientation in time for the astrological project, encapsulate the dual tradition in astrology. The tradition is also divided along the same lines on the question of *how* astrology works. As Geoffrey Cornelius points out:

> There are two approaches found in traditional astrology, often woven together – or muddled – in the attitudes of the same author. The orthodox classical position has an Aristotelian foundation, and is a species of *celestial causation*. The quality of the time moment is determined by the disposition of the influencing heavens 'at that moment'. The second approach is Platonic in its inspiration. It may be characterized as *cosmic sympathy*: the planets and their positions *mirror* the occult quality of the totality of the macrocosm-microcosm 'at that moment'. This sympathy is also mirrored in the knowing that belongs to the soul. The distinction of these two positions tends on

the one hand to an astrology of *causes*, and on the other to an astrology of *signs*, thus giving two different orientations to astrology right down to the present day.[17]

The Hermetic philosophy which underpinned the iatromathematica of the Greek-Egyptian physicians had a major impact on Western Europe in the 15th century, as a result of a translation from Greek to Latin of a collection of writings attributed to Hermes Trismegistos. The translator of these writings, known as the *Corpus Hermeticum*, was Marsilio Ficino, a Christian priest, astrologer, physician, musician and Renaissance magician. By interpreting the philosophical writings attributed to Hermes as a revelation from a remoter period of the coming of Christianity, Ficino assured the acceptability of Hermetic philosophy, (when purged of its magical content) in Christian Europe in the 16th and 17th centuries. Culpeper was one of many who professed this philosophy and who, in addition, wholeheartedly embraced its astrological teachings.

Marsilio Ficino then went on to write his ground-breaking work on medicine and astrology, entitled *Three Books on Life* (1489), of which the third book, *On Comparing Life with the Heavens (De vita coelitus comparanda)*, dealt specifically with astrology. In an earlier work Ficino had criticized the fated attitude of the common astrologers of his day and it is here that Ficino outlined a practice of astrological medicine which, by its recognition of the free will of the human soul, by its identification of natural intermediaries between the celestial and elementary worlds and by its right purpose, that of healing the ills and diseases of human beings, could reconcile an occult practice such as astrology with Christian beliefs.

Ficino called the natural intermediary between the celestial and elementary worlds the 'world spirit' (*spiritus mundanus*), a macrocosmic equivalent of the spirits or pneuma in the human body. In the same way in which the vital spirit, formed from blood and breath (pneuma-containing air), gives life and relation to the whole body and creates the animal and natural spirits of the mind and body, so the world spirit connects the world's body (the Earth, the elementary realm) to its soul (the intellectual realm). As the closing statement of the *Iatromathematica* of Hermes Trismegistos attests: 'Nothing happens in a man that is not connected with cosmic sympathy.' Here then is the medium for 'cosmic sympathy', regarding which

> the later Greek Stoics, the real inventors of the doctrine, had stated
> as if in anticipation of Ficino that the continuity between the human
> medical *pneuma* and the cosmic *pneuma* forms the basis of astrology.[18]

Culpeper's description of this intermediary, the cosmic pneuma
or world spirit, was more simple and down-to-earth:

> Because the beams of the celestial Sun and Moon cannot pass to the
> elementary world but by a medium, viz the air. That's the reason
> animals must breathe and all vegetables and minerals have an aerial
> spirit in them.[19]

This idea, that a medium or cosmic sympathy existed between the
planets of the celestial world and the living beings of the
elementary world, was a widely accepted way of explaining the
astrological effect. It makes the question of whether astrology was
based on signs or causes seem somewhat unimportant. For as S J
Tester notes of a prevailing view:

> what might be called scientific or natural astrology was more or less
> universally acceptable: that is, the uses of astrology in medicine and
> in meteorology and in alchemy. Since the changes of the sublunary
> world were caused by heavenly movements, physical changes like
> chemical reactions and bodily diseases, and the weather [like the
> tides, always accepted as caused by the Moon's movements] were
> clearly linked to the movements of the stars and planets, and no one
> could expect to alter the natures of metals [with their ancient links
> with the planets] or to cure diseases or to understand and forecast the
> weather and related phenomena, storm and flood and earthquakes
> and so on, without a knowledge of astrology. This was not
> superstition; it was good science.[20]

Culpeper often varied in his writings over the question of whether
astrology revealed signs or causes of earthly things below, stating
in one place that 'the gout is caused by Saturn' and then titling
his major work on medical astrology *Semeiotica Uranica* (The Art of
Reading Signs from Astronomy). Ficino, in a more poetic vein,
had variously compared cosmic sympathy and the efficacy
obtained from such occult correspondences with a love that is
inspired by likeness and mutual attraction, with the sympathetic
vibrations of two lutes and with reverberations whereby a wall
gives an echo to a voice. In the end, the important point is that
the possibility of human initiative to intervene, to act in line with

the inclinations of the stars when they promise good and against the trend to avoid or mitigate any evil so promised, was recognized. In discussing that part of Fate which is avoidable, Ptolemy had commented:

> For they [the 'Egyptians'] would never have contrived certain evil-averting sacrifices and vigils and therapies for the universal and particular conditions that come on and abide due to the environing atmosphere, if the opinion of the unchangeability and irreversibility of the future had come into existence among them.[21]

The use of astrology in medicine found great acceptance in past centuries because this understanding of astrology afforded both a scientific explanation of its effect and at the same time a recognition of human free will. Yet, from the modern perspective, this accommodation of astrology within 'science' must have been convenient, though somewhat disingenuous regarding major details of astrological practice, since there is in truth an unbridgeable chasm between rational Aristotelian science and a divinatory art such as astrology. This chasm is no nearer being crossed today.

Although the planets are moving in their courses constantly, and cosmic sympathy allows for a continuous connection between the heavenly and Earth-bound bodies, the actual assignation of significance to planets and zodiac signs is made only when the astrologer plots the planetary positions in a horoscope for a specific inquiry. In medical inquiries, this horoscope may be cast not just at the time of the onset of illness, when the planetary positions and the illness occur simultaneously in time, but also at the time of first consulting an astrologer-physician. Culpeper certainly published judgements on decumbitures arising in both ways.[22] Consequently, the horoscope cannot be simply a mapping of the celestial cause of a disease occurring at a certain moment. It is rather a sign or omen regarding the illness, generated by the desire of the sick person to be healed and dependent upon the free will of that person actually to seek divination on the matter. The important, first consideration in astrology given by the 13th-century astrologer Guido Bonatti states:

> The first, is to observe what it is that moves a person to propose or ask a question of an astrologer; where we must take notice of three motions: the first, of the mind, when a man is stirred up in his thoughts and hath an intent to inquire; the second, of the superior

and celestial bodies, so that they at that time imprint on the thing inquired after, what shall become of it; the third, of the free will which disposes him to the very act of inquiring. For although the mind be moved to inquire, 'tis not enough, unless the superior bodies sympathise therewith. Nor is such motion of the stars enough, unless by the election of his will, the person does actually inquire.[23]

The signs of illness appearing in a decumbiture must match the patient's physical signs and symptoms of disease apparent to the physician's trained eye. Culpeper sought to establish the 'radicality' of the horoscope in this way.[24] He was at pains to downgrade the value of a horoscope cast on the sight of a patient's urine, with the patient absent, a common practice among doctors and lay healers in his day. In his address 'to the astrological physicians of England', he comments:

> I have given you here all my prognostications from the decumbiture of the sick party. And although I ingeniously confess the greatest part of them will hold true in a horary question erected upon the sight of the urine, of which I have now added a compendious treatise, yet this is my judgement at present: that, next the nativity [the natal horoscope], the decumbiture is the safest and surest ground for you to build your judgment upon, and you shall always find it by experience.[25]

The safest and certainty of the decumbiture partly lay in the fact 'that seeing the body [physical examination], hearing the relation [listening to the patient] and feeling the pulse of the sick is a better way to judge than gazing at as much piss as the Thames will hold'.[26]

It is a feature of the mystery, irrationality and inexplicability of the divinatory art of astrology that a decumbiture chart might aptly describe in symbolic terms the physical and mental state of the patient for whom it is cast. Moreover, a thus radical horoscope can be used to elucidate the cause and manner of arising of the disease, its likely course and expected outcome. In fact, the potential, holistic pertinence of astrology to any facet of the context in which it is used means that more than just the patient is represented in its symbols. The astrologer or physician was regularly identified among the planets in the horoscope, for example, and his or her involvement with the patient in the healing process was evaluated accordingly. This is called 'self-referencing' in modern astrology. Culpeper shows as much in a

comment he makes about the aspects of the Moon on a critical
day of the disease:

> But if, when she comes to the quartile or opposition, she meets with
> another planet, be sure the disease changes either to better or worse,
> according to that star she meets withal. And this will appear in the
> sick party, *or else in the physician, or in the course of physick.*[27]

Here the astrological sign is not simply applied objectively to the
patient but may be very material to the conduct, performance or
skill in prescription of the healer at that time. Again, in the one
decumbiture of his own which he left to posterity ('be pleased to
accept this one, in lieu of all the rest'),[28] Culpeper easily identified
his patient's physician (a 'French quack' who diagnosed the plague
in error, terrifying the patient and her household, and abusing her
body with inappropriate and strong purges) with a badly afflicted
Mars in Capricorn, ruler of the 7th house of physicians.

Such irrational features of astrological practice (which in fact
Culpeper did not explicitly discuss or distinguish as problematic)
undermine any attempt to put it on a rational Aristotelian basis.
But it is the case that astrology is an art of revelation and no
amount of argument can persuade a person of its veracity unless
they experience for themselves the power of a symbol to reveal
clearly and irrefutably a truth of a unique situation (for we are not
dealing here with statistical truth nor with probabilities). Both the
physician and the astrologer read signs, the former those of the
human body in a medical context, the latter those in the heavens
for any matter under heaven. This link is barely recognizable in
the modern world but in an older time, when a holistic view of the
cosmos prevailed, the two were much more closely connected.[29]
Consider the following tale from Ancient Babylon and Assyria, in
which the *Baru* carries out the tasks later given to the astrologer.

In his book *The Divine Origin of the Craft of the Herbalist*, E A
Wallis Budge, the famous Egyptologist, describes what happened
when the herbal doctor was called to an important patient.[29] The
doctor or *Asu* questioned the messenger so as to discover the
likely tools and medicines he would need. 'Then with his staff or
rod of office[30] in his hand, and his box, he set out to go to the
house of the sick man. But he did not go alone.' Accompanying
the *Asu* were the *Ashipu*, a priestly official 'learned in exorcisms,
spells and incantations', and the *Baru* or seer who had a great
knowledge of omens. On the road the *Baru* 'watched every

Ruta.

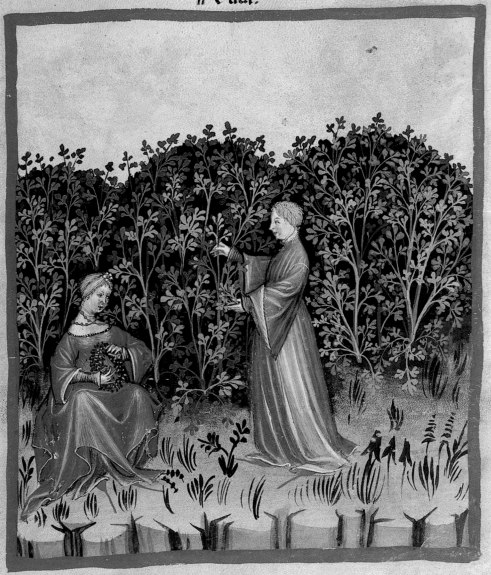

Ruta. complo. cal'a.z.ficca.in̄z. Electio uiridis recens. uuamentum. z feẽr tocicatis z epileñ̄s noccumentum. cat fodam. Remotio nocuiuit. cũ aceto. oleo z fale. Quid geñat humoẽ; acuitum. Conueni- t. frigis z huis. feib; z dcrepitis. hy̆me autumpno.z p̄ncipio ueris.friẽ z huis regionibus.

PLATE 9

RUE (*Ruta*).

The text reads: 'Rue. complexion: hot and dry in the third degree. The fresh green plant is better. Helpful in cases of poisoning and epilepsy. Harmful in causing a migraine, because it produces sharp humours. Take with vinegar, oil and salt to remove its harm. Agreeable to the cold and moist elderly and to those made decrepit in winter, autumn, the beginning of spring and in cold and moist regions.'
From the **Tacuinum Sanitatis in medicina**.

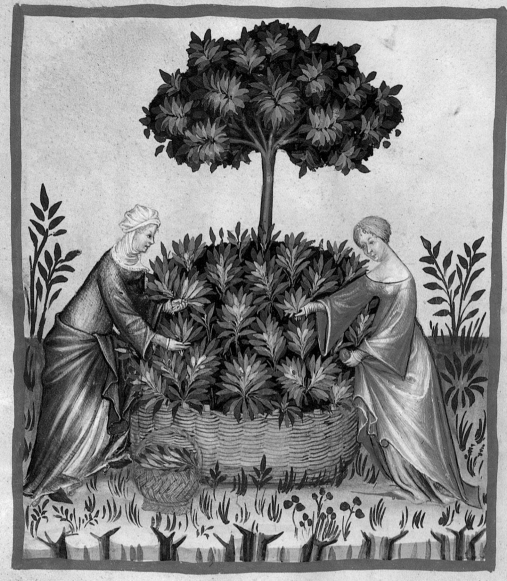

Salum. 2plo.ca. in p. sic. ini. Aecto romestica ortulana. uiridis siluestris. tii.fortio: e ca
lefaciendo. uuamitur. 2fert sto. 7 egritudibz nemox frigis. nocuit tum tarte rescendit.
Remo nocuinti. cu melle rececto. Quid guiat sanguine; grossuz. aliquir calz.ß fert fris
sembz.hueme 7. fris regiombz.

PLATE 10

SAGE (Salvia).

The text reads: 'Sage. complexions: hot in the first degree, dry in the second. Better from a domestic garden
and fresh, the wild kind however is more heating. Helpful in comforting the stomach and in cold diseases
of the nerves. Slowly harmful because it produces thick and somewhat hot blood. Take with purified honey
to remove its harm. Agreeable to the elderly, in winter and in cold regions.'
From the *Tacuinum Sanitatis in medicina.*

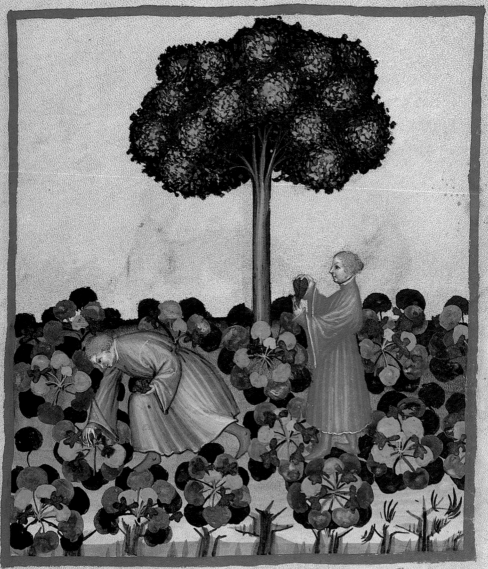

Viole. coplo. fri. in p. hii. in ƚ. Electio lazule. multiplicinu foliozu. iuuantur oloзate.
ad frenesim bibite. puгgant coleram. nocuntium. catro ex.frī noxet. Quid guant. o.
Зuenunt. cal. ƚ. fic. uuenibᴣ. estate ꝛ mīd ꞇoꝉibᴣ.

PLATE 11

VIOLETS (Viole).

The text reads: 'Violets. complexion: cold in the first degree, moist in the second.
The lazuli blue, many-leaved kind are better. Helpful for frenzy. As a drink they purge choler.
Harmful through catarrh from their coldness and because they give rise to lethargy.
Agreeable to hot and dry youths, in summer and in southerly regions.'
From the *Tacuinum Sanitatis in medicina*.

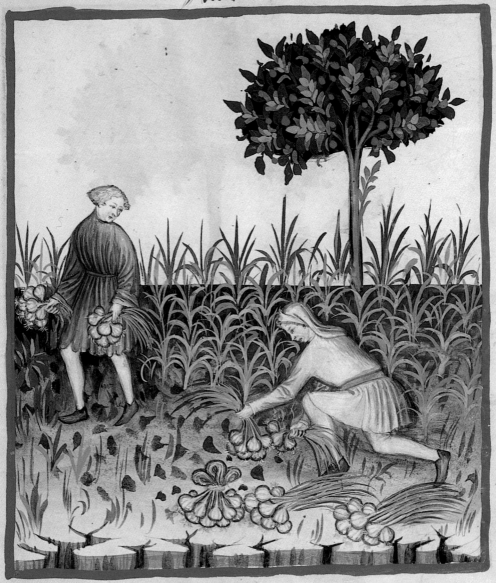

Alea.

Aleum. ợpto. ca. m. iiij. fic m. iij. Et cct arliozes ex co. quõ ẽ modice acutatis. unani. ợt
uenci. frã t mozfus fcozpioni t uipar t infficit umes. Occurrtius nocct ocul t ccrcb zo.
Remo nocti cu acceo t olo. Quid gnũnt humozc; grofflis t acutis: uenit frì decrepi
tis t fcmb; hyeme t montmus t feptentrioalib; :

PLATE 12

GARLIC (*Alea*).

The text reads: '*Garlic. complexion: hot in the fourth degree, dry in the third. Those of
less sharpness are better. Helpful against cold poisons and the bites of vipers and scorpions and
in killing worms. Harmful to the eyes and to the brain, because it produces a thick and sharp
humour. Take with vinegar and oil to remove its harm. Agreeable to the cold, decrepit and
elderly, in winter and in mountainous and northerly regions.*'
From the ***Tacuinum Sanitatis in medicina***.

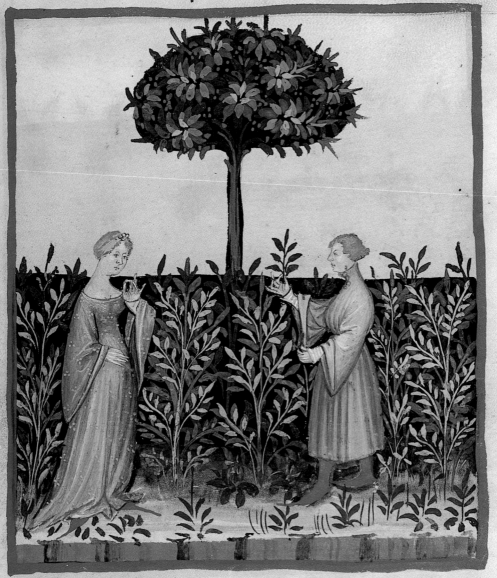

Liquiritia ꝯplo. ca. 7. hu. tpate. Electo reces cui radix ... lme mt grossa 7 sbrilg, lems. cq̄lis sbe
fuuam̄. ꝯfert raucedi. uocis 7 aspitati gutturis 7 pucat urina. apit opillationes nutruozt
renum̄. Nocum̄. ei sue facit abominationice; 7 debilitat appetiti. Remo noeti cu passul. Quod
gnat boni sanguine ꝯuenit oibz ꝯploibz, oi etati tpa 7 regioe.

PLATE 13

LIQUORICE (*Liquiritia*).

The text reads: '*Liquorice. complexion: temperately hot and moist. The fresh root, of a substance
equally between thick and thin, and soft, is better. Helpful to mucus and dryness in the throat and voice,
it provokes urine and opens obstructions of the breasts and kidneys. Its juice harmful in corrupting and
weakening the appetite. Because it breeds good blood, take with dried fruit to remove its harm.
Agreeable to all complexions, and to every age, season and region.*'
From the **Tacuinum Sanitatis in medicina**.

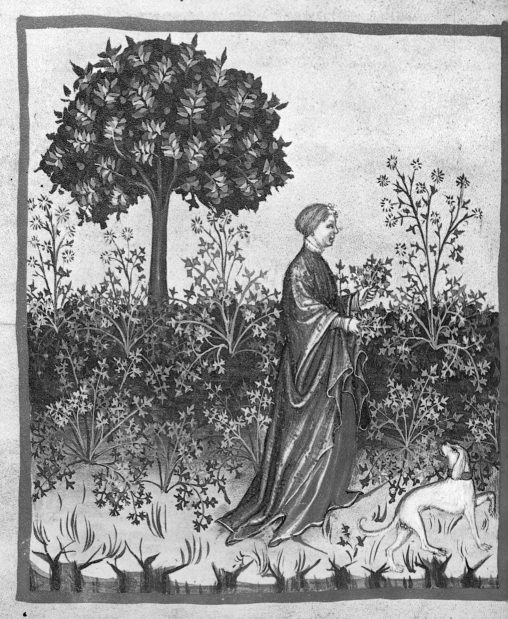

Petrosillum oplo. ca. 7. sic. in². Aceto ortulan 7 domestic'. uuanitum puicat urina. 7 me
strua 7 apt opilatices. nocunitum nimi usus adduct sodam. irmo nocunit eu aceto. Qui
gnat sanguine calin fouem -t. fris 7 huic.sembz. breme. omnibz. regionibz.

PLATE 14

PARSLEY (*Petrosillum*).

The text reads: '*Parsley. complexion: hot and dry in the second degree. Better from a domestic garden.
Helpful in provoking urine and menstruation and in opening obstructions. Harmful in that excessive use
produces a migraine, because it gives rise to hot blood. Take with vinegar to remove its harm to the
disposition. Agreeable to the cold and moist, to the elderly, in winter and in all regions.*'

From the **Tacuinum Sanitatis in medicina.**

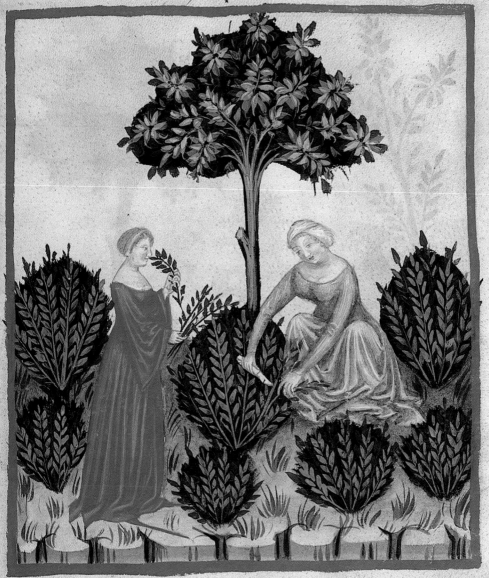

Ysop̄. ca. 7 sic. iii̅. Aecc̄ rices 7 oztulaninn. 7 domestic̄ unam̅. 9 fert pectou̅.hu̅. 7 tuffi.
nocunitu̅ ledit cerebz̄ sua fumositate. Remo̅ nocti cu̅ pendys 7 zuchaio. Quod gn̅at
humores acutos. Conuenut̅ fit̅. 7 hii. na̅ scib̅z 7 decrepitis hyeme. 7 frigis regioib̅z.

PLATE 15

HYSSOP (*Ysopus*).

The text reads: '*Hyssop. complexion: hot and dry in the third degree. The fresh plant from a domestic
garden is better. Helpful in comforting a moist chest and a cough. Harmful to the brain by its vapours,
because it breeds sharp humours. Take with barley sugar and sugar to remove its harm. Agreeable to
those of a cold and moist nature, to the elderly and decrepit, in winter and in cold regions.*'
From the **Tacuinum Sanitatis in medicina**.

· Spinachie ·

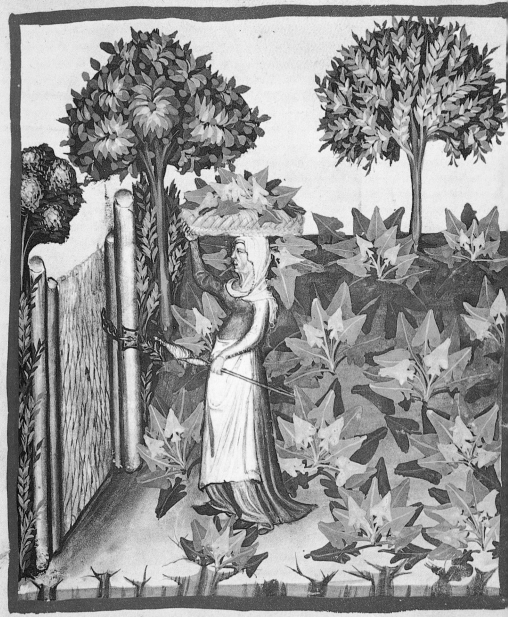

Spinachia. ꝯp̄o. fri. ꝛbu. inp̄. al̄. tp̄ate. Acetō ifuse pluuia. uuanituꝛ. ꝯferuit tu ꝛp̄ctori. noccumtum. corrumpit digōneꝛ. Remo nocuniti suffrissi cum miii aut a ceto ꝛ aromatibꝛ. Quo gn̄ant nutrimitum mediciꝛꝗuenuit calis uuuenibꝛ omni tp̄: omni regior.

PLATE 16

SPINACH (*Spinache*).

The text reads: '*Spinach. complexion: cold and moist in the first degree, others temperate. Those infused in rain water are better. Helpful for the chest and a cough. Harmful in corrupting the digestion, because they give little nourishment. Suffused with honey or with vinegar and aromatic things removes its harm. Agreeable to hot youths, every season and every region.*'
From the **Tacuinum Sanitatis in medicina.**

person, animal or thing which they met, and proceeded to deduce omens from what he saw. He told the *Ashipu* what the omens portended and this man began to recite the incantations which he thought would avert evil from the sick man.' When the three arrived at the house of the sick man, the *Asu* carefully examined the patient. 'Meanwhile the *Baru* continued to deduce omens from the state of the various members of the patient's body, whether his head was hot, or cold, or moist, whether there was foam on his lips, whether he was lying on his right or left side, or on his back' and so on. Once the *Asu* had made his diagnosis and had decided which herbal medicines were to be employed, these were administered. All the while the *Ashipu* had been reciting the appropriate incantations to drive out the evil spirits which these peoples believed was the cause of the disease. 'Thus medicine and magic went hand in hand,' Budge concludes.

Rational Greek medicine put an end to belief in evil spirits as the harbingers of disease. In the Greek community the equivalent of the *Asu* or physician sought out the natural causes of his patient's illness. The work of the *Baru* or seer became divination by astrology, regarding which subject in general I refer the reader to the works of my colleagues.[31] The *Ashipu* was still the magician among the Greeks but, with the advent of Christianity, the incantations or words of power were subsumed under the benedictions, prayers and spiritual healing that were delivered by Churchmen.

Culpeper put into the English language a large part of the teachings of medical astrology as they existed in his day. He wrote nothing on natal horoscopes or horary astrology (the art of judging questions) and only a short work on general astrological elections, the *Opus Astrologicum*, published posthumously. In this respect he was an innovator, seen 'to exemplify the Renaissance insight that practical application is as dignified as theorizing'.[32]

As to the substance of his main work on astrological medicine, the *Semeiotica Uranica* (1651), it follows the layout and largely the content of the principal astrological work of Noel Duret, 'cosmographer to the King of France and the most excellent Cardinal the Duke of Richelieu. 'Tis confessed, in some places I have abbreviated him, in others corrected him. Let another do the like by me.'[33] It is in these corrections that Culpeper inserts the benefits of his own understanding and experience of the practice of medical astrology and enlivens the standard text of medical astrology.

The Astrology of the Human Body

A key component of the application of astrology to medicine depends on the assignation of the planets and signs of the zodiac to the parts of the human body. Culpeper's correlations are as follows:

TABLE OF PARTS OF THE BODY RULED BY THE PLANETS AND SIGNIFICATIONS OF THE PRINCIPLES OF WESTERN HOLISTIC MEDICINE BY THE 7 PLANETS

PLANET	CORRESPONDING PARTS OF THE BODY	QUALITIES	ASSOCIATED HUMOUR	KEY SIGNIFICANT
Saturn	the spleen, bones, teeth, right ear	cold & dry	melancholy	the melancholic humour, spleen & retentive virtue
Jupiter	the lungs, liver, ribs, sides, veins	hot & moist	blood	natural faculty & spirit, digestive virtue
Mars	the gall bladder, left ear	hot & dry	choler	the choleric humour, gall bladder, attractive virtue
Venus	the sexual organs, kidneys, throat, breasts	cold & moist	phlegm	the genito-urinary system, expulsive virtue
Mercury	the brain, 'especially the rational part of it', the tongue, hands, feet, loco-motive power	cold & dry	melancholy	the animal faculty & spirit, the mind
Sun	the heart & arteries the sight & eyes, the right eye of a man, the left eye of a woman	hot & dry	choler	pneuma, innate heat, vital faculty & spirit
Moon	the bulk of the brain, stomach, bowels, bladder, the left eye of a man, the right eye of a woman	cold & moist	phlegm	radical moisture, the humours taken together

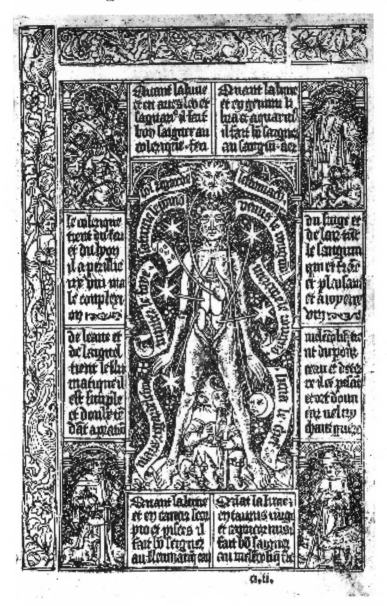

Figure 9 An illustration from Astrological Man from Horai beatissimae
Mariae Virginis, *Paris 1497, showing in the centre the planetary rulership of
the main organs of the body and, in the corners, depictions of the four
temperaments; clockwise from left are the choleric, sanguine, melancholic and
phlegmatic. These are described in the text on each side while above and below are
recommendations about when to bleed each temperament according to the zodiac
sign occupied by the Moon.*

It would seem that Culpeper attributes to the Moon the sensory side of brain and nerve function as well as the activity of the brain in controlling the functions of growth and homeostasis which operate unconsciously. The motor side of nerve function is then governed by Mercury. The Sun claims some rulership over the brain, perhaps particularly in consideration of the spiritual mind (the highest aspects of the rational soul, capable of a knowledge of the oneness of the universe and of God). The physical sight is ruled over by the 'lights', that is, the Sun and Moon together.

TABLE OF ZODIACAL MELOTHESIS, ASSOCIATING THE 12 ZODIAC SIGNS WITH PARTS OF THE BODY FROM HEAD TO FEET[34]

ZODIAC SIGN	CORRESPONDING PARTS OF THE BODY
Aries	the head and everything above the first vertebra of the neck
Taurus	the neck, throat, voice and the seven vertebrae of the neck
Gemini	the shoulders, shoulder bones, arms, hands and fingers
Cancer	the breast, ribs, lungs, pleura, stomach, liver, women's breasts
Leo	the heart and pericardium, back, thoracic vertebrae; the stomach, sides and midriff with Virgo
Virgo	the belly, bowels, navel, spleen, omentum, stomach, sides and midriff
Libra	the kidneys; bladder and buttocks with Scorpio
Scorpio	the sexual organs, bladder, anus and buttocks
Sagittarius	the hips, coccyx and thigh bones
Capricorn	the knees and hamstrings
Aquarius	the legs, tibiae and fibulae
Pisces	the feet, ankles and toes

The 12 signs neatly fall into 4 groups of 3, called triplicities, having correlations with the 4 elements and 4 humours. Thus the Fire signs Aries, Leo and Sagittarius correspond with choler and strong heat in the body; the Earth signs Taurus, Virgo and Capricorn are melancholic and denote the body's solid structure; the Air signs Gemini, Libra and Aquarius signify blood; the water signs Cancer, Scorpio and Pisces are for phlegm and evacuations.

When a horoscope is cast for a particular date and time the zodiac circle, divided into 12 signs each of 30 degrees through which the planets move, is mapped onto the local horizon and meridian of the astrologer. The astrologer has in effect calculated what part of the zodiac circle is rising in the East at that place at the given date and time. The local sky, already divided into quadrants by the horizon and meridian lines, is further subdivided into 12 sections in all, giving six above the horizon, six below, rather like the segments of an orange. Each section is called a 'house' and numbered 1–12 in an anti-clockwise direction from the Eastern horizon. Thus the cusp or starting point of the 1st house, measured as a degree of the zodiac sign on the Eastern horizon, is the *Ascendant* of the horoscope, so called because the whole sky, the zodiac signs and the planets all rise up over the local horizon from this Easterly direction. The cusps of the other 11 houses are shown in a horoscope with their points of intersection with the zodiac wheel, each cusp falling commonly but not always in a different zodiac sign, depending on the method of division of the local sky into 12 houses.

For the purposes of interpretation in medical astrology, the 1st house of the horoscope was associated schematically with the first zodiac sign Aries, the 2nd house with Taurus, and so on. Thus, for example, a planet falling in the horoscope in the 7th house or occupying the 7th zodiac sign Libra can signify a certain condition of the kidneys, depending on the nature of the planet involved and, if in the 7th house, the zodiac sign it occupies.[35]

The cusps of the 1st, 4th, 7th and 10th houses, corresponding to the horizon and meridian lines of the local sky, are called the *angles* of the horoscope and represent important places for planets to occupy. The angles were a particular feature of Greek astrology. In commercial questions, for example, they signified buyer and seller, the commodity and the likely price, and the astrologer Dorotheos of Sidon (1st century AD) used them to describe the nature, qualities and strength of the patient in his current condition, the disease afflicting him, the nature and potential of the astrologer-physician working to heal him and the kind of treatment likely to effect this.[36]

Planets in these angles, or ruling the zodiac signs in which these points fell, were used to describe the nature, qualities and strength of each of these four factors. Sixteen centuries later, astrological significations had become more complex. Culpeper made the following attributions.[37]

1st house and its ruler or 'lord' (the planet ruling the sign on the cusp of the house) represents the patient, his life and health.

6th house and its ruler signifies the sickness. (The 7th and 12th houses may also be considered in this regard, the former because it opposes the 1st house, the latter because, like the 6th, it is an unfortunate house of suffering.)

7th house and its ruler denotes the astrologer-physician.

8th house and its ruler signifies death.

10th house and its ruler, if 'strong' in essential and accidental dignities, symbolizes the required treatment.

4th house depicts the manner in which the treatment will end and may provide a single testimony to the likely outcome of the disease.

Once these significators have been identified in the horoscope, the angular relationships in the zodiac, or 'aspects', of the planets must then be considered. The aspects particularly symbolic of disease situations are the conjunction (0°), square (90°) or opposition (180°). These are best imagined in relation to the lunar phases. When the Sun and Moon are conjunct they are in the same place in the sky (this is when a *new Moon* occurs); when the Sun sets, the Moon sets and there is no Moon to be seen in the sky that night. If the Sun and Moon are in opposition they are in opposite signs of the zodiac (this is when a *full Moon* occurs); the Moon in the East rises as the Sun sets in the opposite place in the West and is visible all night. If the Sun is in square aspect to the Moon it is in a right-angle or 90-degree aspect to the Moon. (This is a quarter of the Moon. The *first quarter* occurs midway between new and full Moon during the Moon's *waxing* phase. She will be half illuminated and in a right-angle or 90-degree aspect with the Sun, to the South as the Sun sets in the West at dusk. She remains visible for half the night. The *last quarter* occurs between full and new Moon during her *waning* phase, when her other half will be illuminated, visible after midnight and in the South before dawn.) The lunar phases (both waxing and waning) which occur approximately every seven days were always held to be evil days in ancient Babylon, the birthplace of astrology, and, as we shall see, were adapted by medical astrologers to denote times of crisis in a disease process. The Moon also formed favourable trine and sextile aspects with the Sun when they were 120 and 60 degrees apart respectively.

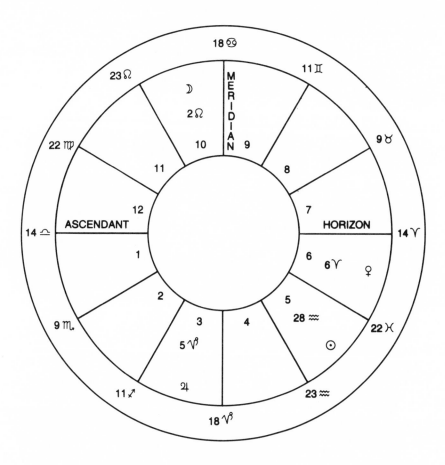

Figure 10 In the horoscope above, an only partially completed decumbiture, 14 degrees of Libra rises in the East. This is the Ascendant or cusp of the 1st house. The whole sky is divided here into 12 houses by the Placidus method. The 1st house contains within it the remaining 16 degrees of the zodiac sign Libra (degrees 14–30) and the first 9 degrees of the following sign Scorpio.

The places where the other house cusps intersect the zodiac are each marked by a degree of the relevant zodiac sign. Venus is passing through the 6th degrees of Aries in the zodiac, a weak place for her because she rules the sign opposite to it, and is thus found to fall in the 6th house of disease. Because Venus rules Libra, the sign on the Ascendant, she signifies the patient, and her weak placing by sign in the house of disease would be very pertinent to a disease situation. Venus in Aries in the 6th house could generally signify heat (Aries) in a part of the genito-urinary system (Venus) or a cold and moist state (Venus) of the head (Aries) or bowel (6th house & Virgo). Venus is in square aspect to, and thus afflicted by Jupiter, who rules Pisces on the cusp of the 6th house and is therefore a significator of disease. His weak placing in Capricorn only makes his potential to symbolize disease the greater. The Moon in Leo in the 10th house of medicine is in a beneficial trine aspect with Venus and may symbolize the nature of the treatment that will lead to recovery.

Table of Rulerships and Places of Strength and Weakness of the Planets

PLANET	SYMBOL	SIGNS RULED	ELEMENT RULED	METAL RULED	STRONGLY PLACED IN	WEAKLY PLACED IN
Sun	☉	Leo ♌	Fire	Gold	Aries Libra	Aquarius &
Moon	☽	Cancer ♋	Earth	Silver	Taurus	Capricorn & Scorpio
Mercury	☿	Gemini ♊ & Virgo ♍	Air	Quick-silver	Virgo	Sagittarius & Pisces
Venus	♀	Taurus ♉ & Libra ♎	Earth	Copper	Pisces	Aries, Virgo & Scorpio
Mars	♂	Aries ♈ & Scorpio ♏	Water	Iron	Capricorn	Taurus, Cancer & Libra
Jupiter	♃	Pisces ♓ & Sagittarius ♐	Fire	Tin	Cancer	Gemini, Virgo & Capricorn
Saturn	♄	Capricorn ♑ & Aquarius ♒	Air	Lead	Libra	Aries, Cancer & Leo

Diagnosis: the Nature, Origin and Location of Disease

All indications from the decumbiture horoscope would be considered in the iatromathematical task of answering important questions for a patient and his physician concerning the disease. Is the patient ill? If so, what has caused it and how did he/she come to fall ill? Which parts of the body are affected? Is the root of the disease in the mind or body? How serious is the condition? Will the illness be long or short? Will it end in life or death? What is the best treatment for the condition? What kind of person is most likely to be able to effect this? When should the treatment or treatments be given?

The first question which must be asked is whether the patient is truly ill. Culpeper seems not to deal with this question, presumably because either the sufferings of his poor, sick patients are clearly manifest or his knowledge of medicine rather than astrology provides him with the answer. It is as if neither he nor his patients have time in their earnestness for such a question. However Lilly, writing as a 'student of astrology' but not yet 'of physick', does consider the question. He looks to see whether the planet signifying the patient is 'out of sorts' either because it is in a sign contrary to its own nature or because either that planet or the Moon is afflicted by the conjunction, square or opposition of Saturn, Mars or the ruler of the 6th house of disease. If such signs are absent and the beneficent aspects or position of Jupiter or Venus are present, Lilly judges that the inquirer is not ill but that 'their mistrust of a sickness was grounded upon some sudden distemper of body, which would presently be rectified'.[38]

Once the presence of disease was established, the horoscopic factors to be considered in trying to discover the nature of the disease were the houses 'of which the sixth, seventh and twelfth signify diseases', the planets and their aspects and 'the nature of the signs, of which fiery signs signify choler and diseases thence proceeding; earthly signs signify the diseases of melancholy; airy signs the diseases of blood and wind; watery signs diseases of watery and salt phlegm'.[39]

The condition of the Moon is central to the astrological judgement of diseases, not least because it signifies the body, as the Sun denotes the spirits or breath (pneuma). If the Moon is afflicted in a certain sign of the zodiac in the decumbiture horoscope, it may be taken as a sign that the corrupted humour, lesion or weakness resides in that part of the body which corresponds to that zodiac sign. Particular attention is paid to the planet from which the Moon separates (or departs) by aspect, and Culpeper stipulates further:

> That place and state of the planet from which the Moon is separated at the decumbiture, and the condition [of] the planet also ... is to be heeded. If you please to observe the state of that same planet, by it you may know the state of the sick, and what the cause of his sickness is.[40]

If either Saturn or Mercury is the afflicting planet (they being reckoned to be cold and dry in quality and effect), the corrupted humour or imbalance will be of melancholy. If either Mars or the Sun (which are hot and dry) afflicts the Moon, expect a disease of choler. Venus and Jupiter, the remaining planets of the traditional seven, were considered benefic, their antagonistic configurations with the Moon therefore much less serious. It is more a case of having too much of a good thing when these planets are significators of disease. Venus was seen to represent harm from too much sex or food (venery and gluttony), and Jupiter excess blood in the body and plethoric conditions in general. We have already seen how excessive sex was thought to deplete the vitality and innate heat and how eating too large a quantity of food resulted in crude, undigested humours entering the body. Both factors caused an increase of phlegm.

The position of the Moon in the decumbiture chart also provides a major point for comparison with the natal horoscope of the patient. Culpeper writes:

> If the Moon be in the place of Saturn or Mars in the nativity, the disease is dangerous; not so if she be in the place where Jupiter or Venus was in them. Or it's possible Jupiter or Venus may hurt in the nativities of such to whose ascendants they are inimical or posited in the sixth or eighth houses.

The patient's natal horoscope could also be used for other purposes, in particular in the assessment of the temperament of the sick person and the calculation of whether the present illness is occurring during a period of life when the vitality is diminished and death is threatened. Culpeper's opinion was that if the astrologer has the natal chart of the patient to compare with the decumbiture and to provide such additional information, 'you shall nor err' in judgement.[42]

In the decumbiture chart, Culpeper groups the Sun, Moon and Ascendant as general significators of disease while the ruler of the Ascendant, the 6th house and its ruler, and planets in the Ascendant or 6th house are the particular indicators. Saturn and Mars also are specific indicators, 'for they naturally hurt the body, whatsoever the matter is'. The combination of a general and a specific significator thus indicates the nature of the disease:

> The sixth house and its lord, and the planets in it, if there be any there, best describe the nature of the disease usually, nay always, if they afflict either of the luminaries [Sun and Moon], or the Lord of the Ascendant.[43]

The Sun, Moon and Lord of the Ascendant should thus be looked on as significators of disease depending on how they are afflicted by other planets. In addition Culpeper points out, 'the Sun is most principally to be looked upon in chronic diseases, the Moon in acute'. This is a reference to the calculation of the critical days in the course of a disease, since the definition of an acute disease, according to Culpeper, is one which is resolved within a lunar month of around 28 days. Otherwise it becomes a chronic condition. Almost all the afflictions of the Moon in Culpeper's version of the *Iatromathematica of Hermes Trismegistos* denote disease conditions which will end in health or death within the lunar month. In regard, then, to chronic diseases, it is worth observing that they often continue because the body is unable to mount a sufficiently vital response to shake off disease once and for all. Since the Sun symbolizes this vital response, its condition in the horoscope may symbolize a reason why the disease grumbles on.

These then are the significators for disease as indicated in the decumbiture chart and the qualities of the afflicting planet denote the nature of the disease. In addition the associations of the planets and zodiac signs were generally made with elemental and humoral imbalances, but their association with specific disease-states was also studied. In the *Iatromathematica* of the Greeks, particular regard was paid to Egyptian lore in relation to the *decans* or ten-degree divisions of the 12 zodiac signs. This lore, older than the casting of horoscopes in Egypt, taught that each of the 36 decans was related to a particular kind of disease, the evil spirit which caused it, a medicinal plant and so on. In all times since, down to the present day, astrologers have made correlations between the planets, planetary configurations, zodiac signs and specific diseases. Culpeper gives the following associations of the seven traditional planets with specific diseases.

ASSOCIATIONS OF THE PLANETS WITH DISEASES

Sun
The Sun, he said, causes 'all diseases of the heart and brain and their attendants, viz the nerves and arteries', heartburn and sore eyes by virtue of its rulership of those parts. Infection with fever and trembling or fainting brought on by a dispersal of the vital spirits are also caused by the Sun's heat.

Moon
The Moon causes all cold and rheumatic diseases, cramps, colic and belly-ache, 'all coagulate and crude humours in any part of

the body', discharges, coughs from chest infections, abscesses, fluid retention, excesses of food and drink and 'all diseases of phlegm', by virtue of her cold and moist qualities or by her general signification of humours, fluids and discharges. She denotes convulsions, epilepsy, palsies and lethargies on account of phlegm obstructing the animal spirits. Her rulership of absent and excessive menstruation and 'all diseases that return often' implies her cyclical nature, and eye problems because she rules those organs. Sciatica, smallpox, measles and tuberculosis are also given.

Saturn
Under Saturn are 'all diseases which come of melancholy, cold and dryness ... all madness that comes of melancholy, fear or grief', and all long diseases. He signifies pain in the bones, broken bones and dislocations, gout, toothache, deafness and leprosy, because he rules the parts affected. His obstructive and corrupting nature brings 'black jaundice', palsies, impotence, hernias, volvulus, whooping cough, pains in the bladder and haemorrhoids. Consumption produces a typically dry and withered state.

Jupiter
To Jupiter is given 'all infirmities of the liver and veins, inflammation of the lungs, pleurisies and empyema', because of his rulership of those parts, also quinsies and fevers.

Mars
Diseases under Mars are 'all diseases coming of choler, anger or passion', burning fevers, burning, scalding, 'all hurts by iron or fire', all wounds, including 'scars and pock-holes in the face', carbuncles, plague-sores, shingles, ringworm and blisters. The brain is affected antipathetically, causing 'frenzy, fury, sudden distempers in the head coming of heat' and migraine. The genito-urinary system is likewise affected, with diseases of the sex organs, dysuria and strangury, kidney and bladder stones and fistulae. The 'yellow jaundice' and haemorrhages are caused by Mars according to the colours manifesting. Plagues and epidemic infections, ergot poisoning and erysipelas are given also.

Venus

Under Venus are all genito-urinary diseases, such as kidney infections, diabetes insipidus and syphilis and 'all diseases coming by inordinate love of lust', because she rules these things.

Mercury

Under Mercury are 'almost all diseases of the brain, as vertigo, madness &c ... all imperfections of the tongue, as stammering, lisping, &c ... snuffling in the nose ... stopping of the head, dumbness, folly and simplicity – the epidemical diseases of the time – and whatsoever hurts the intellectual faculty'. Because of Mercury's antipathy to the respiratory system he signifies 'all diseases of the lungs, as asthma, phthisis, &c', hoarseness and coughs.

Today astrologers are aware of the existence of three other planets in the solar system, Uranus, Neptune and Pluto, which were unknown to Culpeper. These clearly must have some correspondence with the nature of health and disease in the modern world and the knowledge and approach of modern medicine to treat illness. However, these trans-Saturnian planets have been studied by astrologers for much less time than the seven traditional ones and a complete knowledge of their significations is lacking. In my practice, though, I have found Uranus to signify allergy and, with the Sun, problems of electro-conductivity of the heart; Neptune to symbolize generalized weakness and certain hereditary tendencies; and Pluto to represent heart pacemakers, the effects of antibiotics and, with Venus, the contraceptive pill.

The location of a disease will be determined from the sign and house positions of the significators, namely the Ascendant, the Sun or Moon or the ruler of the 6th house or planets in the Ascendant or 6th house.[44] Afflictions to the Ascendant in particular may indicate that the patient is 'troubled in mind'. Culpeper's observations on such a state are tabulated below.[45]

It is apparent that the observations are derived from the general significations which are attributed to each of the planets. In a similar way, as Culpeper makes clear in the horoscope judgement in Appendix 2, it is readily possible to explore with the patient the wider signification of the planets, signs and houses identified as signatures of the disease, with a view to ascertaining

TABLE OF AFFLICTIONS TO THE ASCENDANT

PLANET	STATE OF MIND
Saturn	melancholy, depression, alienation, madness, worry, grief, jealousy, fear, whenever he is 'significator of the disease or in the ascendant or in the sixth house afflicting the lord of the ascendant or either of the luminaries'
Jupiter	'never troubles the mind unless it be that monster which men call religion'
Sun	pride, ambition, vain-glory, when lord of the ascendant, sixth or twelfth house
Venus	love, luxurious expense or something similar
Mercury	strange imaginings and unsupported fears caused by great vexation or long study
Mars	anger, contention, violent passion, etc
Moon	worry, fear, drunkenness

more details of the origin of the complaint. For instance, if Saturn in the Ascendant symbolizes the disease and is ruler of the 3rd house of siblings, some grief or care over a brother or sister may have provoked disease. If Mars is the significator of the problem and is in the 7th house of marriage, the patient may have suffered mental or physical cruelty at the hands of his or her partner. The more fitting the astrological symbolism appears to the context in which it arises, the more certain is the basis of the horoscope on which to extend the judgement to prognosis and treatment.

Prognosis: the Likely Course and Outcome of a Disease

The first question to be answered in iatromathematical prognosis was: will the patient live or die as a result of the present illness? This is apparent in the *Iatromathematica of Hermes Trismegistos*, which dealt with serious acute illness, and in Culpeper's *Semeiotica Uranica*, which gives over 60 aphorisms on the signs of life and death in the decumbiture.[46] However, in *Health for the Rich and Poor, by Diet, without Physick*, Culpeper explicitly rejects the notion of a fixed span of life according to the *anareta* (the planet or place that destroys life) in the natal horoscope:

As for the influences of the planets and their *anareta*, they may go shake their ears. This life is something above their influence, for their influence is only upon the sensual part of man, but this life is rational and far above the pitch of sensuality. We might clear this a little further thus: we all know that there is a starry part within our bodies, as well as without, which, mixing evil influence with that without, causeth diseases. So that if the internal, celestial part were kept pure, there could be no more mixture with any external [as far as it relates to us] evil influence, than is between oil and water.[47]

Marsilio Ficino had said the same in his time. He wrote:

Your lucky stars have decreed for you a life among mortals which is prosperous and fairly long [insofar as I have been able to infer from certain indications]. Without a doubt, your own careful attention and the care of doctors and astrologers can so arrange things that the stars both give faithfully what they promise and even extend it further with a fuller increase. All the learned astrologers and doctors now testify that this can be done by science and common sense.[48]

Thus in no way do the stars announce an inevitable death. In the same way in which preventive medicine, be it hygiene, diet or the avoidance of oppressive physical and mental conditions, can contribute to a long and healthy life, so the whole point of the iatromathematical task is to discover the nature of the illness so that, with the appropriate medical intervention in each specific case, death or continued ill-health can be avoided and the patient restored to well-being. Sometimes, of course, the life of the patient cannot be saved in spite of the treatment received. This was of course much more common in the 17th century but the same concern to ease the sufferings of the dying was shown. Culpeper's amanuensis wrote of him that

As he was an apothecary formerly himself, so he discerned the errors of apothecaries, and was therefore an apothecary to himself and others. He used not to handsel [inaugurate] his experiments, letting loose as some do their mad receipts into sick men's bodies, to try how well nature can fight against them, as one writes, whilst they stand by and see the battle, except it were in desperate cases, when death must be expelled. And when he could keep life no longer, he made an easy passage for it to go out [as his book of the Astrological Judgment of Diseases, where he unites astrology to physick, as they concern the decumbiture of the sick, doth sufficiently discover to the world].[49]

Culpeper wrote his books to give others a full explanation of how to go about treating diseases of all kinds, those which were acute

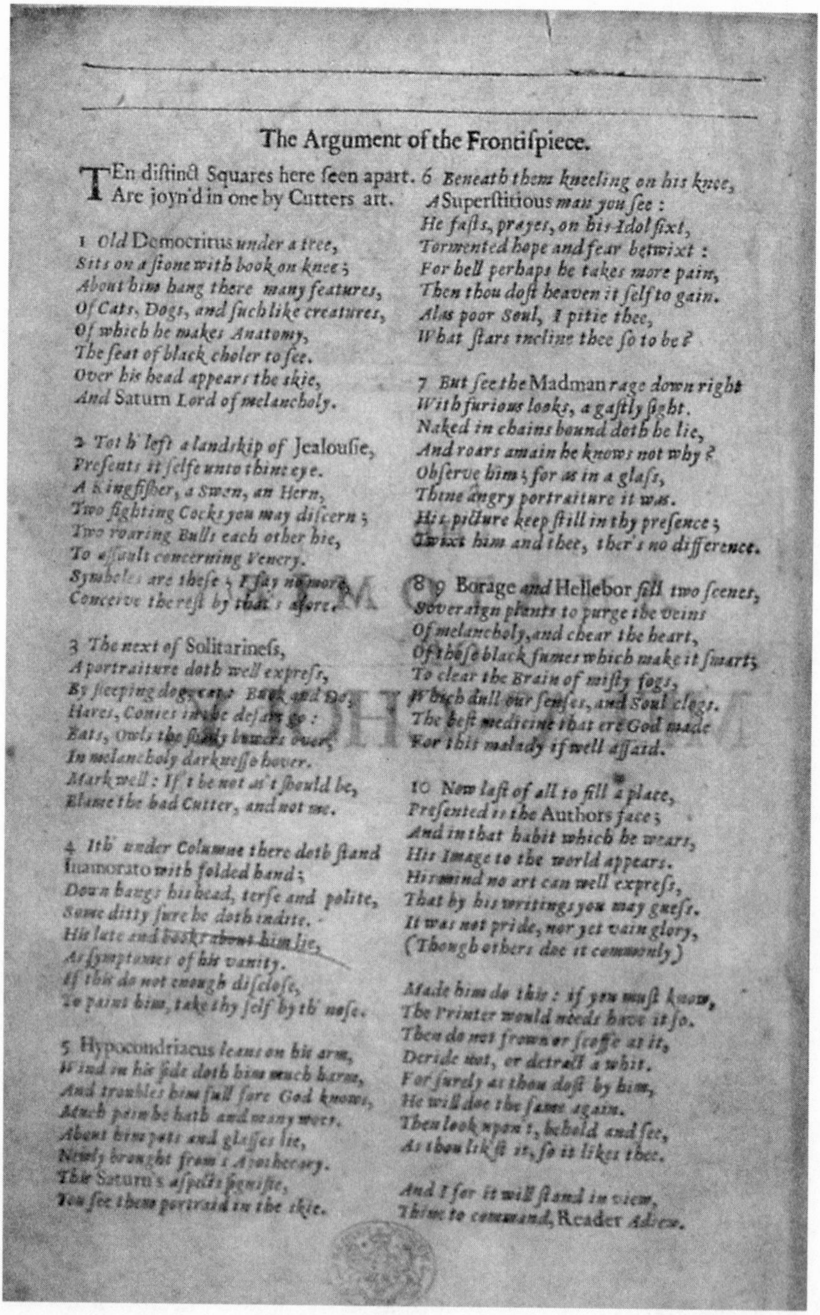

The Argument of the Frontiſpiece.

TEn diſtinct Squares here ſeen apart.
Are joyn'd in one by Cutters art.

1 Old Democritus *under a tree*,
Sits on a ſtone with book on knee;
About him hang there many features,
Of Cats, Dogs, and ſuchlike creatures,
Of which he makes Anatomy,
The ſeat of black choler to ſee.
Over his head appears the skie,
And Saturn Lord of melancholy.

2 To th' left a landskip of Jealouſie,
Preſents it ſelfe unto thine eye.
A kingfiſher, a Swan, an Hern,
Two fighting Cocks you may diſcern;
Two roaring Bulls each other hie,
To aſſault concerning Venery.
Symboles are theſe; I ſay no more,
Conceive the reſt by that's afore.

3 The next of Solitarineſs,
A portraiture doth well expreſs,
By ſleeping dog, cat: Buck and Doe,
Hares, Conies in the deſart goe:
Bats, Owls the ſhady bowers over,
In melancholy darkneſſe hover.
Mark well: If't be not as't ſhould be,
Blame the bad Cutter, and not me.

4 I'th under Columne there doth ſtand
Inamorato with folded hand;
Down hangs his head, terſe and polite,
Some ditty ſure he doth indite.
His late and baskit about him lie,
As ſymptomes of his vanity.
If this do not enough diſcloſe,
To paint him, take thy ſelf by th' noſe.

5 Hypocondriacus leans on his arm,
Wind in his ſide doth him much harm,
And troubles him full ſore God knows,
Much pain he hath and many woes.
About him pots and glaſſes lie,
Newly brought from's Apothecary.
This Saturn's aſpects ſignifie,
You ſee them pourtraid in the skie.

6 Beneath them kneeling on his knee,
A Superſtitious man you ſee:
He faſts, prayes, on his Idol fixt,
Tormented hope and fear betwixt:
For hell perhaps he takes more pain,
Then thou doſt heaven it ſelf to gain.
Alas poor Soul, I pitie thee,
What ſtars incline thee ſo to be?

7 But ſee the Madman rage down right
With furious looks, a gaſtly ſight.
Naked in chains bound doth he lie,
And roars amain he knows not why?
Obſerve him; for as in a glaſs,
Thine angry portraiture it was.
His picture keep ſtill in thy preſence;
Twixt him and thee, ther's no difference.

8 9 Borage and Hellebor fill two ſcenes,
Soveraign plants to purge the veins
Of melancholy, and chear the heart,
Of thoſe black fumes which make it ſmart;
To clear the Brain of miſty fogs,
Which dull our ſenſes, and Soul clogs.
The beſt medicine that ere God made
For this malady if well aſſaid.

10 Now laſt of all to fill a place,
Preſented is the Authors face;
And in that habit which he wears,
His Image to the world appears.
His mind no art can well expreſs,
That by his writings you may gueſs.
It was not pride, nor yet vain glory,
(Though others doe it commonly)

Made him do this: if you muſt know,
The Printer would needs have it ſo.
Then do not frown or ſcoffe at it,
Deride not, or detract a whit,
For ſurely as thou doſt by him,
He will doe the ſame again.
Then look upon't, behold and ſee,
As thou lik'ſt it, ſo it likes thee.

And I for it will ſtand in view,
Thine to command, Reader Adieu.

Figure 11 Title page and frontispiece of Robert Burton's Anatomy of Melancholy *(1628), depicting various states of melancholia, their astrological signatures and the key herbs used to treat them.*

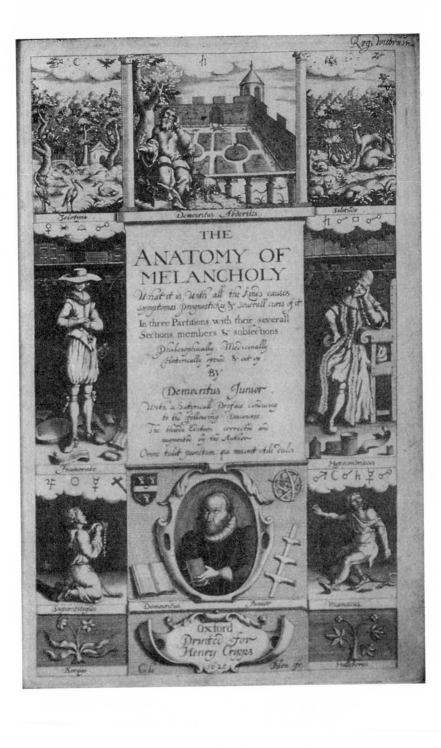

and potentially fatal as much as those which were chronic but not life-threatening. For the poor could not afford medical attention in either event. Nor could serious illness be left to an astrological judgement alone. So, in the final sections of the *Semeiotica Uranica* Culpeper reproduced three books of Hippocratic prognostics, the *Presages of life and death, by the body of the patient being sick*. The reader was to look for these physical signs of impending life or death in a sick person as well as the astrological signs in the decumbiture chart. In such grave matters, Culpeper's first aphorism on the 'signs of death' was certainly to be taken to heart: 'first of all the lord of the Ascendant afflicted in the 8th: the patient is more mad to be *apud inferos* [among the dead], than death is to have him. The man will die and his life will be cast away absolutely *with evil guidance.*'

A judgement on the likelihood of the illness ending in health or death was thus carefully made from the physical and astrological signs in patient and horoscope, and at critical moments in the course of the disease. The moments when there appear signs of worsening or improvement in the patient's condition, 'whereby the sick is either brought to recovery or death', are called *crises* meaning 'outcome', 'decision' or 'judgement'.

> The cause of the crisis is twofold: inward, outward. The internal cause is taken from its own proper principle, if you will believe Hippocrates, and that is double or twofold. For either nature labours to expel the humour that causeth the disease, or else the humour itself being drawn to a place, and not fit for excretion, by its own weight or quality burdens nature and so breaks out ... Nature, if she be strong, is a good physician for all diseases and separates that which is good from that which is bad, and having done so, prepares that which breed annoyances for excretion and at last makes a shift to cast it out. The external cause of the crisis is caused by an alteration of the air, whence ariseth an alteration of the breath a man draws in, from cold to heat, from dry to moist, or the contraries to them both.[50]

Culpeper adds to this an opinion of Hippocrates that sometimes ill diet replaces air as a cause of a crisis. Next, he identifies two kinds of crises: those in acute diseases, which are to be judged from the Moon and her configurations with other planets at the time of the crisis, and those in chronic diseases, which are judged from the Sun. The question of the expected time and nature of a crisis in a given disease is very complex.[51] Generally, however, there is agreement in the medical-astrological tradition that 'the particular influence of the Moon – whether it is for the good or for the bad – is concluded to be stronger in seven-day periods.'[52] This is because in seven days the Moon traverses roughly a quarter of the zodiac so that she is in 'square aspect', 90 degrees or three whole signs from where she started. This means that she now falls in an element different from that of the sign position she occupied in the decumbiture and this alteration in her qualities denotes the first lunar crisis in the course of the disease. The second lunar crisis, if the patient still languishes with an illness, is when the Moon is exactly 180 degrees from her position in the decumbiture, around 14 days later. The third, when she has traversed 270 degrees of the zodiac, after about 21 days, and the fourth crisis when she returns to the position she occupied in the decumbiture chart. After this, if the disease still persists, it is regarded as chronic and the crises will be judged from the motion of the Sun in roughly 90-day periods. The Sun will be in square to its position in the decumbiture after approximately 90 days and this constitutes the first solar crisis, and so on.

The astrological method of judging crises is added to by consideration of the Moon or Sun at two other positions in their courses which are termed the *judicial and intercidental days*. The former occur when the position of the Moon or Sun is advanced 30, 120, 210 and 300 degrees from their places in the decumbiture. The latter, as its name suggests, lies between the positions on the judicial and crisis days, namely at 60, 150, 240 and 330 degrees from the decumbiture position. Culpeper defines them as follows:

Of days, some are called by their own nature, *critical days*. Others are called *judicial days* and they are so called because upon them dame nature and her son Dr Reason would make manifest what the disease is, and Dr Experience tells me 'tis true. Another time is called *intercidental*, which is a time [which] falls out between the judicial days and the critical. Upon these intercidental days the disease is usually remitted. If so, then a good crisis may be expected; if not, an evil. I shall explain these terms before I go further. A man falls sick, there is the first crisis [the decumbiture], let the cause of the disease be what you will. When the Moon comes to the same degree of the next sign she was in at the decumbiture, there is the judicial day. For in that time the disease shows itself in its colours, with bag and baggage. When the Moon comes to her sextile, it brings the intercidental day, and should mitigate the disease. If she do not, she is aspected to evil planets, and if she be aspected to ill planets, an ill crisis is to be expected, and so the contrary.[53]

Thus the astrological consideration at each of these times concerns the aspects of the Moon, as Culpeper makes clear:

> Your fastest way then to judge of the disease is by the aspects of the Moon to the planets. When the Moon meets with the inimical or hostile beams of Saturn or Mars, have a care of your patient. And if you know what hinders, by the same reason you may know what helps.[54]

At the crises the condition of the Moon or Sun is to be noted, for 'if on a critical day she behold a good star, there is no question of recovery to be made', whilst 'if she be afflicted on the critical day, a good crisis cannot be expected: sickness keeps his old house, unless death dispossess him'.

Other factors to be assessed from the decumbiture chart which have a bearing on prognosis are the strength of the illness and whether it is likely to be long or short in duration. The strength of the illness naturally has a bearing on its duration and is signified in several ways. Culpeper advises the astrologer to 'consider if the Sun, Moon, Ascendant and their lords be much or little afflicted'[55] for the greater the affliction, the more severe and protracted is the disease. On the other hand, if the planet signifying the patient is stronger in the horoscope than that representing the disease, nature will soon pull through. 'Never forget this general rule,' adds Culpeper later, 'the stronger the Moon is at the decumbiture, the better it is for the sick; the weaker she is at that time, the worse,' for the Moon signifies nature. Then, 'consider the age of the sick party, for old age brings longer sicknesses than youth', and also 'the time of year, for Autumn and Winter bring longer sicknesses than Spring and Summer'. Next, 'consider the complexion of the patient, for a melancholy man is more subject to retain a sickness than a choleric'. Note also that it is only a small step from his normal *eucrasia* or healthy temperament for a choleric man in his thirties to fall ill in Summer with a hot disease. More serious would be a similar 'distemper' in a phlegmatic type of the same age in Winter, since the alteration of the quality is greater.

Finally, 'consider the planet afflicting, for Saturn produceth longer sickness than Mars'. Mars signifies short but acute diseases and is more severe when he afflicts the Moon in the waxing phase.

Saturn indicates chronic diseases of some duration, made all the more intransigent if he afflicts the Moon in a waning phase. The Sun and Jupiter indicate short diseases and Venus those of middling length. If Mercury signifies the disease, its course will vary according to the planets Mercury aspects. The Moon symbolizes episodic diseases which come and go. Other testimonies concerning the length of illness are taken from the sign on the cusp of the 6th house of disease. A cardinal sign on the cusp (Aries, Cancer, Libra and Capricorn – the signs in which the equinoxes and solstices fall and which therefore mark the change in seasons) indicates a short disease, especially if the cusp falls at the end of the sign. Fixed signs (Taurus, Leo, Scorpio and Aquarius – the signs in which the seasons are firmly established) suggest a long disease; and mutable signs (Gemini, Virgo, Sagittarius and Pisces – the signs in which the seasons are starting to change) remission and relapse. In addition, Culpeper ends this chapter with a commonsense observation:

> Judge of the length or shortness of the disease according as the disease is. For it is not to be expected that a fever should last seven years. And it is as little to be hoped that a consumption should be cured in a day.

A final note on astrological prognosis of disease involves the planet to which the Moon applies by aspect in the decumbiture chart. It is a general rule in astrology that the separating aspects of planets indicate what has already happened, the applying aspects what is to come. We have seen how the nature of an illness now present may be judged from the separating aspect of the Moon. So the planet to which the Moon next applies has some bearing on what may happen next. Its strength or weakness in the decumbiture chart is assessed to see how well it may perform what it threatens, be it good or ill. If it is one of the benefic planets, Venus or Jupiter, it will symbolize hopes of recovery and the use of medicines and treatments of the nature of this planet becomes a part of the treatment to bring this about. If it is one of the malefic planets, Saturn and Mars, its potential harm must be countered by the use of treatments contrary to this. The question of *sympathy* and *antipathy* is the key to iatromathematical therapeutics and it is this we must consider next.

Sympathy and Antipathy

Culpeper's maxim stands that 'as the cause is, so is the cure, sympathetical or antipathetical'.[56]

In Galenic medicine, the basis of medical treatment is that contraries are cured by contraries. This means that, if a disease is present which is hot and dry in quality, so that the body is made hotter and drier than its normal balance or *eucrasia*, the treatment must be cooling and moistening in order to restore the balance. This is the original meaning of allopathy, or antipathy, to use Culpeper's word. In astrological medicine, however, the more important principle is treatment by sympathy. This is what is meant by homeopathy, that like cures like (*similia similibus curantur*), although Culpeper performed this with herbal medicines. Using the occult (hidden from view) correspondences of herbs and other medicinal agents, change is effected by sympathetic magic.

The question of treatment by sympathy or antipathy therefore requires some careful examination especially as it is for Culpeper 'the whole key of physick'. In the introduction to his herbal, in which 'the herbs, plants, &c are now ... appropriated to their proper planets', Culpeper gives the following 'instruction for the right use of the book':

- Firstly, consider what planet causeth the disease.
- Secondly, consider what part of the body is afflicted by the disease, and whether it lie in the flesh, or blood, or bones or ventricles.
- Thirdly, consider by what planet the afflicted part of the body is governed.
- Fourthly, you have in this book the herbs for cure appropriated to the several diseases ... whereby you may strengthen the part of the body and its like; as the brain by herbs of Mercury, the breast and liver by herbs of Jupiter, the heart and vitals by herbs of the Sun, &c.
- Fifthly, you may oppose diseases by herbs of the planet opposite to the planet that causeth them: as diseases of Jupiter by herbs of Mercury, and the contrary; diseases of the luminaries [Sun and Moon] by herbs of Saturn, and the contrary; diseases of Mars by herbs of Venus, and the contrary.

- Sixthly, there is a way to cure diseases sometimes by sympathy, and so every Planet cures his own disease, as the Sun and Moon by their herbs cure the eyes, Saturn the spleen, Jupiter the liver, Mars the gall and diseases of choler, and Venus diseases in the instruments of generation.[57]

In a given case, with the decumbiture chart aptly symbolizing the presenting sickness, the planets governing the disease and the part of the body afflicted are identified to meet the first three requirements. Let us assume the disease is a urinary tract infection and, appropriately, Mars afflicts Venus in the decumbiture chart. We know that Venus governs the part affected and we have identified Mars as the afflicting planet. Culpeper says 'be sure always [to] fortify the grieved part of the body by sympathetical remedies'. Thus herbs of Venus with an affinity for the urinary system are indicated, fulfilling the fourth requirement and constituting treatment by sympathy. Next, it must be asked whether the disease itself comes by sympathy or antipathy. Culpeper asks us to

consider whether the planet afflicting do govern the part afflicted. And if he have any dominion in that part of the body, he causes it by sympathy ... as suppose diseases in the bones, spleen, &c. If Saturn be the cause of it, it's by sympathy because he governs those parts. If by antipathy, consider what part of the body any planet afflicts, either by his presence [ie in the zodiac sign corresponding to the part afflicted] or aspects [to the planet ruling the part affected]. And then secondly consider who or what planet governs that part. If the planet afflicting be an enemy to the planet governing that part, then the disease is caused by antipathy.

As is the disease, so is the cure. If by antipathy, then apply those medicines proper to the place affected and governed by the afflicted planet. So here is a cure by antipathy: as suppose Saturn afflicts some parts that the Moon governs. Here the disease is cured by antipathy because Saturn is an enemy to the Moon. To cure which, apply things proper to the part affected and governed by the Moon, because they are antipathetical to the disease caused by Saturn.

If the disease be caused by sympathy, then you must apply medicaments to the part affected, or disease affecting, and governed by that planet afflicting. Here is [a] cure by sympathy; here the planet that kills or strikes is repelled or is beat by his own weapons.[58]

In our example it is clear that not only does Mars, the afflicting planet, not rule the part of the body affected, but is also an 'enemy' to the planet which does rule that part, namely Venus. Thus the disease comes by antipathy and so its treatment, in this respect, must be by antipathy to Mars. So, once again, herbs of Venus are indicated. Mars, being a hot and dry planet, will signify a hot disease, which is to be expected in such a case of infection and inflammation. Thus the indications for treatment are to employ cooling and soothing herbs of Venus which are appropriate to the urinary system and which have the power to heal the inflammatory effects of Mars. This fulfills the fifth requirement above. As to the choice of medicinal agents, the herb yarrow (*Achillea millefolium*) is one to consider in this instance, since it is cold in the first degree and 'is most fit for those that have inflammations, it being an herb of Dame Venus'. (The qualities and actions of commonly used herbs are tabulated at the end of Part 4.) Not only is yarrow proper for the genito-urinary system by occult correspondence (ie a herb of Venus) but also by medicinal quality, since the herb is indicated for vaginal discharge and excessive menstruation ('stoppeth ... the terms in women'), genital problems in men ('helps inflammations and excoriations of the yard') and kidney infections and excessive diuresis ('helps the running of the reins' and 'helps such as cannot hold their water'). Thus the choice of herbal medicine is made according to the plant's therapeutic properties as well as its occult correspondence.

It should be apparent from this example that the treatment is consistently by sympathy to the part affected (as if a weakness of the part is implied by its being dis-eased), even when it is by antipathy to the planet afflicting. This is still the case if the disease comes by sympathy, ie if Venus symbolizes the disease and the sixth requirement above has to be met. Culpeper, using his example of Saturn as the significator for the disease, sums it up thus:

> If Saturn cause the disease by sympathy, cure it by the sympathetical herbs of Saturn. If he cause the disease by antipathy, note whether it be antipathy to Sun or Moon. Or if it happen to the instruments of generation, be sure it is by antipathy to Venus. Make use of the sympathetical herbs of those planets for cure.[59]

What of purely antipathetical remedies, that is, those which not only oppose the significator of a disease coming by antipathy but also having no sympathetical strengthening of the part affected? Here Culpeper gives us a warning:

> Do not forget that sympathetical cures strengthen nature; antipathetical cures, in one degree or another, weaken it. And now your own mother wit [if you have any] will teach you that antipathetical medicines are not to be used, unless to such patients whom Doctor Ignorance or Doctor Carelessness hath had so long in hand, that sympathetical will not serve the turn.[60]

There is here, in the treatment of existing disease, an analogy with preventive medicine, where the most important thing is to keep the human being strong so that he or she can resist disease. So too in treatment, the physician, who 'is nature's servant, or at least should be so', seeks to employ the 'healing power of nature' to support the body of the sick person in its task of throwing off the illness. Only where this has failed, or in a potentially life-threatening situation where the effects of the disease must be rapidly countered, are antipathetical remedies to be considered. Among such medicinal agents are to be reckoned modern chemical medicines whose side-effects are sufficient testimony of their ability to weaken nature as their therapeutic power is to combat disease and to suppress symptoms.

The indications for the use of herbal medicines according to occult correspondences, by sympathy with the part afflicted and/or by antipathy to the disease, are not restricted to the significations of their ruling planets only but can also apply to those planets to which they are in aspect. Culpeper introduces the matter with an example. Take Mars, the 'lesser malefic', as the afflicting planet. It is noted in the decumbiture chart that he is conjunct (in the same part of the zodiac) with Jupiter, the 'greater benefic'. If the illness proved to be a liver disorder, the liver being ruled by Jupiter and here afflicted by Mars, the treatment would simply be by sympathy to the part affected and herbs of Jupiter are indicated. However, for an illness in another part of the body not ruled by Jupiter, then Jupiter, being configured with Mars and a benefic, can mitigate the effects of the illness. In this example, therefore, herbs of the nature of, and in sympathy with, Jupiter would have the power to correct the harmful qualities induced by a disease of Mars. This is another method of cure by sympathy.

Cure can also be effected by antipathy in this manner. If, for example, Mars was the afflicting planet and was conjunct with Saturn, and the disease was not in a part of the body ruled by Saturn, herbs which are in antipathy to Saturn would have to be used since Saturn will aggravate a disease of Mars. Such an approach greatly extends the indications for use of a herbal medicine according to its occult correspondence. Culpeper states:

> By the foregoing rules it seems all or most of the planets do govern some one or more particular things proper to all or most diseases. By which it will follow that every planet hath a share in every particular member there by sympathy or antipathy, as to the member itself or planet governing it. I answer in general, every particular planet has a compound or mixed share in every part, like as has the four elements. But, particularly, every planet has [a] share in every part, either sympathetically or antipathetically. Hereby you see without any College-light that one medicine may cure or be good for more diseases than one, and so may cure one disease by sympathy, another by antipathy.[61]

The matter of sympathy and antipathy is thus made more complex. The basic principle is that although every planet has some share in most diseases, in most herbal remedies and in each part of the body that share is based on a sympathy or antipathy. This is the factor to be determined, because 'as the cause is, so is the cure, sympathetical or antipathetical'. Although the doctrine of signatures was based on curing like with like, the question of sympathy and antipathy in Culpeper's medicine rests largely in the use of astrology and in the occult correspondences of the planets and zodiac signs, with its determination established by astrological rules.

The planets can therefore be antipathetical to each other in three ways.

- *According as they rule opposite signs.* So Venus and Mars are antipathetical or 'enemies', likewise Mercury and Jupiter, and Saturn and 'the lights' (Sun and Moon). This is detailed in the fifth of Culpeper's instructions listed above. In addition, planets found to be in opposition in their signs of exaltation (the place in which the planet is supposed to exert its greatest influence) are also counted. In this way, since Mercury is exalted in Virgo and Venus in Pisces, Mercury is an enemy to Venus, the former being a significator for the studious – an activity which induces melancholy – and the latter for the sport of love, the desired qualities for which are heat and moisture. Furthermore, a planet is antipathetical to another if the sign of its fall is ruled by that other planet.

- *By virtue of their opposite temperaments or qualities.* 'And so Jupiter is an enemy to Saturn, he being hot and moist, Saturn cold and dry. So Mars is an enemy to Venus, he being hot and dry, she cold and moist.'

- *When their conditions differ.* 'So there is enmity between Sol and Saturn for one loves the court and the other the country. Jupiter is enemy to Mars, for he loves peace and justice, Mars violence and oppression. Mars is enemy to Venus, for he rejoiceth in the field, she in the bed; he loves to be public, she plays least in sight.[62]

The antipathy of planets is provoked 'accidentally' (in other words because of their position in the horoscope rather than their inherent qualities) when they are in difficult angular relationships. The case of an afflicting planet in conjunction with a benefic or malefic has already been given, and indeed the consideration of Jupiter and Venus as beneficial and of Mars and Saturn as harmful is a judgement applicable at every stage of the medical-astrological endeavour, no matter what these planets specifically signify in a given decumbiture chart. Moreover, while Jupiter particularly opposes Saturn, and Venus Mars, Culpeper advises to 'make use of that fortune which is the strongest'. Thus the opposition of planets is said to be an aspect of perfect enmity and the square aspect between planets means that each is in a zodiac sign of opposite (active, if not also passive) quality. For instance, the square from Aries to Cancer is from a hot and dry sign to one that is cold and moist and these are quite different. The square from cold and moist Cancer to hot and moist Libra is then an example where only the active qualities, hot and cold, differ. Moreover, this change from one quality to another is not only the basis for the critical days (as discussed earlier) but also represents the transmutation of elements in nature.

If there is no antipathy between planets, as described above, then there is to be found some sympathy between them. So the Sun and Mars agree in that they are both hot and dry. A 'trine' aspect between the Moon and Venus can only mean that Venus will benefit the Moon since they have similar qualities and are in good aspect to each other. In *Culpeper's Herbal,* the author explains the application of these rules to the prescription of herbal medicines in his description of the herb *Carduus benedictus* (blessed thistle).

> It is an herb of Mars and under the sign Aries. Now in handling this herb, I shall give you a rational pattern of all the rest and if you please to view them throughout the book, you shall to your content find it true. It helps swimmings and giddiness of the head or the disease called vertigo, because Aries is the house of Mars. It is an excellent remedy against yellow jaundice and other infirmities of the gall because Mars governs choler. It strengthens the attractive faculty in man and clarifies the blood because the one is ruled by Mars. The continual drinking the decoction of it helps red faces, tetters and ringworms, because Mars causeth them. It helps plague-sores, boils and itch, the bitings of mad dogs and venemous beasts, all which infirmities are under Mars. Thus you see what it does by sympathy.
>
> By antipathy to other planets, it cures the french pox, by antipathy to Venus who governs it. It strengthens the memory and cures deafness by antipathy to Saturn who hath his fall in Aries which rules the head. It cures quartan agues and other diseases of melancholy and adust choler by sympathy to Saturn, Mars being exalted in Capricorn. Also it provokes urine, the stopping of which is usually caused by Mars or the Moon.

Treatment by sympathy is applied another way, too, in consideration of the planet signifying the patient in the decumbiture. For if he or she is appropriately symbolized as Saturn in the context of the illness, then herbs indicated for the condition and ruled by Saturn are to be administered to strengthen the sick person. These horoscopic considerations for the decumbiture chart are fully laid out in Appendix 2. It should also be noted that if the ruler of the natal ascendant is, say, Saturn, diseases signified by this planet will prove less harmful to that person, 'for the devil will not hurt his own; the like of Mars'.

The Favourable Moment for Treatment

Astrological symbolism is employed not only for diagnosis and prognosis according to the positions of the planets in the decumbiture chart and at the judicial, intercidental and critical days, but also for choosing or 'electing' the most favourable moment for a given treatment. In the *iatromathematica* of the Egyptians, there are injunctions against surgery and the cutting 'with iron' of that part of the body associated with the zodiac sign which the Moon occupies at a given moment. This is a key factor in an astrological election for the best time to undergo a surgical operation. Likewise each of the four administering virtues is best strengthened by giving medicines for the purpose when the Moon occupies a zodiac sign of the same qualities. For example, when a person subject to continual vomiting (but where the usefulness of this mechanism of the body to cleanse itself of some noxious matter is working against the health of the sufferer) is made weak by the inability to keep anything down, there is a need to strengthen the retentive faculty. The appropriate medicines should be given when the Moon is in an Earth sign which corresponds to the retentive faculty. Likewise, to purge the body by the use of a laxative, or an emmenogogue to induce menstruation, the required medicine will be best administered when the Moon is in a Water sign which corresponds to the expulsive faculty. Another example is to

> diminish a humour when the Moon diminisheth in light [wanes]. Increase when she increaseth in light. Phlegm opposeth choler, melancholy opposeth blood. 'Tis none of the worst ways to diminish choler by increasing phlegm.[63]

It may be the case, however, that the treatment strategy is one of longer-term resolution of a chronic disease. The patient then simply needs to follow a course of treatment with slight adjustments to the prescription as his or her condition improves, and in view of the astrological signs on the judicial, intercidental and critical days. With the treatment being conducted from the astrological as well as the medical point of view, the indications obtained from astrology may be something like 'give cooling and moistening herbs of Venus which strengthen the womb and cordials of the Sun for the heart'. The astrologer-physician will want to give medicines which truly carry the qualities of Venus and the Sun from the macrocosm into the microcosm of the patient's body. This will have been done if the herbal medicines to be prescribed have been gathered and prepared at those times when Venus and the Sun are particularly strong. This then represents another key addition of astrology to medical practice. Culpeper, at the end of his herbal, under directions for making medicines, gives a key to gathering medicines according to the state of the heavens so that their occult virtues are made as strong as possible.

The first rule is to gather a herb in the hour of the planet which rules it: 'Our present division of the day into 24 hours of 60 minutes each is the result of a Hellenistic modification of an Egyptian practice combined with Babylonian numerical procedures.'[64] The Egyptians gave us the 24 hours of the day, 12 during daylight and 12 at night. These hours were unequal and seasonal. An hour of daylight was longer in the summer months, shorter in the winter months and exactly equal with the hours of night on equinoctial days.

The appropriate planetary hour is calculated as follows. For any day, divide the time between sunrise and sunset by 12, which produces the length of each of the 12 hours of daylight. If the day, reckoned as the 24-hour period from dawn to dawn the next day, is a Monday, the day of the Moon, then the first planetary hour belongs to the Moon. If it is a Wednesday (Woden's day, which is Mercredi in French) the first planetary hour after dawn belongs to Mercury. Each of the seven days of the week belongs to one of the seven planets. The planetary hours follow one another in a set order which continually repeats itself, namely Saturn, Jupiter, Mars, Sun, Venus, Mercury, Moon. Thus the second planetary hour on a Monday belongs to Saturn and, on a Wednesday, to the Moon. It will be found by following this order of the planets through the 12 hours of daylight and the 12 hours of night on a Monday that the unbroken sequence gives us the correct planetary ruler for the first hour after dawn on a Tuesday (the day of Mars, or Mardi), namely Mars.

The calculation of the planetary hour can be made without needing to cast a horoscope. But a complete horoscope is considered in this practice and Culpeper gives the following rules:

> Let the planet that governs the herb be angular and the stronger the better [ie in essential and accidental dignities]. If they can, in herbs of Saturn, let Saturn be in the Ascendant; in the herbs of Mars, let Mars be in the Midheaven, for in those houses they delight.[65]
>
> Let the Moon apply to them by good aspect and let her not be in the houses of her enemies [ie the signs ruled by Mars and Saturn].

On this second point Culpeper is nothing if not practical. It

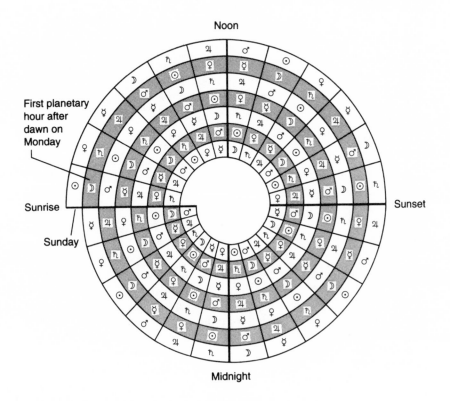

Figure 12 The snail begins at sunrise on a Sunday. The first planetary hour from sunrise on a Sunday belongs to the Sun. The rest of the 12 daylight planetary hours, 6 before noon, 6 after noon, are attributed to the planets in the repeating order of Saturn, Jupiter, Mars, Sun, Venus, Mercury, Moon. The sequence continues through the 12 planetary hours of night until sunrise on Monday (the Moon's day) is reached, when it is revealed by the "snail" that the first planetary hour from dawn on Monday belongs to the Moon. This sequence continues through the rest of the days of the week.

would be folly for the treatment to be delayed for a languishing patient while the astrologer-physician is waiting for the Moon to come to the required place. So, he adds, 'If you cannot well stay till she apply to them, let her apply to a planet of the same triplicity. If you cannot wait that time neither, let her be with a fixed star of their nature.' Culpeper gives instructions for the right time to pick a couple of herbs. In his herbal, under 'angelica', he states that

> it is an herb of the Sun in Leo. Let it be gathered when he is there, the Moon applying to his good aspect. Let it be gathered either in his hour or in the hour of Jupiter. Let Sol be angular. Observe the like in gathering the herbs of other plants and you may happen to do wonders.

For the herb greater celandine, Culpeper writes:

> This is an herb of the Sun and under the celestial Lion and is one of the best cures for the eyes that is. All that know anything in astrology know as well as I can tell them: that the eyes are subject to the luminaries. Let it then be gathered when the Sun is in Leo, and the Moon in Aries applying to his trine. Let Leo arise. Then you may make it into an oil or ointment which you please to anoint your sore eyes withal. I can prove it both by my own experience, and the experience of those to whom I have taught it, that most desperate sore eyes have been cured by this only medicine. And then I pray, is not this far better than endangering the eyes by the art of the needle? For if this do not absolutely take away the film, it will so facilitate the work that it may be done without danger.

Culpeper specifies here that the Moon should be in Aries at the time of gathering this herb for the eyes because Aries rules the head. It should be further observed that, to carry out Culpeper's instruction, the herb must be gathered at dawn. Note the same consideration of the position of the Moon in another election for the gathering of a herb used to treat a condition of the brain. In order to treat epilepsy he recommends mullein, because, 'they say that the herb being gathered when the Sun is in Virgo and the Moon in Aries and in their mutual antiscions [the various mirror-image positions relating to the Cancer-Capricorn axis in the zodiac] helps'.

The astrologer-physician will therefore look at the state of the heavens at the time of a person falling sick or first consulting him for signs of the cause, nature and location of the disease. He will make an initial prognosis according to these signs and watch carefully the disease process and the patient at 'critical' and other days for further signs of improvement or deterioration. Treatment is conducted according to the medical indications and these astrological signs. If a certain treatment is necessary to avert an expected downturn in the patient's condition, the moment for administering or beginning this treatment can be identified. So, too, can the moment most favourable for the gathering or preparation of the required medicines calculated. Furthermore, these considerations based around the decumbiture chart can be augmented by signs taken from the natal horoscope, since from this the temperament of the patient[66] and the propensity to suffer certain kinds of diseases can be obtained and compared with the present sickness, the age and sex of the patient and the season in which the illness came on. Thus, in Culpeper's words:

> the natural philosopher ... inquires into the causes, effects, times, places, fashions, events; the whole and every part of the whole in the mineral, animal and vegetable kingdoms, and how nature produced them by the elements. The astrologer is, or at least ought to be, very well versed in every part of natural philosophy ... from there he inquires and searches the motion and course of the celestial bodies, and what effects such motions must naturally produce upon minerals, animals and vegetables. Then comes in the Divine, who being admirably skilled in both these arts ... teaches what God is, what the spirit and soul of man is, what the angels are and what religion is. He also teaches how man should glorify God in his life and conversation.[67]

PART 4

The English Physician: Herbal Medicine and Therapeutics

His Arts to him, when great Apollo gave
He did nor augury nor arrows crave
Nor the melodious lute, but to prevent
His father's death who now with age was spent
To be a herbalist, and medicine
To learn he rather did his thoughts incline.

Culpeper's rendition of Virgil,
The English Physitian (1652)

The teaching on diseases in Western holistic medicine was called the Doctrine of the Three Contra-Naturals.[1] This was divided into a study of the diseases themselves, their causes and their sequels. Inquiry into the nature of diseases, which is now called pathology, was rather undeveloped from the modern perspective. This is because of a change in the basic concept of disease in the 19th century from symptom complexes of the kind which Culpeper describes to lesion-anatomical syndromes elucidated by developments in pathology. Then, with the discovery of germs or disease-producing micro-organisms, a great emphasis was put on the aetiological (the investigation of the causes) and usually bacteriological origin of diseases.[2] The disease in itself, therefore, became more interesting to doctors and scientists than the type of person suffering from it.

In Western holistic medicine, however, the emphasis was on what kind of person had the disease. Diseases themselves were distinguished according to what kind of body tissue was affected: whether the disease was organic, that is, affecting compound tissues such as the liver or kidneys (including congenital diseases existing from birth as well as disease-induced malformations and abnormalities in the size, position or number of a given organ);

or whether the whole body was suffering a distemper or imbalance of the humours (with or without morbid matter or abnormal humours present in the body) known as a *dyscrasia.*

The Nature and Causes of Diseases

Practitioners of the Western holistic tradition divided diseases into simple and composite disorders. A **simple disorder** was constituted by a disorder of **temperament** in a simple part or throughout the body, where the qualities of the part or the whole were altered and in a state of imbalance.

It was shown earlier that eight imbalances of temperament existed, four simple imbalances involving only one quality in excess, either heat, cold, dryness or moisture, and four compound imbalances with two qualities altered, namely an excess of heat and moisture and of the blood humour, of heat and dryness (choler), of cold and dryness (melancholy) and of cold and moisture (phlegm). Each of these imbalances, beyond or different from the *eucrasia* of the person, constituted a disease state. Morbid matter (a 'peccant' or 'depraved' humour) might also be present in the body at the same time, so that another eight possible forms of imbalance – ie those just named but accompanied by the presence of an abnormal humour responsible for the imbalance – were added, making 16 in all.

The treatment of dyscrasia or a disorder of temperament differed according to whether an abnormal or 'peccant' humour was present or not. For, if present, it had to be concocted and voided from the body. If the dyscrasia was general, with no particular part or organ dis-eased by the presence of such a humour, the disorder should prove to be mild, so long as it was not much removed from the natural temperament or eucrasia of the patient. A *cachexia* or ill condition of the whole body was therefore believed to be present only when accompanied by an underlying serious disease such as cancer

Where a simple dyscrasia was present, without signs of excess or abnormality of humours, the diagnosis was made according to the following indications:[3]

Table of Signs of Temporarily Acquired Temperaments

ABNORMAL HEAT	ABNORMAL COLD	ABNORMAL MOISTURE	ABNORMAL DRYNESS
feeling of uncomfortable heat	weak digestion	signs similar to those of abnormal cold	dry skin
excessive thirst	less desire for drinks	laxity	insomnia
quick exhaustion of energy	laxity of joints	excessive salivation & nasal secretions	wasting
undue discomfort in fevers	tendency to catarrh & phlegmatic fevers	tendency to diarrhoea and dyspepsia	intolerance of dry foods, a like of moist things
burning & irritation in pit of stomach	aversion to cold foods	intolerance of moist foods	discomfort in autumn
bitter taste in the mouth	greater discomfort in winter	excess of sleep	hot water & light oils readily absorbed
weak & rapid pulse		puffiness of eyelids	
intolerance of hot foods			
comfort from cold things			
distress in hot weather			

These signs were considered together with the signs associated with the temperament of the person. Brock wrote in 1923 that the disorders that modern pathologists attribute to hormonal disequilibrium were formerly and similarly explained as a dyscrasia of the temperament and humours.[4] It is interesting to note, then, certain clinical features attributed to an overactive and underactive thyroid gland, for instance: the intolerance of heat, rapid pulse, diarrhoea and weight loss of hyperthyroidism, and the intolerance of cold, depression, weight gain, cold skin, dry hair, and swelling of the hands and feet seen in hypothyroidism.

Since the root of disease was found in a state of plethora, in which symptoms were directly related to an imbalance within the body (when excess humours obstructed the flow and distribution of blood and spirits), such a state of the body denoted a condition more serious than an imbalance in the four qualities. The symptoms and signs were considered under six headings:[5]

Functional disturbances
These were assessed in terms of impairment, for instance, defective vision or a weakness of the stomach with slow or insufficient digestive power causing acid belching;[6] dysfunction (visual hallucinations; abnormal digestion or decomposition in the stomach); and loss of function (loss of vision; complete absence of digestion).

Excretions
There may be a lack of normal excretions, ie faeces and urine, or the excretions may be abnormal in substance (tissue, cartilage, stones, healthy blood), quantity (polyuria or excessive urine passed), quality, including colour (mucus in stools or black stools, called melaena, due to altered blood) and passage (eg vomiting faeces).

Pain, its site and quality
Pain was thought to arise as the sensation of contrariety produced by a contrary thing. Avicenna listed 15 types of pain:[7]

- *boring* pain, caused by the retention of gas or gross matter within the folds of a hard organ such as the colon, continually goading and tearing it
- pain of *compression,* produced when fluid or gas is confined in too small a space
- *corrosive* pain, caused by material trapped between the muscle fibres and their sheaths and resulting in a disturbed temperament of the muscle
- *dull* pain, from an overly cold temperament of a part, from closure of the pores or from the overfullness and distension of the cavities of the body, as in a plethora, preventing the spirits from reaching an organ
- pain of *fatigue,* caused by undue toil or by a composite

disease manifesting as lassitude and due to an ulcerating humour, an overabundant humour under tension or a gaseous substance

- *heavy* pain, due to inflammation in an insensitive organ such as lungs, liver or kidneys, or in an organ which has had its sensation destroyed by inflammation, so that the organ drags on the surrounding structures and fasciae and causes them to feel a heavy pain
- *incisive* pain, caused by a humour of sour quality
- *irritant* pain, due to a change in a humour to a harsher, rougher nature
- *itching* pain, owing to an acrid, sharp or salt humour
- *pricking* pain, similar to a boring pain, when matter enters an organ for a time and tears or ruptures it
- *relaxing* pain, caused by matter accumulating in and stretching the belly of a muscle, making it lax while the tendon is taut
- *stabbing* pain, due to a transverse stretching and separating of the membranes of an organ, or sometimes in the whole body
- *tearing* pain, due to a humour or gas entering between the bone and the periosteum, or from cold strongly constricting the periosteum
- pain of *tension*, caused by a humour overstretching nerve or muscle fibres
- *throbbing* pain, due to a hot inflammation

Pain was said to dissipate bodily strength and to interfere with the normal functioning of organs. Pain from an organ signalled that the organ was hot but the ensuing dissipation of its vitality would afterwards render it cold. 'Depraved' humours caused pain by their acrid quality or by their abundance in an organ, stretching its fibres.

Inflammatory swellings
These were of six kinds, the 'peccant' humour being one of the four humours, or else a 'watery' humour or gas. Resolution of such conditions came about by digestion and excretion of the offending humour, by the formation of pus or by the conversion of the humour into a hard mass (eg a fibroid). When blood was involved, the swelling was called a phlegmon (haematoma). A

swelling of choler was an erysipelas, inflaming the skin and manifesting with severe constitutional symptoms. Black bile was considered responsible for hard tumours when cold and dry, and as 'bile burned black' (adust choler) it caused cancers. Haemorrhoids[8] and some glandular swellings were attributed to black bile, others to hardened phlegm. Watery swellings manifested as dropsies, due to heart failure or portal obstruction, and oedema, hydrocoeles and cysts. Swelling by gas was seen in the pain of flatulence in the gut, the bloating of the belly and by general puffiness of tissues.

Special symptoms
These included symptoms such as wasting, a black tongue, a burning fever, etc, and were duly taken into account.

Relations between organs
It was believed that organs and sites could be secondarily affected by sympathy or *consent*.[9] Adjacent parts were thought to be easily affected, one by another, and, similarly, parts of the same type, eg the nerves. This was considered true also of subservient parts: for example, in the way that a disease of the liver affects the veins and vice versa. The same applied to arteries and the heart, and to the nerves and the brain. The hotter organs, the heart and liver (but not the stomach, bladder or womb), were also said to sympathize with the affected part because they easily attract noxious humours and vapours. This was true also of soft organs, such as the skin and lungs, because, by virtue of their attraction of moisture, they offered little resistance. However, if one of the principal organs was affected, namely the brain, heart or liver, then the whole body would manifest the distemper.

Otherwise, connections between organs were recognized for a variety of reasons, such as the relation of breasts and womb, and bladder and kidneys. Regarding the head, the highest organ in the body, any intemperate heat or noxious vapours could rise in the body to affect that organ. The brain would be particularly affected by an over-hot stomach or womb, resulting in hysteria, or by vapours rising from an overheated spleen which produced strange and melancholy thoughts. Treatment would be directed to the organ primarily affected and the improvement in symptoms from the organ affected by consent (the brain in this example) due to such treatment was regarded as evidence of the truth of secondary affections by consent.

TYPES OF PLETHORIC STATE

Of the above groups of symptoms any plethoric state may produce pain, due to stretching of vessel walls or organ capsules, while functional disturbances were more typical of the effect of abnormal humours. Thus the physician had to determine whether the obstruction was due to the quantity or quality of the offending or 'peccant' humour, which humour was imbalanced or in excess, and how far removed the patient was in the disease state from his or her normal temperament.

With **quantitative plethora**[10] (excess of normal humours), blood vessels and other channels are distended and overfull with humours. This may lead to rupturing of a vessel and the escaping of the humour into surrounding structures, thereby choking them. In this case, prompt bleeding or venesection was used to draw off the excess of humour in the blood vessels, because there was a danger of heart attack, stroke (apoplexy) or epilepsy. Signs of a quantitative plethora are:

- feeling of heaviness in various parts of the body
- sluggish movement or lassitude
- loss of appetite
- redness of complexion
- distension of blood vessels
- tightness of skin
- a full pulse
- high-coloured and dense urine
- subjective sense of weak vision
- dreams of carrying heavy weights, being paralysed and unable to move or speak

The condition we call hypertension was also considered an early stage of quantitative plethora.

In **qualitative plethora** (excess of abnormal humours), the spirits and faculties and the vitality as a whole will be compromised depending on the site of the abnormal humour. The danger in such a case is from putrefaction. Chronic, degenerative conditions fall into this category of disease. The signs of a qualitative plethora are:

- feeling of heaviness
- lassitude
- loss of appetite
- redness of complexion, distension of blood vessels, tightness of skin, a full pulse and a high-coloured and dense urine – only present if the quantity of humours is also in excess
- dreams of itching, stinging or burning of the body and the smell of bad odours

In a case of qualitative plethora, the 'peccant' humour must be identified for treatment, according to the following signs:[11]

TABLE OF SIGNS OF A DOMINANT HUMOUR

BLOOD	YELLOW BILE	BLACK BILE	PHLEGM
heaviness of body especially behind eyes	frequent attacks of tingling of the skin	excessive hairiness	flabbiness of body
frequent stretching & yawning	yellow colour of eyes and complexion	dark complexion, skin dry & dark	excessive pallor, skin cold & moist
drowsy & sleepy	dry nostrils		excessive sleepiness
dull mind with poor perception	burning/irritation from hot bath or Sun	anxiety	mental dullness
sweet taste in mouth	bitter taste in mouth	burning in epigastrium	weak digestion with acid eructations
red tongue	rough & dry tongue		flabby muscles
boils & ulcers on tongue common	excessive thirst	false appetite	reduced thirst unless phlegm is acid
fatigue without exertion	rapid pulse		soft, slow pulse
bleeding from gums, anus & nostrils	nausea/vomiting: green or yellow bile	thick & turbid urine: blue, black or red	pale urine
	irritative diarrhoea	thick & dark blood	excessive salivation
	desire for cool breezes		viscid saliva
dreams of red things & of blood flowing	dreams of fire and flags coloured yellow	dreams of dark places & fearful objects	dreams of water, ice, rain & hail-storms

It was generally the view that diseases of blood and phlegm were milder than those of yellow and adust (black) bile, which, owing to the toxicity of these humours, caused more serious and malignant conditions. It was also held that diseases of choler and adust choler could manifest suddenly as acute diseases as could diseases of blood, for these were often infections. Diseases of phlegm, however, were usually chronic.

Signs of abnormal choler in the body, according to Riviere,[12] were those of ordinary choler but manifesting with much more intensity and caused by long use of foods of a 'vicious juice' in the diet such as garlic and onions. Otherwise it could be caused by the effect of vehement heat on an existing choleric state of the body. He described abnormal and adust choler (black bile), the cause of cancers, as insufferably acrimonious while melancholy arising as a residue from the putrefaction of blood was a milder form of such a disease process and so the splenetic symptoms were less vehement.

Normal phlegm which in abundance gives a phlegmatic temperament, was said to be either tasteless (insipid) or slightly sweet, while an abnormal salt phlegm arose from putrefaction by extraneous heat or by the retention in the body of watery dampness because of overuse of salt in the diet. Riviere gave the signs of a salt phlegm in the body as a great thirst, itchy scabs on the skin, a salt taste from catarrh flowing down the throat and certain dysenteries. The phlegmatic humours condensed by extreme cold into a 'glassy' or vitreous phlegm found only in the digestive tract manifested with a biting or stabbing colicky pain, fixed in the same spot. Riviere distinguished this from the wandering and unsettled colic arising from flatulence. Another extremely hardened form of phlegm, called 'gypseous' phlegm, manifested as kidney and bladder stones and in the chalky deposits or 'tophi' found in gout sufferers. Occasionally such hardened humours were coughed up from the lungs 'like hail'.

A purely **watery humour** abounding in the body manifested as 'distillations' flowing from the cold and moist brain to various parts of the body, and as dropsies and watery swellings. This humour could arise in the body from a moist diet, from eating an excess of summer fruits or from drinking water excessively. The failure of the body to deal adequately with such food and drink indicated a cold and moist liver, a melancholic temperament or obstructions of the liver, spleen and kidneys. The signs presented would be oedema, ascites and other watery swellings, frequent sweating and the need to spit often.

Gas was thought to arise from the effect of a weak heat on crude and thick chyle and other matter in the digestive tract. It was seen in those of a melancholic temperament and in obstructions of the spleen. The failure to digest the humours properly allowed their decomposition and the production of gas. This gas caused a tensive, moveable pain in a part but there was no sense of heaviness there. Foods particularly implicated in the production of gas were: chestnuts, turnips, beans, peas and pulses. Other symptoms and signs included noises in the ears, fasciculations (muscle twitches), belching and retching, rumblings of the belly and bloating with wind. Those suffering flatulence may dream of things light in weight and quick in motion.

Fever

In the Doctrine of the Three Contra-Naturals, fever was classified as a disease in itself, not just a symptom, although the Hippocratic view that fever was nature's way of ridding the body of noxious humours meant that it constituted a healing crisis also. Culpeper's statements on fevers in an early piece of writing simply followed the tradition in distinguishing fevers according to the parts of the body they affected and in prescribing a treatment by contraries, to oppose either the cause of the fever or the fever itself.[13]

Fevers were divided into different types. The fevers that harmed the spirits were called ephemeral. Fevers which arose from the putrefaction of humours and threatened to continue the process of putrefaction either within the blood vessels or else outside in the fleshy parts of the body were called putrid fevers. The putrefied blood which caused the fever had to be evacuated by venesection or concocted and purged by medicine. A fever which was not resolved was called a continuous fever and was known to be particularly dangerous. Fevers which were caused by a putrefying phlegm and which lasted roughly a day were called 'quotidian'. Fevers which became acute every third or fourth day were termed tertian and quartan fevers respectively and were judged to be caused by putrefaction of choler and melancholy respectively. Malarial infection is the prime example of these kinds of fevers, which were chronic with acute episodes. Finally, a fever which was thought to be located in the solid parts of the body, wasting the radical moisture and causing a consumption was called a hectic fever. Tuberculosis falls in this category, with its chronic pyrexia and night sweats.

OTHER SIMPLE DISORDERS

Beside the disorders of temperament, other states counted as simple disorders were:

A disorder of **structure**. A part or organ may undergo a change of form of either its overall shape or a part of it, such as ducts, cavities and surfaces. Included in this group were such conditions as a sixth finger and other errors of development, varicose veins, ankylosis of the spine, fibrosis of the lungs, warts and atrophy of the mucous membranes of the digestive tract. The size of a part might be changed, as in elephantiasis of the legs or general emaciation and the wasting of the flesh seen in the aged as part of the overall decline. Further, a change in position might affect locomotion of the body, as in dislocations, hernias, gross tremors of the limbs and gout.

A **'solution of continuity'** or loss of integrity of a part or organ. This covered abrasions and excoriations of the skin, wounds, including traumas such as the severing of a nerve or a bone fracture, and ruptures of blood vessels and membranes. In such cases the cause of disease was obvious and the medical treatment beyond question. Culpeper recommends, for instance, butcher's broom (*Ruscus aculeatus*) for 'knitting and consolidating broken bones or parts out of joint'; tormentil (*Potentilla tormentilla*) 'to stay all kinds of fluxes of blood ... whether at nose, mouth, belly or any wound in the veins or elsewhere', and comfrey (*Symphytum officinale*) in either eventuality. Herbs for wounds were a mainstay of treatment for a solution of continuity.

Some other abnormalities were classed as disfigurements and, though not actually diseases in many cases, they were regarded as such, often because they were said to arise from an abnormal temperament. Under this heading came alopecia and baldness, vitiligo [abnormal pigmentation of the skin], a sun-tanned or wind-wrinkled skin due to environmental effects, body odour, pock marks and excessive fatness or thinness.

COMPOSITE DISORDERS

Composite disorders were defined as the conjoining of several morbid states into one disease. The disorders of temperament in an organ were included here because the disease might involve a solution of continuity or a change in size together with the alteration of qualities. Likewise an abscess on the leg represented a loss of integrity to the skin as well as an inflammatory process. In this case abnormal humours had been discharged into the tissue spaces of the leg which nature had sought to expel by creating an abscess. The pus discharged was said to be that particular humour, altered from a nutriment which the weakness of the tissues in the leg had been unable to use. This was demonstrated in the change from the leg's healthy temperament to one of excess heat, with inflammation.

WEAKNESS OF ORGANS

A diminished faculty or weakness of an organ in the body may arise because its temperament has been upset. Otherwise the weakness was said to lie in either the substance of the organ or in the vital force responsible for its activity.[14] The substance of the organ may be affected by a persistent abnormality of the organ's temperament. Usually this was undue cold, so that the faculty and the activity of the organ were diminished, but an abnormally hot temperament of an organ could disperse the vital spirit flowing to it and render it numb. Excessive dryness could bring on weakness by increasing the density of the organ and interfering with the free play of its faculty. Likewise, an overmoist state weakened the organ because the over-relaxed state of the tissues obstructed the flow of spirits. Thus there is an optimum, balanced state of an organ denoted by its healthy temperament, just as the string on a lyre is at the correct degree of tension to produce its pure tone. Structural disease in the substance of the organ would, of course, weaken it also.

The vital spirits vivifying an organ could fail in their task if these spirits were dispersed because of undue heat in the body. This comes about through external heat, eg the weakness felt through a dispersal of the vital spirits after a hot bath, or from heat generated by certain emotions. Also, the vital spirits could be dispersed indirectly in a state of depletion. The causes of depletion were given as haemorrhage, true diarrhoea, ascites, the incision or rupture of a large abscess, dilatation of the pores and profuse sweating, excessive exertion, pain, fever or starvation. Finally, persistent activity of an organ or overactivity weakened the organ, because this activity heated the organ and dispersed once again the vital spirits flowing to it.

The weakness of an organ had consequences beyond its own disability.[15] If the stomach was weak by being abnormally cold while the temperament of the liver was normal, the improperly concocted chyle (full of phlegm) from the stomach could cause obstructions in the liver. Likewise, these crude humours passing to overhot kidneys could become hardened and so produce kidney stones. The kidneys were thought to become weakened, and kidney stones more likely, by excessive sex which consumed much of the radical moisture of the body. A person could also inherit some weakness, or predisposition to disease, such as gout, from the parents.

The Causes of Disease and Their Diagnosis

The causes of disease were divided into those factors exciting or bringing on the disease state, those predisposing the sufferer to such a disease, and those which were coincident with the disease. The predisposing causes of disease were the temperament and any disorders of structure of the body. The exciting cause was that which brought on the disease as opposed to predisposing the sufferer to it. Today these causes are often attributed to infection. Generally, the exciting cause was identified as a dysregulation of one of the Six Non-natural Things, such as the quality of food and drink taken, excessive exertion, poor sleep or some great emotional upset. Such a cause could act directly, as the heating effect of garlic, or indirectly, such as the production of heat in the body from cold water which closes the pores of the skin. Furthermore, a hot condition would not be helped by its occurrence at the height of the Summer, the heat of the season constituting in this case a coincident cause. Overall, to consider something as a cause of disease, that agent had to be sufficiently powerful and in prolonged contact with the body, and the body suitably predisposed, to make the person ill. Since the individual temperament was central to the predisposition to disease, it was thought possible that the same cause might lead to the appearance of different diseases in different people at different times.

The **sequel** to a given disease is its associated symptoms and signs. Symptoms were said to follow the disease 'as the shadow follows its substance', and patients might complain of the effects of impaired functions or altered and corrupted qualities of the body. Signs were regarded by physicians as reliable, objective indications of the actual condition.

DIAGNOSIS

The physician, on being consulted by his patients, would consider their age and sex, their occupation, where they lived and what kind of air they breathed, at home and at work. The patients' temperament or 'habit' had to be assessed and the following ten 'classical' questions were put to them:[16]

- what is the main complaint?
- when was it first noted?
- what made the patient ill?
- is it getting worse or better?
- what is his or her diet?
- what is the state of the bowels?
- has any natural evacuation stopped?
- how is the patient's energy (whether laborious or idle)?
- what is his or her disposition?
- does the patient tend 'naturally to breed bad humours'?

The physician would then examine the patient's body, feeling for masses in the abdomen and paying attention to superficial rashes, swellings and lumps. It was important to feel the patient's skin and to determine whether, for his or her given temperament, it was too hot, cold, dry or moist. The secondary qualities of the skin, such as softness or hardness, together with its colour were assessed at the same time. The pulse was felt to judge the state of the vital faculty, and the urine examined for evidence of waste products of the various concoctions or digestions of the body. Attention was paid to other evacuations from the body in terms of their colour, smell and taste.

Although Culpeper knew it to be important to feel the pulse of each patient in order to assess his or her vital faculty, he never wrote at length from his own experience. His translation of Jean Fernel's

Treatise on Pulses,[17] published posthumously, covered the basics of what is a very complex part of diagnosis. Of the pulses to be found among the different temperaments and intemperaments,

- a **great** pulse was one which felt long, broad and high and a **little** pulse was short, narrow and low, with a mean existing between the two extremes
- a **vehement** pulse beat hard upon the fingers, and was **faint** if its beat was weak, again with a mean between them
- the frequency of a pulse in time was indicated by the terms **swift** and **slow**, and, if neither, then it was moderate
- the quality of the artery was reflected in the **soft** and **hard** pulses with a mean between them
- the spreading or perfusion of the artery gave either a **full** pulse, which was large, swollen and full of humours, or an **empty** pulse, swollen with wind rather than blood

Beyond these five key points, the rest between beats was of note and then the varieties of abnormal and irregular pulses.

Culpeper wrote only a few 'useful observations' on diagnosis from the urine. Urinalysis was considered very important in Western medicine. However, in his short *Urinal Conjectures,*[18] although Culpeper conceded that some of this tradition was 'worthy of serious consideration',[19] he expressed concern over the uncertainty of diagnosis from the urine on the grounds that if the bladder is diseased all such judgement is in vain, and because urine may appear to be healthy in a patient near death when the disease is affecting the spirits of his body.[20]

Culpeper said of his description of the condition of the urine (typical for each of the simple and complex temperaments given in Part 2) that 'such as have any wit in their heads may hereby come to all the judgement of urine that I as yet know of'.[21] In addition, wrote Culpeper, the colours of the urine in the presence of disease must be strictly observed. Residue settling at the bottom of the urinal then rising as a cloud, pear-shaped or pyramidal and white, denoted health. Other colours denoted a corresponding distemper, with black the most ominous. If the urine was white or pale but clear, it signified melancholy, so the disease was likely to keep its hold on the body since the retentive virtue was allowing little to leave the body in the urine. If the urine was clear but yellow, in other words looked normal, it could be an indication that the disease would continue because there was no sign in it that the body had concocted the 'peccant' humour as necessary for recovery.

Culpeper took his lead from Hippocrates in writing that in fevers 'gross resolutions, like dust or bran in the bottom of the urine' and 'slimy, muddy, tawny, dirty, filthy, stinking urine' were signs of imminent death. Generally, deposits were also to be judged by their colours and, overall, the colour and smell, even the taste of the urine were to be assessed in terms of a predominant humour and in the context of the other signs of disease and the temperament, age, place of habitat, diet, etc, of the patient. As Culpeper wrote:[22]

> If a child's urine be brought to you and it looks pale and clear, like conduit water, it is very bad ... I told you before such a humour was the badge of a melancholy disposition. Youth is naturally hot and moist, melancholy cold and dry. Ergo, extreme inimical to youth.

The Treatment of Diseases

Treatment for various diseases was called 'taking the cure' and all treatment strategies aimed to restore the dynamic balance of health in the human body. All diseases were reckoned to have four stages: an initial stage with few or no signs of disease; a period when the disease was increasing; an acme when the disease had reached its full height; and then the final resolution of the condition. In both acute and chronic diseases, the Hippocratic pattern of indigestion, concoction and crisis formed the basis for medical intervention. Abnormal humours arising from faulty digestion had to be treated with medicines so that the body could then concoct them. This process was distinct from normal digestion or *pepsis* and was termed *pepasmos*. Once the abnormal humours had been concocted, nature could then evacuate them from the body. Signs of concoction were to be seen in the production and expulsion of pus via the normal excretory pathways, by means of a formation of an abscess or in the state of the urine. This evacuation of the disease-causing humour constituted the crisis: a successful cleansing of the body by the

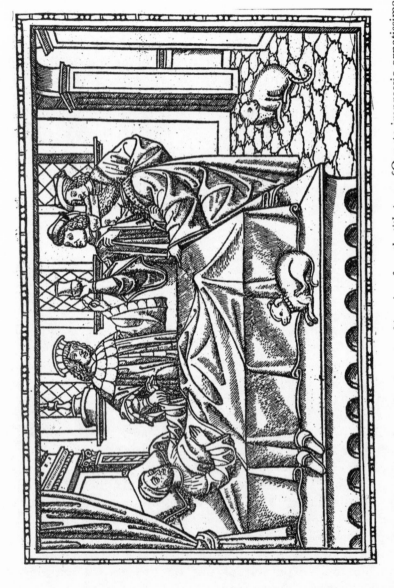

Figure 13 A physician taking a patient's pulse and viewing his urine, from the title page of Quarto impressio ornatissima: continens omnes Galeni libros alias impressos. … *Pavia (1515–16).*

healing power of nature ensured a return to health, although this might be aided by nature's servant, the physician, who could help to restore strength and function to the part of the body affected by the disease through the prescription of tonic medicines.

The basis for selecting remedies for the correct preparation of abnormal humours was the same as that for the treatment of the simple dyscrasias and imbalances of healthy humours, namely allopathic treatments of opposites by opposites. Thus, if the dyscrasia or excess humour was cold and moist in quality, the treatment had to be hot and dry to prepare the humour or to restore that patient to his or her eucrasia. The degree of the heating and drying quality of the regime had to match the degree of excess cold and moisture of the imbalance, always with regard to the age and sex of the person, and the time of year. If the medicine was too heating and drying, another dyscrasia of just these qualities could arise from the treatment. If the medicine was not sufficiently heating and drying, the treatment would be ineffective. If the imbalance was a simple one, a constipation, say, with only dryness in excess while heat and cold were in a healthy balance, food and medicines which moisten the body were indicated. If the body was hot but not dry, only slightly cooling foods and medicines were thought to be needed, the regime reflecting the fact that dryness and moisture were in balance and that the excess of heat in the body was not extreme.

In a case of excess cold and moisture in the body, the strategy might be to purge the body of excess of normal phlegm as much as to prescribe a diet of more heating and drying foods, medicines of similar quality and exercise. Similarly in chronic conditions the aim might be a gradual resolution, or *lysis*, of the imbalance along these lines rather than the provoking of a healing crisis. This gradual resolution of the condition was thus similar to the regime for preserving health in a like temperament, except that the intention was to return the patients to their eucrasia, rather than to proceed from that state towards an optimum balance and state of health.

A third strategy of treatment in Western holistic medicine was *apostasis*, the driving away of the disease into other parts. This might be actively undertaken if the disease was centred in or near a vital organ since it would be less threatening to life and health if the abnormal humour moved to a peripheral and less noble part of the body. The principles of *revulsion* and *derivation* in venesection or blood-letting embodied this strategy.

The Role of Diet

The prescription of a correct diet for a given state of disease was seen as essential. What would be the point of correcting abnormal humours with medicines if the diet, or any other of the Six Non-natural Things, caused their continued production in the body? Consequently, diet represented the first stage of treatment and indeed it was found that a good regimen of diet and lifestyle factors could on its own remedy some cases of dyscrasia and plethora, by correcting the temperamental imbalance according to its qualities and by ending the production of abnormal humours by ensuring that only that quantity of food which could be properly digested was eaten.

The physician would ask about the existing diet of the patient in relation to his or her disease. For example, thick, 'clammy' humours from certain cold and moist foods or arising from the poor digestion of a phlegmatic type could cause obstructions to the free passage of blood and spirits in an organ or vessel, leading to local congestion and impaired organ function. Sharp and acrid foods or medicines might induce a dryness of the digestive tract and predispose it to ulceration. On the other hand, a diet containing too much fatty and oily food could produce a *lienteria* or difficulty of the intestines. Then, food would speedily pass undigested through the digestive tract as a diarrhoea or, conversely, if partially digested, would remain long enough in the tract to ferment. A diet of too many astringent foods (eg in heavy tea drinkers) could bind and narrow passages in the body.

The question of whether the diet should be full, moderate or sparing had to be decided. A **full diet** was indicated where bodily strength and vitality or the power of digestion were low. Fish, eggs and other meats (proteins) which are digested slowly were included in a liberal selection of foodstuffs. A **moderate diet** simply preserved the strength of the body in its condition. A diet based around white meat and a little fish and eggs was in all probability sufficient. In a **sparing diet** emphasis was then put on fruit and vegetables, as bulky foods of little nourishment, when crude humours were being created in the body. This was especially required if the pores were choked with dense matter. Such a diet also preserved strength in cases where the digestion or the functioning of the body was impaired and light foods such as soups, broths and porridge were eaten. Complete fasting was appropriate in acute conditions, for nature was deemed unable to carry out *pepsis* at the same time as *pepasmos*. The period of fasting could be ended at the next critical day, a few days later, if signs of concoction were present. Generally, it was observed that the less work nature had to do in expelling the disease, the more plentiful the diet could be. Where there was doubt, a full diet was recommended unless the disease was acute.

Therapeutic Strategies

In **dyscrasias**, if a hot condition was also dry by virtue of the heat, as was often the case in older individuals and always in chronic conditions, treatment was by diuretics and purgatives. Wormwood was cited as a typical aperient. The treatment had to be effected very slowly and lifestyle changes made for the duration. Exercise was to be reduced, easily digestible foods eaten, daily hot baths some time after a meal were recommended, and all things which increase heat in the body were to be avoided.

The strategy for cold dyscrasias was to administer hot foods and medicines. Honey mixed with powdered warming herbs was recommended, together with massage using warming oils[23] and hot baths and exercise, to induce sweating. In a cold and moist dyscrasia, rheumatic and plethoric conditions were likely. Consequently phlegm had to be evacuated from the body and diuretics given before meals. The digestion needed the assistance of an increase of heat for concoction and of a reduction in the amount of food eaten.

The regime for a cold and dry dyscrasia was that adopted for the aged. They should eat hot and moistening food and drink, take hot baths and gentle exercise such as walking, get plenty of sleep and avoid constipation. The bowels should be opened daily. Diuretics and herbs purging phlegm were indicated, along with massage using warm oils to stimulate the vital faculty. The diet should be based on small, frequent meals. Fruit and vegetables and milk were recommended and a little ginger or garlic occasionally if the person was used to such things, to increase heat without producing any dryness. Heavy, sharp and astringent foods had to be avoided, along with young white or sweet wines. Mature red wines were reckoned good in a small quantity, because of their heating and diuretic effect. Persons of this dyscrasia had to avoid tiring exercise, exposure to the Sun, prolonged wakefulness, worry and excessive sex.

If **obstructions** due to a plethora were present, contributing to the excess of heat of the body by the resulting dysregulation of the vital spirits and the innate heat, these required opening medicines. Much caution was required here lest the application of cooling herbs hardened the thick matter causing the obstruction. On the other hand, the application of heating, attenuating medicines could aggravate the hot condition. Treatment therefore began with cold, cutting and cleansing substances such as barley and endives, gradually increasing the heat through the appropriate herbs temperate with respect to heat and finally making use of diaphoretic herbs. The same applied to cold dyscrasias where a cooling effect could be increased by the use of diaphoretics because of their ability to disperse the innate heat and vital spirits. However, this was done only to a certain degree because the reduction in innate heat represented the loss of vitality, while coldness implied its destruction.

The humours causing obstruction were thought to be either over-abundant, thick (like clay) or viscid (like melted glue). The treatment for over-abundant phlegm was purgation. This was always performed first by stool, to rid the body of thick humours which might block the narrower passages of the urinary tract and the pores of the skin, and then by diuretics and diaphoretics via urine and sweat respectively. Thick humours had to be made thin with attenuating medicines and viscid humours had first to be cut up and cut away from vessel walls by incisive, cutting and cleansing medicines. Glutinous and unhealthy humours sticking to the walls of the digestive tract were often also treated with lubricant laxatives, typically aloes.

Thick humours which had been made thin but had still not been evacuated in sufficient quantity only changed the obstruction from one type to another, more watery in consistency. Diuretics were used to purge watery humours, thin phlegm (ie not thick enough to cause obstructions) and choler. However, diuretics were avoided when any part of the urinary system was inflamed, since the waste matter leaving the body by that route might aggravate the inflammation.

Diaphoretic herbs (those that induced sweating) were used to purge thin or thinned humours and, being heating medicines, were deemed very appropriate for chronic conditions which were usually found at root to be cold in nature. However, the attenuating action of diaphoretic herbs could, by their injudicious use, thicken gross humours by dissipating the thinner portions of them. This could bring obstructions in the body and close the pores of the skin, resulting in the putrefaction of the humours and the development of hard tumours in organs. Thus any gross matter had to be reduced first by purgation via the bowels. This was sometimes sufficient to restore the body to a healthy balance. Otherwise, to avoid thickening the humours, pure attenuants had to be combined with softer herbs of a thin matter.

Obstructions occurring in cold dyscrasias were remedied by pungent foods such as pepper, garlic and onions, followed by bathing and a little massage, avoiding any weak or painful parts of the body, as well as cleansing herbs such as celery for the urinary system and hyssop for the lungs. Honey was also said to help prevent such obstructions and joint pains.

In diseases of the blood which were thought to be more prevalent in sanguine types with an excess of this humour, bleeding was the usual treatment, to evacuate the noxious blood and to cool the body. In such a hot and moist condition, the moisture could overcome the innate heat to cause putrefaction. Therefore some gentle exercise in those accustomed to it was deemed of value in dispersing the humours, as was bathing before meals. The purging of waste matters from the body was recommended routinely in those of a sanguine humour in early Spring each year. The quantity of food eaten also had to be limited to avoid overproduction of sanguine humour.

The medicines used in cases of **inflammatory swellings** were called discutients. They had the power to draw the matter away to a different part and were astringent in action. In hot or acute swellings cold discutients were used, in cold swellings, hot and dry ones. In the second stage of the disease (that of increasing inflammation), resolvent (thinning) medicines had to be added to the discutients, in equal proportions at the height of the swelling. In the final stage of resolution, only attenuants and relaxant remedies were used, cold relaxants being more drying than hot ones.

If there were signs of swollen lymph nodes, no discutients were to be used. For it was believed that the swollen glands indicated morbid matter in the vital organs which had to be dealt with first, the cervical glands relating to the brain, the axillary to the heart and the inguinal to the liver. Such cleansing would then further swell these glands as they worked.

Hard inflammatory masses needed softening with hot and moist medicines, after which attenuating medicines were applied to disperse the matter. For gaseous swellings, hot medicines which rarefied the gas and opened the pores of the body for its dispersal were indicated. The diet had to be corrected to avoid the recurrence of the gas. External inflammatory swellings with ulceration or erosion, such as the vesicles of weeping eczema or herpes, needed cooling and drying medicines. Internal inflammatory swellings required evacuation of the offending humour, followed later by discutient and astringent remedies, while bathing, wine, exercise and emotional excitement or upset were to be avoided. If maturation towards abscess formation was taking place, emollient and opening medicines were given. Internal ulceration required purifying agents like honey and herbs with an affinity for the part affected as target remedies, together with astringent styptic medicines.

Herbal Medicines

If the nature of a malady was unknown, it was thought best to leave it to nature either to cure it or reveal clearly what the problem was. If medicines were to be prescribed in such a situation, it was borne in mind that cooling medicines could be more harmful than hot, that drying medicines could be given without harm for less time than moistening medicines, and that, anyway, these passive qualities were altered by alteration of the active ones. Furthermore, a dyscrasia more intense or more removed from the natural temperament of the patient needed stronger medicines and vice versa. For example, if an old man needed cooling and moistening medicines to restore him, treatment had to go beyond reducing his temperament to equability since the hot and dry disease was very removed from what would be natural for an old man.

Three rules were applied to the prescribing of medicines. Firstly, the medicine had to be selected according to its qualities, so that for a cold condition, heating medicines were given, and so on.

Secondly, the nature of the part to be treated had to be considered when deciding on the quantity and quality of the medicine. Once again, if an organ normally hot was made cold by disease, the heating power of the medicine had to be greater than in the case of a cold organ made colder, because of the severity of the symptoms associated with the former. Dense organs with small channels such as kidneys needed stronger preparations than loose organs with wide orifices such as the lungs. The more remote an organ was from the stomach and liver, where all internal medicines were first destined to go, the stronger the medicine had to be, for it underwent two concoctions before reaching the part affected. The physician also had to be mindful that a strong cooling of a vital organ would have the effect of cooling the whole body. In this respect the order of nobility of organs came into play. Injurious medicines such as vesicants (those which cause blisters) and pungent (hot) herbs were not put on sensitive organs and caution was exercised in mixing medicines of contrary qualities. However, it was usual to mix at least one medicine of a contrary quality into a patient's prescription, so that, for instance, vinegar was added to hot prescriptions and saffron to cooling herbs for the heart to aid penetration or to make the medicine something in sympathy with the part to be treated. (Culpeper, in general, advocated including a remedy for the heart in all prescriptions.) Also, it was observed that a dyscrasia could be corrected by a medicine but the effect was not lasting because the herb, being of thin parts, was soon dispersed. The addition of other herbs of a thicker substance was found to give more stability and an increased period of efficacy.

Thirdly, medicines were to be administered according to the stage of disease, with adjustments continually made to the prescription. For instance, a disease due to active fermentation of humours (rendering them sour) demanded early evacuation before the humours matured, unless the fermentation was only moderate. Gentle medicines were to be used first and stronger ones later, unless such delay threatened a loss of vitality. Delay in direct treatment was to be avoided, though it was often better late than never. It was the opinion that medicines should be interchanged at intervals and reliance on just one agent be avoided, because tissues were thought to become accustomed to one medicine and might therefore fail to respond to the treatment. Furthermore, the part to be treated might respond to a medicine at one time and not at another. This is one situation in which astrology was most valuable, by its ability to indicate the most appropriate treatment at a given time.

A gentle treatment was followed where two maladies were found to be present. For instance, colic arising from glutinous humours in the digestive tract needed cooling anodynes for the pain and heating, cutting medicines for the humours causing it. Again, fever required cooling medicines but the obstructions in the channels which gave rise to the heat needed hot attenuating medicines. The strategy was to proceed gently in both directions.

Sometimes, moving to a different climate had to be advised, for good, clean air was a most important factor to aid healing. Finally, anything which pleased, calmed and gratified the patients was recognized to contribute to their healing, although it was felt right to shame or embarrass the patients if it would stop them continuing what was harmful to them.

TEMPERAMENTS OF MEDICINES

Herbal medicines were classified as either temperate, hot or cold, in respect to their active qualities, and with or without a drying or moistening quality. In '*A Key to Galen and Hippocrates' Method of Physick*', Culpeper gives the following analysis of the manifest qualities of herbal medicines.[24]

- Temperate herbs were used to strengthen a weak part where there was no manifest imbalance of heat and cold, or in fevers due to phlegm, the cause being cold and moist and the effect hot and dry. Temperate medicines would avoid increasing the fever by heat or condensing the phlegm by cold.

Herbs with a manifestly hot temperament were categorized according to the degree of heat.

- Herbs hot in the 1st degree were said to impart a moderate and natural heat to a part cold by nature or cooled by accident. In this way heat was restored when lacking or cherished when weak. The effects of such medicines were to thin offending humours and expel them by sweat and insensible perspiration through an opening of the pores of the skin. In addition to helping mild fevers, they promoted proper concoction and the production of good blood by cherishing the natural heat required for these processes, and they removed weariness. Many anodynes (which relieve pain) come under this heading, such as chamomile. Overuse of these medicines was said to consume the substance and strength of the spirits of the body.

- Herbs that are hot in the 2nd degree were judged hotter than the natural temper in man. Their use was to cut and scatter tough humours, to clear obstructions to the pores of the skin, and to correct stomachs full of phlegm.

- Herbs hot in the 3rd degree were more powerful yet in cutting tough and compacted humours and in promoting sweating. Many of them were used to resist poisons in the body but their injudicious use was said to cause fevers.

- The 4th degree of heat was reserved for herbs so hot that they can burn. Their external application could cause blistering and inflammation.

No cold medicines were accounted naturally friendly to the body. They removed heat indirectly and were not so frequently used as hot medicines.

- Herbs cold in the 1st degree were used to qualify the heat of food in the Summer, as many salad herbs do, to ease heat in the bowels and to cool the blood in fevers. Children and those with weak stomachs, Culpeper says, are easily hurt by cold medicines.

- Herbs cold in the 2nd and 3rd degrees were to be used in people with strong stomachs and hot livers to ease the heat of choler, to treat insomnia and frequent fainting (which was done by closing the pores of the skin, repressing sweats and thus stopping the spirits from being dissipated) and externally for inflammatory swellings.

- Herbs classified as cold in the 4th degree are narcotic. They ease extreme pain by stupefying the senses and, Culpeper says, are only to be used when there is no other option.

Herbal medicines said to be moistening did not go beyond the second degree of moisture because, if the herb was also hot, the moisture was reduced by its drying action, and if cold, this reduced the moisture by condensation. In addition, care was taken with the use of moistening medicines as they were believed to dull the activity of the body and take away its natural strength.

- Herbs moist in the 1st degree softened the body by emollient action and strengthened the expulsive virtue. They were used to ease coughs and dry throats.
- Herbs moist in the 2nd degree thickened the blood and spirits, counteracted sharp and acrid humours and aided the expulsion of matter via the bowels.

Drying medicines were known to consume moisture, arrest discharges, diarrhoea and loss of blood, and render the body and its organs firm so as to restore proper function in lax tissues. Their use was for bodies and organs full of moisture. However, if such herbs were inadvisedly given, especially those dry in the third and fourth degrees, they were reckoned to dry up the radical moisture of the parts, causing under-nourishment and consumption in them.

THE DOCTRINE OF SIGNATURES

As well as their qualities of heat, cold, dryness and moisture, other 'manifest' aspects of a herb were considered. By 'manifest', Culpeper means 'such as are obvious to the senses, especially to the taste and smell'.[25] Liquorice, in fact, is named after the Greek for 'sweet root' (*Glycyrrhiza*) and the name bittersweet (*Solanum dulcamara*) speaks for itself.

Other 'manifest' aspects of a herb were considered apart from its taste and smell, such as what it looked like or where it grew. Herein lay the doctrine of signatures. Culpeper wrote 'because out of thy thoughts God shall not pass, his image stamped is on every grass'.[26] In this way, the visual appearance of a plant was often believed to reveal its medicinal use by its likeness to a part of the body. As Culpeper said of the lesser celandine (*Ranunculus ficaria*), 'Behold here another verification of that learning of the ancients, viz that the virtue of a herb may be known by its signature, as plainly appears in this; for if you dig up the root of it, you shall perceive the perfect image of that disease which they commonly call the piles.'[27] Lesser celandine is thus commonly named pilewort, meaning the herb for piles.

By the same doctrine of signatures, eyebright, whose diminutive white flowers with a splash of yellow resemble inflamed eyes, was used to treat such a condition. Culpeper attributed this plant to the Sun, which rules the eyes, and to Leo, for it is in July and August, when the Sun passes through the zodiac sign Leo, that this herb can and should be gathered. All three sorts of centaury (*Centaurium erythraea*) are 'under the dominion of the Sun, as appears in that their flowers open and shut as the Sun either sheweth or hideth his face'. Culpeper advocated that 'in diseases of blood, use the red centaury; if of choler, use the yellow, but if of phlegm or water, you will find the white best'.[28]

MEDICINES PROPER TO EACH PART OF THE BODY

Head

The most important medicines for the head were those used for treating the brain. These were called cephalic medicines. The brain was deemed cold and moist but easily affected by temperature. More often the brain was troubled by cold (a 'head cold'), with signs of heaviness, much phlegm in the nose and mouth, dulled wits and sleepiness.[29] Herbs of a gently warming and drying quality which cut and cleanse these humours were then indicated and after this purging was done, the brain could be strengthened. Since the brain is in the highest part of the body, it was also judged to be affected by hot vapours rising from other over-heated organs, causing such things as insomnia, headaches and congestion of the head with little phlegmatic discharge. In this case, cooling cephalic medicines were called for, but the over-heated organ or excess heat in the body had also to be treated. The herbs willow, plantain, sweet violet and rose are examples of medicines which cool the head, while rosemary, betony, cowslips, vervain and feverfew heat the head.

Culpeper gives advice, too, for the treatment of other organs in the head. Herbs given internally which strengthen the sight should be those ruled by the Sun or Moon, and as examples he mentions eyebright and moonwort. For the mouth and nose, no ill-tasting or foul-smelling medicines should be used since these may upset digestion. The ears and the faculty of hearing were reckoned cold and dry in quality and easily affected by cold. Therefore hot and dry medicines should be used to treat them. As to the teeth, they are affected by excessive heat or cold and particularly by sharp and sour-tasting things (whilst sugar rots them). Treatment was by cleansing and binding remedies.

Chest and Lungs

Medicines to treat the chest and lungs, internally or externally, were called pectorals. Such herbs, which were said to strengthen the lungs and encourage easy breathing and good expectoration (the discharge of phlegm from the chest and lungs) while soothing a rough and dry respiratory tract, were soft, mild and gentle in character. Sweet-tasting medicines and syrups were often used but this had to be done in moderation, says Culpeper, in case these provoked obstructions in the lungs. A rough and hoarse voice was indicative of dryness and, along with soothing pectorals, such as liquorice, coltsfoot and sweet violet, salty and sour foods had to be avoided. Some pectorals described as cutting and cleansing in action were used when tough and compacted phlegm was present in the lungs. Other herbs were thought to thicken mucus found too thin to be easily expectorated, or to thin them if they were too thick. Pain on the inspiration of cold air and difficulty in expectoration were signs of cold lungs and an indication for warming pectorals such as betony, balm, hyssop, elecampane and liquorice. Among the herbs cooling over-heated lungs are coltsfoot, sweet violet and plantain.

Heart

The heart nurtures life in the body and adds vigour to the emotions by virtue of its innate heat. Excess heat, as in fevers, poisons and melancholy vapours rising from a hot spleen, was judged to affect the heart adversely. Medicines used to treat the heart were called cordials. Cordials were made sweet with sugar and medicinal by use of the four cordial flowers, namely borage, viper's bugloss, sweet violet and rose. Cooling cordials, such as viper's bugloss, wild lettuce and white pond lily were only used in fevers and other cases of extreme heat, for the heart is naturally the hottest organ in the body and cold medicines were therefore considered detrimental. For poisoning of the body, 'pestilential' fevers and infectious diseases, herbs resisting poison, such as rue, juniper, angelica, blessed thistle, elecampane, centaury and

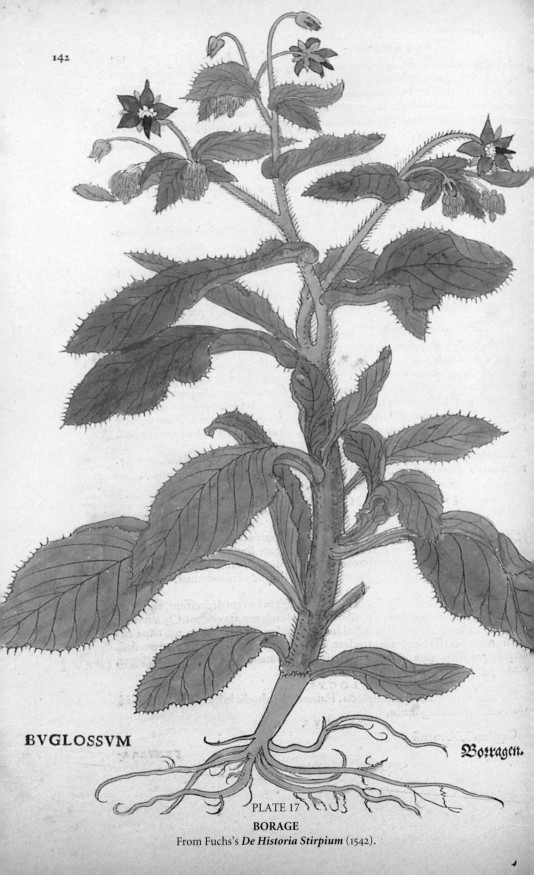

142

BVGLOSSVM   Borragen.

PLATE 17

BORAGE

From Fuchs's *De Historia Stirpium* (1542).

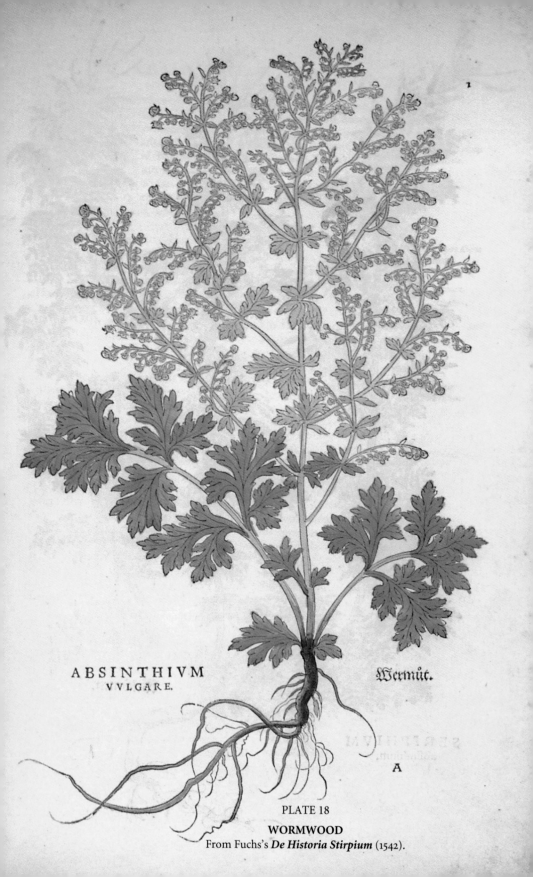

ABSINTHIVM
VVLGARE.

Wermůt.

A

PLATE 18

WORMWOOD

From Fuchs's *De Historia Stirpium* (1542).

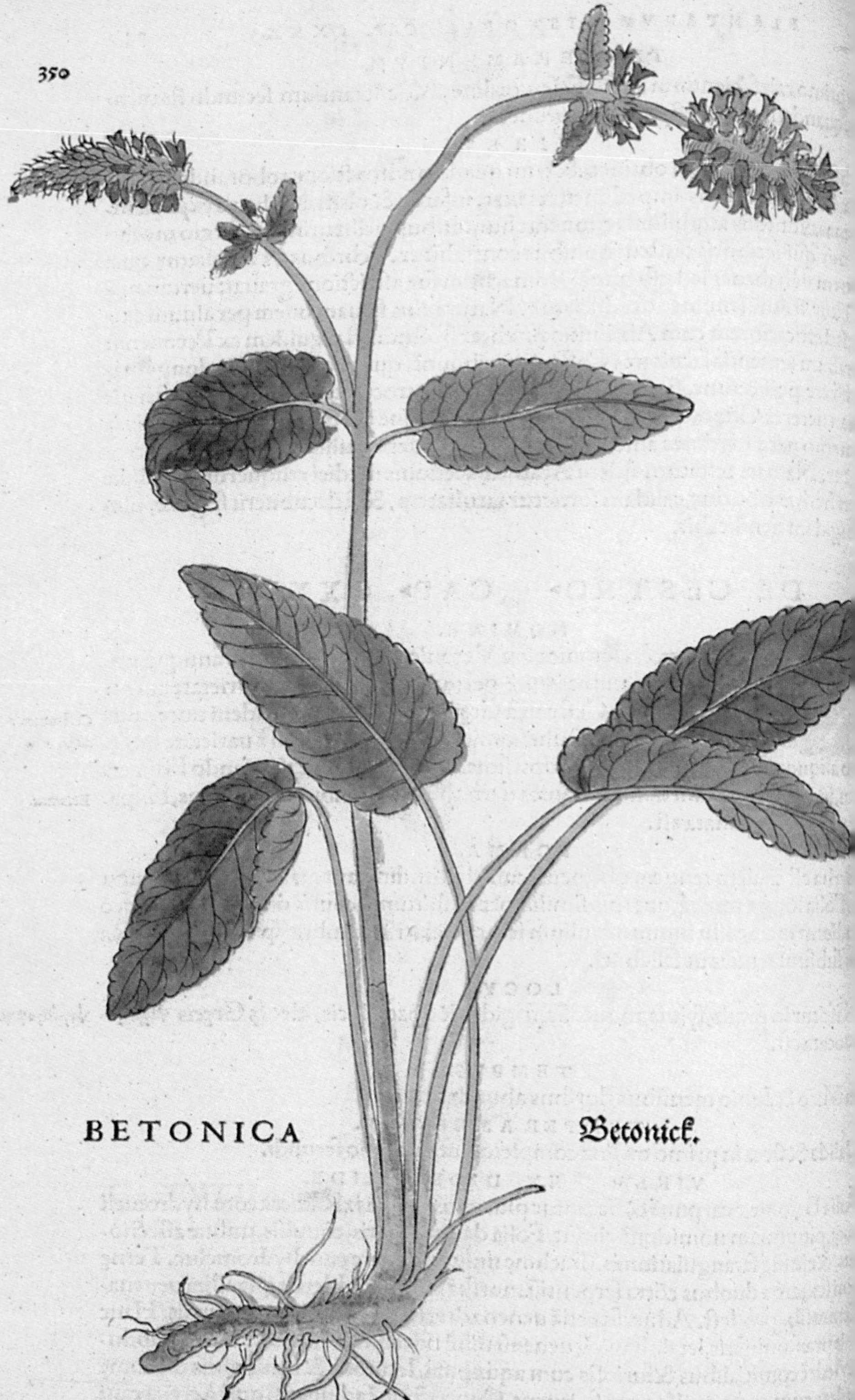

BETONICA   Betonick.

PLATE 19

BETONY

From Fuchs's *De Historia Stirpium* (1542).

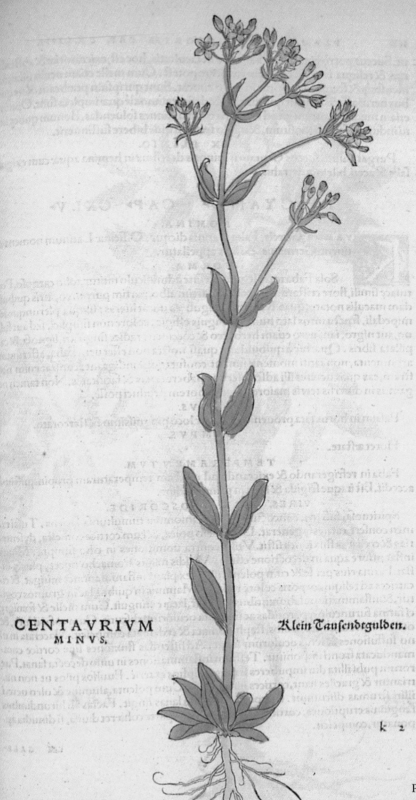

CENTAVRIVM
MINVS.

Klein Tausendgulden.

PLATE 20

CENTAURY
From Fuchs's *De Historia Stirpium* (1542

PLATE 21

EYEBRIGHT
From Fuchs's *De Historia Stirpium* (1542).

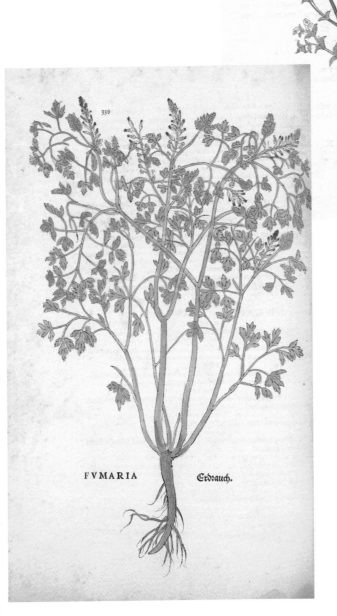

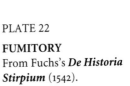

FVMARIA   Erdrauch.

PLATE 22

FUMITORY
From Fuchs's *De Historia Stirpium* (1542).

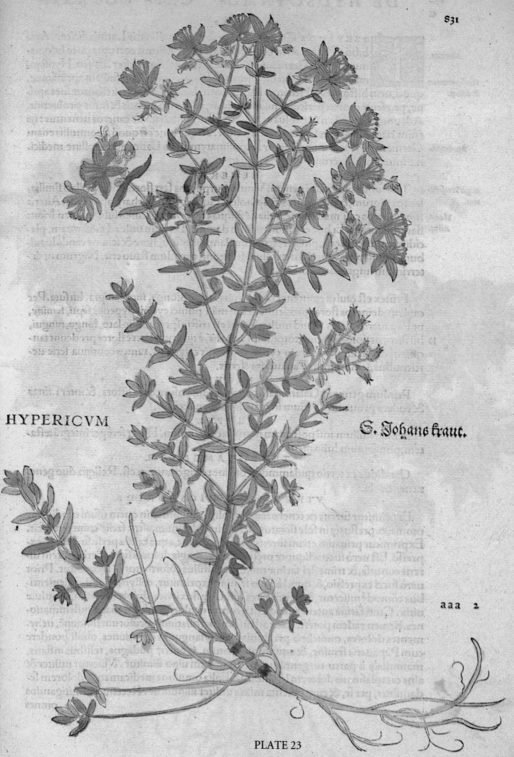

HYPERICVM

S. Johans kraut.

PLATE 23

ST JOHN'S WORT
From Fuchs's *De Historia Stirpium* (1542).

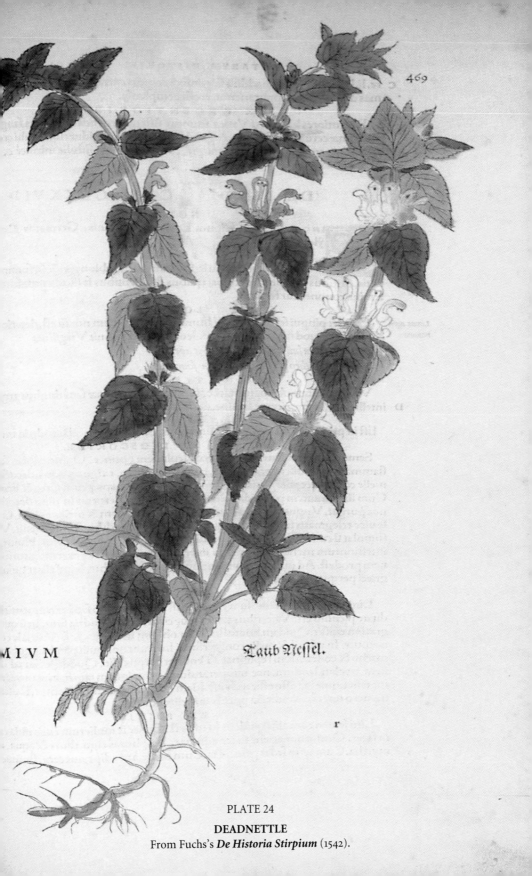

MIVM

Taub Neffel.

r

PLATE 24

DEADNETTLE

From Fuchs's *De Historia Stirpium* (1542).

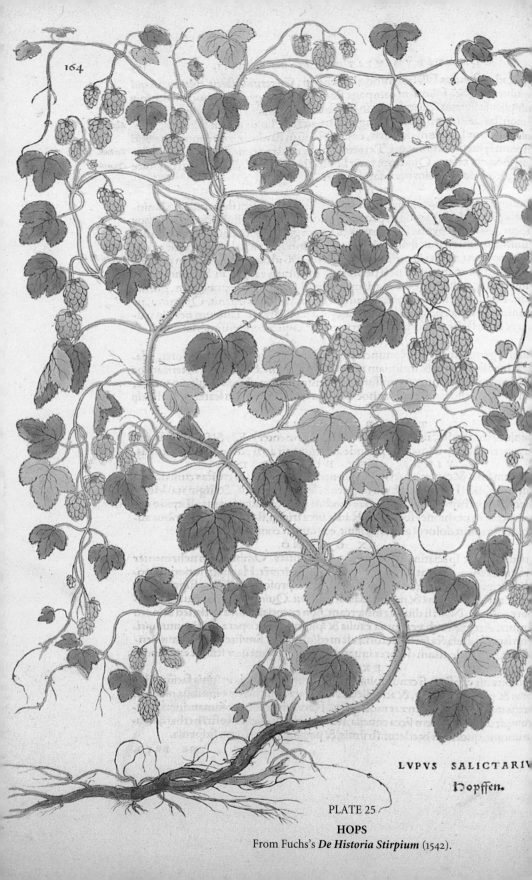

164

LVPVS SALICTARIV

Hopffen.

PLATE 25

HOPS

From Fuchs's *De Historia Stirpium* (1542).

especially garlic were used. In the case of the heart being troubled by melancholy vapours, herbs which cherish and refresh the vital spirit were called for. Culpeper lists among these borage, balm, rosemary, citron peel and the spices, for spices were said to refresh the vital spirits (as sweet-smelling herbs do the animal spirits). These medicines also kept back melancholy vapours from the heart. Cordials generally had the effect of cheering the heart and mind in a person suffering some mental anguish and emotional upset.

The signs of an excessively hot and dry heart were: a pulse that is swift, full and hard (ie does not easily yield to pressure by the fingers), difficulty in catching the breath, and a furious, angry or rash manner. For this state of the heart Culpeper recommends borage, sorrel, wild lettuce and purslane. If the heart was hot and moist, the inclination to anger would be more easily appeased, expiration would be longer than inspiration and the pulse found to be swift and full but soft and easily yielding to pressure. There would be a susceptibility to putrefaction or bacterial infections of the body. Sweating and bleeding were therefore recommended, to rid the body of the excess of moisture, and for sweating the cordial herbs rue, balm and angelica could be employed.

When the pulse was slow, weak and soft, the person fearful or unusually timid and unable to be roused to anger or to put up much of a fight over things, the condition of the heart would be judged to be cold and moist and the body as a whole was expected to be phlegmatic in temperament. The usual heating cordials such as angelica, cinnamon, saffron, marigold, balm and rosemary were given in these circumstances.

Stomach

The stomach was reckoned to be naturally hot and dry. In health people were said to have an appetite for foods of the qualities of their temperament, so the phlegmatic drank milk, for 'every like is maintained by its like'. But when they were unwell people were thought to choose foods opposite in quality to the nature of the disease. Appetite could be lost due to the presence of abnormal humours in the stomach, such as choler or the results of the putrefaction of undigested food, the latter being also a sign of weakened digestion. Furthermore, the retentive virtue, by which food is held long enough in the stomach for digestion to be completed, could be deranged, causing recurrent vomiting or diarrhoea.

Culpeper calls those herbal medicines which purge humours from the stomach *orectics* and those which strengthen the stomach after purging *stomachics*. In the latter group were all the spices, which are warming, aromatic medicines. Bitter herbs which stimulate the appetite were not to be given before the stomach had been cleansed of offending humours, and were commonly prescribed before meals. Herbal medicines which strengthen the retentive virtue, such as yarrow, were stomachics. These possessed a binding quality and were prescribed before meals to remedy diarrhoea, or after meals if vomiting was the problem. If the stomach was hot, digestion was easy and food which was accounted difficult to digest, such as red meat, cheese and oily fish, could be taken. A stomach which was cooler than its usual state meant an increased appetite but a poorer digestion, resulting in 'sour belching'. Warming herbs for the stomach were given to rectify this, such as ginger, fennel, calamus, mint, wormwood, cinnamon and other spices. An over-moist stomach produced a reduced thirst and appetite but required the same herbal medicines. An excessively dry stomach increased the thirst and the enjoyment of over-cooked meats. Moistening and slightly cooling medicines were then needed such as many fruits and vegetables, syrup of violets, wild lettuce and barberry.

Liver

Herbs for the liver were called hepatics. Those which strengthened the liver were very gently astringent and helped to retain food in the liver during the second concoction. However, excessively astringent herbs troubled the liver through causing obstructions and hindering the distribution of blood by narrowing the vessels and passages. Other hepatics, the true ones, were held to open the obstructions that the liver could often suffer by a cutting and attenuating quality without any excessive heat. Included in this number were wormwood, milk thistle, white horehound and agrimony. Such herbs are also gently astringent (binding and drying) and cleansing.

Inflammation of the liver subsequent to obstruction demanded the use of cooling, cleansing and attenuating medicines, mixed with some heating herbs so as not to spoil the liver's digestive virtue. Excessive cooling of the liver was thought also to render the adjacent diaphragm cold, with the result that breathing was made more difficult. An excessively hot and dry liver (which was made evident by choler in the body) caused dry scabbing of the skin (eczema), a dry and rough state of the bowels with likely constipation and visibly large and hard veins. For this cooling herbs were indicated, such as fumitory, dandelion and sweet violet. A hot and moist liver approximated to its normal temperature and, if excessively so, was treated by sweats and bleeding typical of the management of dyscrasias of blood.

When the liver was deemed cold and moist, the blood was full of phlegm, because the liver had not been hot enough to concoct it all into blood. The bowels would be loose in this case, the veins narrow, the person phlegmatic in temperament and liable to dropsies. Heating hepatics were recommended here, such as hyssop, centaury, chamomile, cinnamon, hops and fennel. If the liver was cold and dry, the complexion of the whole body would be melancholic, the physique lean, and treatment would focus on the spleen.

Spleen

The spleen was believed to be the receptable for the melancholic humour. This thick and earthy humour could cause obstructions in the bowels, leading to a diminished efficiency of digestion, or it could harden into tumours. The melancholic humour was cold and dry, unless it was the burned or adust type of choler, in which case it would be hotter. Cooling and moistening herbs proper to the spleen were needed for the latter type of melancholy, but they should not be too cold, for there is not the same degree of heat present as exists with pure choler. Cordials had to be added to repress the vapours rising from the hot spleen. If the offending humour was the thick, cold and dry kind of melancholy, cutting and opening medicines were required.

Herbs which opened obstructions of the liver usually did the same in the spleen, but the less astringent medicines were regarded as most appropriate, since astringency was thought to hinder rather than help the spleen. Fumitory and wormwood were mentioned by Culpeper. If the spleen was not only obstructed but hard as well, emollient medicines were used externally over the spleen. Some of a melancholic temperament were apparently full of a watery humour and this had to be purged by those herbs which evacuate phlegm and moisture from the body, such as elder or senna. Generally, the lean type of melancholic needed more flesh on their bodies.

Kidneys and Bladder

According to Culpeper, herbs proper to the kidneys and bladder rectified either stones present in the organs (the anti-lithics), inflammations or thick humours by their cutting action. Very astringent medicines were not used, for fear of preventing the passage of urine. The bladder was thought to need stronger medicines than the kidneys because it is further away from the centre of the body. Among the remedies which Culpeper gives for stones and gravel of the kidneys and bladder are birch, goldenrod, hawthorn, nettles and milk thistle.

Womb

Medicines proper to the womb were supposed to regulate menstruation and to correct absent, scanty or excessive bleeding. It was a principle of gynaecology in Greek medicine that the womb could move around in the body, and the use of certain herbs to treat such conditions as the 'rising of the mother' and the 'suffocation of the mother' reflected this principle. However, it may be useful now to regard these afflictions only as disruptions to the normal functioning of the body due to a distempered womb. The womb, like the brain and stomach, was said to be attracted by sweet smells and repelled by foul. Thus Culpeper's universal remedy for an overheated womb, arrach, which 'smells of old rotten fish, or something worse' may have been deemed so effective because it 'drove away' diseases from that organ. Again, for the 'rising of the womb' sweet-smelling things were to be applied to the vaginal area and the foul-smelling asafoetida to the nose. For prolapse of the womb, the opposite approach was taken. The importance of smell thus linked the womb and the brain, so that when the womb was afflicted, the brain suffered (today's pre-menstrual syndrome). Culpeper reasoned that since both the womb and the brain were associated with signs of the zodiac (Aries and Scorpio) ruled by the same planet, Mars, cephalic medicines (those used for the head) could also be used to treat the womb. Moreover, of burdock, a herb associated with the womb and made to be a herb of Venus, he says, 'by its leaf or seed you may draw the womb which way you please, either upwards by applying it to the crown of the head, in case it fall out, or downwards in fits of the mother, by applying it to the soles of the feet; or if you would stay it in its place, apply it to the navel, and that is one good way to stay the child in it'.

Culpeper imparted a knowledge of herbs which in his experience regulated the cyclical activity of the womb, whatever the reason for their action. He also laid out the treatments indicated for the various distempers of the male and female genitalia. Excessive heat was said to provoke lust and sexual activity in a person, and cold to kill it off. Excessive heat also caused dryness and this state, indicated by a lustful habit and much pubic hair, was remedied by wild lettuce, white pond lily, plantain, rose, silverweed and cooling foods such as cucumber and melon. The natural state of the male and female genitalia was reckoned to be hot and moist, and abstinence from sex to be more harmful for those of such a sanguine temperament. It would appear that an excessively hot condition of the genitals was the more troubling. The genitals in a cold and moist state made a person averse to sexual intercourse, and the relevant signs were little pubic hair and a failure to conceive or father a child. To remedy this, Culpeper advocates, among other herbs, mugwort, pennyroyal, juniper, tansy, vervain, feverfew, galangal, nutmeg and cinnamon. Those whose genitals were cold and dry were expected to be more infertile, these types preferring study to sex. To promote their fertility, they would be required to follow a more hot and moist diet by eating 'windy' foods such as peas, beans, parsnips, figs and pine-nuts and 'lustful, fruitful' animals such as crabs and prawns.

The Joints

Culpeper called medicines for the joints 'arthriticals'. He described the joints as 'nervous', so that cephalic medicines, such as cowslips or rosemary, were deemed best suited to them (although in a stronger dose, because of the distance of some joints from the centre of the body), as were other heating and drying medicines which are gently astringent. With pain and inflammation in a joint, the strategy was to give anodynes (pain killers) like chamomile, and cooling medicines, such as willow, or henbane externally, to counteract the heat of the inflammation. Heating medicines would then be administered, usually of a cutting and drawing action, to rectify its cause. Finally, gently astringent remedies were applied to strengthen the joints.

THE ACTIONS OF HERBAL MEDICINES

Herbal medicines were divided by Culpeper into the following categories.

Emollient medicines

According to Culpeper, emollient or softening medicines were used to reduce a hard substance such as an organ or swelling to its proper temperature. To do this, emollient medicines were in effect hot and moist and not at all astringent, despite some being categorized according to their taste as dry in some degree. In taste, emollient medicines were judged to be slightly sweet and fatty or oily, never sharp, sour or salty, with neither a rough nor a sticky feel. They were often used with cutting or attenuating medicines hot in the 2nd or 3rd degree. Examples:

- marsh mallow, sweet violet leaves and pellitory of the wall were accounted among the five emollient herbs, also white pond lily, linseed and fenugreek

Hardening medicines

Opposite to emollients were hardening medicines. Culpeper classified these as cold and dry in quality, with the action of *thickening* humours and, for any herb very cold in quality, of *congealing* them, as cold freezes water to ice. These were seen to have the power to close the pores and to stop insensible transpiration. All these medicines are astringent, with the power to soak up moisture like a sponge does water, or to balance the moisture with dryness. Examples:

- (*warming*) bistort, chaste free, balm
- (*temperate*) tormentil
- (*cooling*) rose, shepherd's purse, horsetail, plantain, comfrey and willow

Loosening medicines

Loosening medicines were said to have a relaxant effect on muscles, tendons, ligaments, and membranes and capsules over organs, when these are distended or stretched by dryness, cold, fullness of humours or swellings. Culpeper says they are indicated for 'cramps and convulsions'. They were judged hot and moist in quality but less hot and more moist than emollient medicines. The analogy of hard wax being softened was applied to the action of emollients and that of the stretched strings of a violin being loosened to the effect of loosening medicines. Examples:

- chickweed, cowslips, lavender, motherwort, St John's wort, betony, mullein, juniper, briony, pennyroyal, southernwood, centaury, gentian and elecampane

Attenuating medicines

Culpeper acknowledges that there was little difference between attenuating, drawing and discutient medicines, save that drawing medicines were hotter than discutients. Attenuating medicines *cut* and *thin* humours. They were judged to be sharp, sour or bitter in taste, with a 'dilating', as opposed to astringent, effect on the tongue. They were used to open obstructions of the bowels by cutting and thinning tough and viscous humours sticking to the walls of the digestive tract, to cleanse the lungs of phlegm, to encourage menstruation, and to promote other natural activities of the body impeded by the presence of thick humours. These herbal medicines were accounted hot and dry but some cooling medicines, such as vinegar or dandelion, were seen to have a cutting and therefore an attenuating action. They were prescribed after the body had been purged of the grossest of the humours, lest in dispersing some of the lighter parts of a humour by their heat, they left behind a harder obstruction to the free flow of the vital spirits and thus provoked a fever. Examples: *see under* 'Discutient medicines', below.

Drawing medicines

Drawing or 'attractive' medicines were perceived to be hotter than attenuating medicines. Culpeper says 'As all cold things bind and harden, as is apparent by the frost binding and hardening water and mire, so all things very hot and drying draw, as is clear by the Sun, who is the original of heat, drawing up the dew.' Drawing medicines could be used to remedy deranged humours in the bowels and were specifically employed externally to draw humours to the periphery of the body, to draw out poisons, splinters and thorns, to warm and to draw the vital or animal spirits to a part paralysed or in danger of becoming gangrenous. Examples: *see under* 'Discutient medicines', below.

Discutient or diaphoretic medicines
Discutient or 'discussing' medicines were also called diaphoretic. They worked by means of insensible transpiration through the promotion of sweating. All diaphoretic herbs were regarded as hot, even though their effect may be to cool the body by allowing heat to escape, and were credited with a drawing action also. They were found to have a burning or biting (pungent) taste. They were employed to treat plethoric conditions, along with blood-letting, and to cleanse the body of thin or watery humours or swellings and of vapours arising from over-heated organs. They were often indicated when the disease was past its peak, or certainly after the thicker humours causing the disease or swelling had been purged and attenuated, but sometimes they were applied in the rising stage of a disease due to heat of the blood. Examples of herbs with attenuating, drawing and diaphoretic actions:

- chamomile, melilot, marsh mallow, pellitory of the wall, mugwort, mint, lavender, hyssop, thyme, briony, rue, pepper, garlic
- for the 'discussion' of swellings, Culpeper particularly mentions cleavers, dock, balm, linseed and fenugreek

Another opening action belonged to those herbal medicines with the power to 'open the mouths of vessels'. These were used to remedy congestion by opening the blood vessels and allowing easy passage and flow of blood. They were easily recognized by their hot, sharp, piercing and biting or pungent taste, such as pepper, and were opposed in nature by cold and astringent remedies which close blood vessels. Examples:

- garlic, onions, pepper, and, among the 'five opening roots', fennel, parsley and celery

Repelling medicines
Repelling medicines were drawn from the cold, dry and astringent *hardening* herbs. They arrested 'fluxes' (discharges) such as diarrhoea and blood loss and were also used to divert humours elsewhere in the body. Their indications included hot swellings, headaches and fevers (vinegar of roses, for instance, would be applied to the head to drive away heat), and they were said to be tart or sharp in taste and were usually administered at the start of diseases. In the treatment of swellings they would be

used first, as diaphoretics were used last, with the warning not to overuse them in case the pores were overcontracted and the diaphoretics would not work later on. These repelling medicines were not administered in the presence of poison or great pain in the body. Examples: *see under* 'Hardening medicines', above.

Burning medicines

Burning medicines included *rubefacients*, which were used to draw blood and spirits to wasted or paralysed limbs, and the true *pyrotics* or burning medicines, employed to dissolve hard and callous tumours, to remove warts and polyps, to draw humours to the periphery of the body, and to treat gout and lethargy. They also had a use in the management of fistulae and malignant ulcers. They were not to be administered before the body had been purged. Rubefacients were to be tempered with milder medicines. Examples:

- (*rubefacient*) ginger, mustard
- (*true pyrotic*) cuckoo-pint

Cleansing medicines

Cleansing medicines were found to be either hot or cold and of a rough, earthy quality. They differed in medicinal effect from diaphoretics in that they carried away humours with them, while diaphoretics scattered the humours by their heat. Internally, some of them were used as purges, while externally they were applied to ulcers, to cleanse them of pus. Examples quoted by Culpeper:

- elder, agrimony, tansy, willow, horehound, southernwood, wormwood and pellitory of the wall

Glutinative medicines

Glutinative medicines were used to ripen ulcers by their heat, or to restore flesh to them. They were reckoned to be insipid, fatty or slightly sweet in taste, with a viscous or mucilaginous quality. After the application of glutinative medicines, astringent or *scarifying* herbs were put onto an ulcer as the final part of the cure. So-called *suppuring* medicines (gently warming to ripen a swelling) were applied externally to treat phlegmones (haematomas). Examples:

- (*glutinative*) comfrey, gentian, centaury, horsetail and plantain
- (*suppuring*) marsh mallow, briony and white pond lily

Diuretics

Diuretics were classified as either hot or cold. Hot diuretics, with a biting and cutting action, were used to help the kidneys separate out the waste from thick and viscid blood. Cold diuretics helped open the urinary passages by correcting their excessively dry, hot or inflamed state. Such a distemper had to be corrected before using diuretics in the treatment of hot dyscrasias or watery humours. Examples:

- (*heating diuretics*) ground ivy, betony, juniper, nettles, tansy and wormwood
- (*cooling diuretics*) burdock, dandelion and plantain, the 'greater cold seeds' of melons, gourds and cucumber and the 'four lesser cold seeds' of succory, endive, lettuce and purslane

Emmenogogues

Emmenogogues, or herbs promoting menstruation, were said to have an affinity with diuretics in as much as they too were classified as hot and attenuating. The retention of menstrual blood was reckoned to make the body diseased and liable to such things as dropsies, epilepsy and derangements of the mind. Culpeper says that, ideally, emmenogogues should be hot in the 3rd degree, in no way astringent, and administered when the period was due (or else nature would be weakened) to thin the blood and promote menstruation, along with pungent herbs to open the mouths of blood vessels to the womb. A body full of humours had first to be purged. Many herbs were counted as emmenogogues. Examples:

- southernwood, mugwort, rue, sage, thyme, nettles, rosemary, St John's wort, centaury, parsley, horehound, basil and even chamomile, valerian and calamus
- herbs used to curb excessive menstrual flow were taken from the astringent medicines and included bistort, shepherd's purse, plantain, white pond lily, comfrey and tormentil

Medicines to promote fertility

'Most herbs that are hot and moist and breed wind' (ie flatulence) were regarded as medicines to promote fertility or 'breed seed', for fertility depended on good blood. These had to be hotter for people of a phlegmatic temperament and more moist for the melancholic. Otherwise, excess heat in such medicines encouraged lust and if they were also very drying they would hinder fertility. Pungent medicines were said to stimulate the genitals but their constant use would 'scatter the seed' and reduce fertility. Examples:

- (*promoting seed*) galangal, raisins, sweet almonds, pine-nuts, figs, rocket, chick peas, beans and the 'keys' (the fruit) of the ash tree.

Galactogogues

The production of breast milk was also thought to be dependent on a supply of good blood, since the creation in the body of milk or seed represented a fourth concoction of the blood. Thus any abundance of humours had to be purged before using galactogogues, or herbs to promote the production of breast milk. Such herbs were usually temperately hot. Examples:

- wild lettuce, fennel and marsh mallow to promote milk, (and mint to repress its production).

Carminative medicines

Herbs used to expel wind were called carminative. They were known to be hot and biting or pungent. Examples:

- (*hot*) fennel, anise, cumin and caraway
- (*less hot*) celery, wild carrot and cardamom
- (*others*) chamomile, pepper, wormwood, garlic, angelica and parsley

Anodynes

To ease pain, anodynes were used externally. These would not heal a disease but would bring relief from painful symptoms. To do this, in either a hot or cold condition, they had to be fairly temperate in quality, for pain was seen to be an effect of a sudden and extreme change of quality in a part. Temperate medicines which were slightly attenuating could let out the hot vapours causing the pain through the pores and restore the part to equilibrium. Narcotic herbs eased pain by numbing the part and dulling the senses. Examples:

- (*temperate*) chamomile, linseed, fenugreek, wormwood, fennel, dill and rosemary
- (*narcotic*) henbane

Purging medicines

Purging medicines were distinguished according to their gentle or violent manner of operation and whether they purged by stool or by vomiting. Purging by vomiting was reckoned generally more violent and was never administered to someone with a weak stomach. Culpeper urges his readers to use 'vomits' as little as possible. Purging in general was not carried out if the patient was weak in any of the three primary faculties, was excessively thin, obese or anaemic, was experiencing spasms or fluxes such as diarrhoea, or was engaged in hard manual labour. Purging was avoided in Winter and Summer, in the very young or very old, and usually in those of choleric temperament. The powerful purges of Culpeper's day were scammony for choler, black hellebore for melancholy, and colocynth for phlegm and watery humours. However, Culpeper warns that these can kill and recommends gentler purging wherever possible. Such remedies were taken regularly to have a gradual effect, as is often the practice today. This was necessary with tough and viscous humours of long continuance, for instance, especially melancholic humours. Examples:

- (*for purging choler*) wormwood, hops, aloes, prunes and rhubarb
- (*for phlegm and water*) hyssop, elder and broom
- (*for melancholy*) senna and fumitory

PHARMACY

In his herbal,[30] Culpeper recommends that if leaves are needed, they should be green and full of juice, the blemished ones discarded, and must be picked where the plant likes to grow and where it is prolific. Thus, 'betony which grows in the shadow is far better than that which grows in the Sun, because it delights in the shadow.' Herbs which like to grow by water should be picked by water, and so on. Leaves from flowers which run to seed should be picked before the plant is in flower, otherwise the flowering tops of the plant ought to be used. Culpeper recommends all herbs to be dried in the Sun, then kept in a dry place. Herbs which grow on dry ground or are dry in quality should keep longer than those that grow in damp places or are full of juice. The signs of a dried herb past its best are loss of colour and loss of smell.

The above also applies to the gathering of flowers. Seeds should be gathered when fully ripened and are easily kept for quite some time but are best in the year after their collection. As for roots, Culpeper thinks they can be taken at any time in the growing season, preferably on a dry day when the roots are whole and free of rottenness; they should then be hung up to dry. Barks are to be collected in the Spring when they are most easily removed from a tree. Roots and bark are usually boiled or decocted to extract their qualities more easily. Such decoctions, Culpeper says, 'are of most use in such diseases as lie in the passages of the body, as the stomach, bowels, kidneys, passages of urine and bladder, because decoctions pass quicker to those places than any other form of medicines'. Decoctions can be sweetened with sugar or an appropriate syrup and kept only for a few days, and 'if the weather be hot, not half so long'. In making compound decoctions, using various parts of different herbs, each must be added in sequence according to the length of time taken to extract their qualities. Thus roots and barks are cooked first, then herbs, seeds, flowers, and finally spices.

If the juice of a plant is required, it should be pressed out of the plant and then set over a fire. This will cause the scum to rise to the surface, which can be skimmed off leaving a clarified juice. Culpeper then advocates two methods of preserving the juice. One way, used particularly for the juice of fruits, is to boil the juice down to the thickness of honey. This was called a *rob* and was used in treatments of the mouth. The other way was to put oil on top of the juice in its container, to a depth of two fingers. In dispensing a juice preserved this way, a little oil would come out of the bottle also. This was spooned off and any juice taken in excess of the immediate requirement could be put back into the bottle where it would sink below the oil once again.

Herbal medicines were administered in a variety of forms. Easiest of all was a **simple**, a single herb infused in boiled water to make a tea or boiled, strained and drunk as a decoction. A 'convenient' measure, Culpeper says, is a handful of the herbs to a pint of liquid for a simple infusion and the dose for a decoction was from 2 to 5 fluid ounces at a time, ie up to a wineglass full.

Compound preparations involved using a number of herbs to make these and other forms of medicines.

Simple or distilled waters were produced by the distillation of herbs in water, the distillation being fractionated to separate out the essential or 'chymical' oil if the plant possessed such a volatile component. Culpeper judged such simple waters 'the weakest of artificial medicines, and good for little unless for mixtures of other medicines'. Many herbs were prepared in this way (and rose water and elder flower water are still made today), or mixed together to make compound waters. Herbal infusions have taken their place today. As for the *essential oils* of single herbs, Culpeper warns his readers that they 'generally are not to be taken alone by themselves by reason of their vehement heat and burning, but mixed with other convenient medicines ... The general way of taking them is to drop two or three drops of them in any convenient liquor or other medicine.' He mentions the essential oils of wormwood, hyssop, marjoram, the mints, oregano, pennyroyal, rosemary, rue, sage, thyme, chamomile, lavender, orange and lemon. Of rosemary, he comments that 'the chymical oil drawn from the leaves and flowers is a sovereign help ... to touch the temples and nostrils with two or three drops for all the diseases of the head and brains spoken of before'. **Spirits** were also prepared by distilling one or more herbs in wine, or by macerating spices in alcohol or 'spirit of wine'.

Single herbs, such as dried wormwood, rosemary and eyebright, were also steeped in wine and set in the Sun for 30–40 days to make a *physical wine*. Other herbs such as squills were similarly prepared in *vinegar*. A posset drink, made from hot milk and curdled with cold ale, was regarded as temperate in quality and taken as a medicinal drink with the addition of fresh herbs, usually of a cooling quality to treat hot conditions.

Syrups were made from the decoction, infusion or juice of one or more herbs, heated with sugar or honey to make a thick liquid. Generally, Culpeper thought this vehicle for herbal medicines good for the weak and for those with queasy stomachs. Syrups were usually either alterative (that is, they alter the qualities of heat, cold, dryness and moisture in the body), cordial or purging, sugar being a suitably moist addition to cherish the innate heat of the heart or, for purges, to encourage the expulsive virtue. Culpeper reckoned that a well-made syrup should last a year. The addition of two fluid ounces of a suitable syrup to a pint of the simple water of a herb made a **julep**, for immediate use only. They were commonly used to prepare the body for purging, to open obstructions and the pores, to digest tough humours, and to temper imbalances of heat. Syrups were also made with vinegar and honey instead of sugar. These were called **oxymels**.

Culpeper named a thicker sort of syrup a **lohoch**, although we know it by its Latin name of *linctus*. He used it for 'roughness of the windpipe, diseases and inflammations of the lungs, difficulty of breathing, colds, coughs, etc' and suggested it should be taken on the bruised end of a liquorice stick and held in the mouth to let it melt of its own accord. An **electuary**, on the other hand, was made by the addition of powdered herbs to a syrup or clarified honey, the product needing to be well mixed. These were often cordial or purging in action, the dose being a half to two drams (drachms) (about 2–8 grams) and a half to one ounce respectively. Herbs were powdered and added for immediate use.

Conserves and **preserves** represented another vehicle for herbal medicines. Conserves were made by beating together sugar and the leaves or flowers of herbs, while preserves were syrups containing pieces of fruit, like our jams, or roots. Preserves were seldom made from flowers or barks. Culpeper says that some conserves, such as conserve of roses, can keep for many years, while others made from borage or cowslips will only last a year and must be regularly checked for signs of spoiling, namely the formation of a hard crust on top 'with little holes in it, as though worms had been eating there'. Once again, these preparations were suitable for 'sick and squeamish stomachs'.

Pills were regarded as an appropriate vehicle for very bitter medicines because they could be swallowed without tasting them. They were, according to Culpeper, originally invented for purging the head, since 'they are longer in digestion and therefore the better able to call the offending humour to them'. They were made either by the addition of powdered herbs to a syrup and rolled into balls or else the herbs were boiled and reduced to a soft extract and shaped into pills to harden. Both pills and **troches**, or 'little cakes', could be made by mixing powdered herbs with the mucilage of gum tragacanth and left to harden. Troches of wormwood or galangal were carried in the pockets of those with cold and weak stomachs, to take as the need arose. **Pessaries** were another similar vehicle for the administration of herbal medicines to particular parts of the body.

Fixed **oils** were made by steeping and gently boiling herbs in olive oil or by adding herbs steeped in wine to oil in a water bath which was heated to evaporate the wine. Some oils were made by steeping a herb in olive oil and by leaving it in the Sun for a certain number of days, this last being an oil made by infusion rather than by decoction. Other oils were obtained by pressing it out, such as olive oil itself or oil of almonds. These and other oily liquids made from boiling the herbs in hog's grease could be mixed with turpentine and wax to make an **ointment**. There were, in fact, many different ways to make an ointment depending on what it was to contain. Thus there were both *simple* and *compound ointments.* Ointments could be spread upon a suitable cloth to make a **plaster**.

TABLE OF SOME COMMONLY USED MEDICINAL HERBS SHOWING THEIR QUALITIES AND ACTIONS

Definitions are taken from Culpeper's herbal, *The English Physician Enlarged* (1656), and from the catalogue of 'simples' in the old and new dispensatories in *Pharmacopoeia Londinensis* (1669).[31]

PLANT NAME	LATIN NAME	PLANET RULER	QUALITIES	PARTS AFFECTED	MAIN ACTIONS
Agrimony	*Agrimonia eupatoria*	Jupiter in Cancer	hot 1 dry 1	heats liver/ spleen, kidneys/joints	cleansing, cutting, binding
Angelica	*Angelica archangelica*	Sun in Leo	hot 3 dry 3	heats heart, stomach & womb	resists poison, carminative
Lemon Balm	*Melissa officinalis*	Jupiter in Cancer	hot 2 dry 2	heats & dries lungs, heart & stomach	cheers heart & mind by purging melancholy
Betony	*Betonica officinalis*	Jupiter in Aries	hot 2 dry 2	heats head, lungs & kidneys; dries heart	diuretic, opens obstructions
Borage	*Borago officinalis*	Jupiter in Leo	hot 1 moist 1	heats & moistens heart	comforts heart, expels melancholy
Greater Celandine	*Chelidonium majus*	Sun in Leo	hot 3 dry 3	heats head & liver; treats eyes	sharp, cutting, cleansing, discutient

PLANT NAME	LATIN NAME	PLANET RULER	QUALITIES	PARTS AFFECTED	MAIN ACTIONS
Chamomile	*Matricaria chamomilla*	Sun	hot 1 dry 1	heats head, liver & joints	anodyne, purges choler
Chaste Tree	*Vitex agnus-castus*	Mars	hot 3 dry 3	consumes procreative seed	astringent, sharp, discutient, carminative
Cinnamon	*Cinnamomum zeylandicum*	Sun	hot 2 dry 2	heats lungs, heart, stomach & womb	attenuating, cleansing, softening, diuretic
Coltsfoot	*Tussilago farfara*	Venus	cold 1 dry 1	cools lungs	treats inflammations
Dandelion	*Taraxacum officinale*	Jupiter	cold 2 dry 2	cools stomach & liver	opening, cleansing, healing, diuretic
Eyebright	*Euphrasia officinalis*	Sun in Leo	hot 1 dry 1	heats head	restores sight, strengthens brain
Feverfew	*Tanacetum parthenium*	Venus	hot 3 dry 2	heats head & womb	emmenogogue, purges choler & phlegm
Fumitory	*Fumaria officinalis*	Saturn	cold 2 dry 2	cools head, liver, bowels & spleen	opening, clears skin & purges melancholy
Garlic	*Allium sativum*	Mars	hot 4 dry 4	heats body extremely	resists poison, diuretic, carminative, binding
Gentian	*Gentiana lutea*	Mars	hot dry	heats liver & spleen	opening, cutting, cleansing, glutinating
Ginger	*Zingiber officinale*	Mars	hot 3 dry 3	heats stomach, bowels & joints	carminative, digestive, discutient, diuretic

PLANT NAME	LATIN NAME	PLANET RULER	QUALITIES	PARTS AFFECTED	MAIN ACTIONS
Henbane	*Hyoscyamus niger*	Saturn	cold 4	cools joints & inflammations	narcotic, poisonous, external use only
Hops	*Humulus lupulus*	Mars dry 2	hot 2 bowels &	heats liver, choler & spleen	purges phlegm, diuretic, opening, cleansing
White Horehound	*Marrubium vulgare*	Mercury	hot 2 dry 3	heats lungs, liver & spleen	cutting, opening, cleansing, discutient
Juniper	*Juniperus communis*	Sun	hot 3 dry 1	heats heart, stomach kidneys & bladder	opening, cutting, diuretic, carminative
Lavender	*Lavandula officinalis*	Mercury	hot 3 dry 3	heats head	opening, diuretic, not used in plethora
Wild Lettuce	*Lactuca virosa*	Moon	cold 2 moist 2	cools most parts of the body	hypnotic, galactogogue c/i lung disease*
Mallow	*Malva* spp.	Venus	cold/ moist 1	cools bowel/kidneys	purges choler
Marsh Mallow	*Althaea officinalis*	Venus	hot/dry 1	kidneys, heats	emollient, glutinating
Mint	*Mentha* spp.	Venus	hot 3 dry 3	heats stomach & womb	binding, digestive, stops milk, discutient
Mugwort	*Artemisia vulgaris*	Venus	hot 2 dry 2	heats womb	emmenogogue, attenuating, for women

* c/i means 'contra-indicated in'. Most herbs heating or cooling the kidneys affect the bladder similarly.

PLANT NAME	LATIN NAME	PLANET RULER	QUALITIES	PARTS AFFECTED	MAIN ACTIONS
Stinging Nettle	*Urtica dioica*	Mars	hot 3 dry 3	heats lungs, kidneys, womb	opening, diuretic, astringent, antilithic
Parsley	*Petroselinum crispum*	Mercury	hot 2 dry 2	heats stomach, liver & spleen	diuretic, carminative, cutting, emmenogogue
Plantain	*Plantago* spp.	Venus	cold 2 dry 2	cools head, lungs, bowels, & kidneys	cleansing, glutinating, astringent, repelling
Rose	*Rosa* spp.	Jupiter/ Venus	cold 1 dry 1	cools head, lungs heart & stomach	strengthening animal & vital virtue, astringent
Rosemary	*Rosmarinus officinalis*	Sun in Aries	hot 2 dry 2	heats and dries head, heart & joints	astringent, carminative, helps memory
Rue	*Ruta graveolens*	Sun in Leo	hot 3 dry 3	heats lungs, heart & joints	emmenogogue, resists poison, cutting
Sage	*Salvia officinalis*	Jupiter	hot 2 dry 2	heats stomach, liver, spleen, womb, joints	astringent, diuretic, emmenogogue
Senna	*Cassia* spp.	Mercury	hot 2 dry 1	heats head, heart, liver & spleen	purges melancholy, choler & phlegm
Blessed Thistle	*Carduus benedictus*	Mars in Aries	hot 2 dry 2	heats head & heart	opening, cleansing, resists poison
Thyme	*Thymus vulgaris*	Venus	hot 3 dry 3	heats head, lungs, stomach & womb	diuretic, emmenogogue

PLANT NAME	LATIN NAME	PLANET RULER	QUALITIES	PARTS AFFECTED	MAIN ACTIONS
Valerian	*Valeriana officinalis*	Mercury	hot 1 dry 2	heats heart, bowels & kidneys	astringent, diuretic & emmeno-gogue
Vervain	*Verbena officinalis*	Venus	hot 2 dry 2	heats head, kidneys & womb	opening, cleansing, healing & strengthen-ing
Sweet Violet	*Viola odorata*	Venus	cold 1 moist 2	cools head, lungs, heart & stomach	cleansing, cooling, cordial, purges choler
Willow	*Salix* spp.	Moon	cold 2 dry 2	cools head & joints	cleansing, astringent without sharpness
Worm-wood	*Artemisia absinthium*	Mars	hot 1/2 dry 1/2	heats stomach & spleen	cleansing, purges choler, strengthen-ing
Yarrow	*Achillea mille-folium*	Venus	cold 1 dry 1	cools kidneys and bladder	astringent, healing, glutinating

The table above lists two sorts of qualities of the herbs – both their *manifest* qualities of heat, cold, dryness and moisture, and their *hidden* qualities by virtue of astral influence. Culpeper's assignation of a planetary ruler, and thus a hidden quality, to each plant in his herbal was comprehensive. He was critical of 'the practice of most physicians [I say not of all] in these later ages as well as ours, to say when they cannot give, nor are minded to study a reason why a herb, plant, etc hath such an operation or produceth such an effect in the body of Man, it doth it by a hidden quality', because they failed in 'not minding the whole creation, not knowing what belongs to *astral influence,* not regarding that excellent harmony the only wise God hath made a composition of contraries [in the knowledge of which consists the whole ground and foundation of physick], no more than a horse that goes along the street regards when the clock strikes.'[32]

Astrology thus illuminated and aided Culpeper's practice of physick and he wanted to reveal its benefits to others. He wrote: 'Wormwood is a herb of Mars ... I prove it thus. What delights in Martial places is a Martial herb. But wormwood delights in places (for about forges and iron works you may gather a cart load of it) ergo it is a Martial herb.' Stinking arrach (*Chenopodium olidum*), also named vulvaria or stinking motherwort, is 'a herb under the dominion of Venus and under the sign Scorpio. It is common almost upon every dunghill.' This example shows how Culpeper sometimes found grounds to associate not only a planet but also a sign of the zodiac with a plant; the latter specifying which part of the body the herb has a particular affinity with. For although in the case of stinking arrach its planetary ruler refers to those parts of the body ruled by Venus, namely the kidneys and organs of reproduction, the connection with Scorpio indicates the herb's use for diseases of the latter. Culpeper therefore commends it as a universal medicine for the womb because it corrects excess heat in that organ by qualities of coldness and moisture.

In the case of motherwort (*Leonurus cardiaca*), a herb of Venus in Leo, the calming, soothing qualities attributed to the planet are made apparent in the herb's use as a sedative affecting the nerves, but its particular affinity is for the heart. It is a tonic for that organ and used to treat palpitations. Rosemary (*Rosmarinus officinalis*), a herb of the Sun in Aries, which flowers each year when the Sun passes through that sign, has a particular relation to the head since Aries is associated with the head. It is hot and dry in the 2nd degree, a nerve and heart tonic, good for the memory and certain kinds of (cold) headaches. Fennel (*Foeniculum vulgare*), ruled by Mercury in Virgo, has an affinity for the brain (Mercury) and bowels (Virgo).

It was Culpeper's intention, by associating a planet, and in some cases a zodiac sign, to each herb, that his readers should understand which remedies strengthened the various organs and parts of the body according to cosmic sympathy. He wrote in the introduction to his herbal:

> I knew well enough, the whole world, and everything in it, was formed of a composition of contrary elements, and in such a harmony as must needs show the wisdom and power of a great God. I knew as well, this creation, though thus composed of contraries, was

one united body, and man an epitome of it. I knew those various affections in man in respect of sickness and health were caused naturally (though God may have other ends best known to himself) by the various operations of the microcosm. And I could not be ignorant that as the cause is, so must the cure be. And therefore he that would know the reason of the operation of herbs must look up as high as the stars. I always found the disease vary according to the various motions of the stars. And this is enough one would think to teach a man by the effect where the cause lay.

Culpeper thus put astrology at the heart of his herbal because the study of the natural world by which to attain the knowledge to heal extended 'as high as the stars'. For the opinion prevailed that 'what many physicians have failed to accomplish with the most potent drugs, an astrologer has effected by use of a simple herb through intelligent observation of the access and recess of the signs'.[33] This, then, is Culpeper's medicine: a practice of Western holistic medicine that draws on all the natural powers in the cosmos to relieve and heal the sufferings of the sick and to teach the preservation in health of body, mind and soul.

APPENDICES

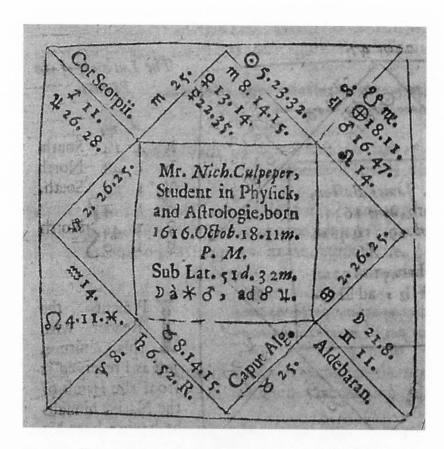

Figure 14 The natal horoscope of Nicholas Culpeper, as cast by John Gadbury, from his Collectio Geniturarum *(1662).*

APPENDIX 1

The Natal Horoscope of Nicholas Culpeper

Culpeper's School of Physick, published in 1659, contained a 13-page calculation and judgement on Nicholas Culpeper's natal horoscope,[1] shown opposite,[2] by the astrologer John Gadbury. I will use this to show the calculation of the temperament from a natal horoscope, to augment what is known of Culpeper's use of the symbolism of his nativity and to examine and improve upon Gadbury's own rectification of Culpeper's horoscope.

Gadbury's reading of Culpeper's temperament from his natal horoscope was as follows:

> His temperature, according to astrologers, should be melancholy-choleric, as is plain by an earthy sign ascending and Saturn's position in an earthy sign also. And the Moon being among Martial fixed stars, and stars of the same nature in the ascendant are very strong testimonies of choler prevailing over this native. But the greatest argument of choler predominating I take to be the Sun's reception with Mars from violent signs, which seems to signify that choler should overpower the humour of melancholy, notwithstanding an earthy sign ascending &c.
>
> He was indeed of such a temperature. I remembered to have heard him confess that melancholy was an extraordinary enemy unto him, so great at some times that, wanting company, he would seem like a dead man. And at other times would his choler macerate him very strangely, yea, more often than the distemper of melancholy.

Culpeper offered the opinion that 'complexion, or temperature of body is better judged by an argument *a priore* than by an argument *a posteriore*, from the nativity than from the effects of it, for foreign climates and sickness alter the colour.'[3] Consequently, the astrological assessment of temperament is most necessary. A method of determining the temperament from the natal horoscope is given by Lilly in his *Christian Astrology* (1647).[4] The qualities of the following factors must be noted.

- The sign ascending. Example: if Gemini, a hot and moist sign, ascends, it is marked hot and moist in the calculations.
- The planet ruling the ascendant. Example: if Mercury is the Ascendant ruler, he is cold and dry.
- The sign positions of planets in aspect to the ascendant degree. Example: if Mars in Pisces is square to the Ascendant, this is from a cold and moist sign.
- The sign position of the Moon. Example: Moon in Taurus is in a cold and dry sign. If the Moon is also in the Ascendant, these qualities are doubled, eg cold 2 and dry 2 when rising in Taurus.
- The sign positions of planets in aspect to the Moon.
- The sign position of the dispositor of the Moon. Example: Moon in Taurus is in a sign ruled by Venus. She is thus the Moon's dispositor. If she is in Aries, she is in a hot and dry sign.
- The season of the year. Example: when the Sun is between the Spring equinox and the Summer solstice, in other words falling in either Aries, Taurus or Gemini, he is given the qualities of that season, namely hot and moist. When between the Summer solstice and the Autumn equinox, he is hot and dry, etc.
- The sign position of the planet in the horoscope which, according to its placing, is strongest in essential and accidental fortitudes. *See* Lilly's tables.[5] If this planet is also the Ascendant ruler, the qualities are tripled.

To the total for each of the qualities from these factors are added the qualities of the planets according to their relationship with the Sun, as follows:

Table of Qualities

PLANET ASPECTING MOON OR ASCENDANT	USUAL QUALITIES	IF ORIENTAL OR RISING BEFORE SUN	IF OCCIDENTAL OR SETTING AFTER SUN	MOON PHASE	QUALITIES
Saturn	cold & dry	cold & moist	dry	from new to 1st quarter	hot & moist
Jupiter	hot & moist	hot & moist	moist	from 1st quarter to full	hot & dry

PLANET ASPECTING MOON OR ASCENDANT	USUAL QUALITIES	IF ORIENTAL OR RISING BEFORE SUN	IF OCCIDENTAL OR SETTING AFTER SUN	MOON PHASE	QUALITIES
Mars	hot & dry	hot & dry	dry	from full to last quarter	cold & dry
Venus	cold and moist	hot & moist	moist	from last quarter to new	cold & moist
Mercury	cold & dry	hot	dry		

Clearly there is much complexity in the determination of the temperament from the natal horoscope, and in the final analysis it depends on sound astrological judgement. For if either Saturn or Mars, the intemperate malefics, aspect by conjunction, square or opposition the Moon or Ascendant (and I would include the Sun as well), they strongly tip the temperament towards melancholy or choler respectively.[6] In Culpeper's horoscope both Saturn and Mars are thus configured with the Sun, emphasizing his choleric-melancholic temperament. The calculation of the temperament from his horoscope runs as follows:

TABLE OF CALCULATION

SIGNIFICATORS OF TEMPERAMENT		HOT	COLD	DRY	MOIST
1 the sign ascending	Capricorn		1	1	
2 the Ascendant ruler	Saturn		1	1	
3 sign positions of planets aspecting Ascendant					
Saturn by trine	Taurus		1	1	
Sun by sextile	Autumn		1	1	
4 Moon sign	Gemini	1			1
5 sign positions of planets aspecting Moon					
Mars by sextile	Leo	1		1	
Jupiter by opposition	Sagittarius	1		1	
6 sign position of Mercury, dispositor of Moon	Scorpio		1		1

SIGNIFICATORS OF TEMPERAMENT		HOT	COLD	DRY	MOIST
7 season denoted by Sun sign	Autumn		1	1	
8 sign position of strongest planet, Mercury	Scorpio		1		1
SUB-TOTAL		3	7	7	3
Saturn occidental				1	
Mars oriental		1		1	
Jupiter occidental					1
Moon phase			1	1	
TOTAL		4	8	10	4

The cold and dry qualities of melancholy stand out here. Culpeper wrote in 1650:

> I am exceedingly melancholy of complexion, subject to consumptions and chilliness of my vital spirits, a slavish and sickly life being allotted to me in this city. I had the Sun opposite to Saturn in my nativity, which probably may be the natural cause of it.[7]

Saturn as Ascendant ruler befits a scholar and Puritan such as Culpeper but he was not dour or mean-spirited because of it. Saturn's conjunction with Pluto may undermine the tendency to strict orthodoxy and self-discipline, while Mars in square to and in mutual reception with the Sun provides the spark of choler, as Gadbury attests, which frequently inflamed Culpeper's tinder-dry melancholic temperament.

From another point of view, the mutual reception of Mars, ruler of his house of achievement and honour, with the Sun in Scorpio culminating there, is a powerful testimony to his fame and reputation lasting way beyond his own death and even into the present day, as if the potency of his life's work is continually renewed. Moreover, Culpeper was a revolutionary and innovator, which the trine of this Sun in Scorpio to Uranus aptly symbolizes, whose infamy among the politicians and doctors was far outweighed by his popularity among the population at large (Uranus in the 7th). Through it all, his compassion for and struggle in support of the common man and woman shine through, as perhaps the close, challenging square from Neptune in Libra to the rectified Ascendant, and his own melancholic temperament, denote.

The strength of Mercury natally in square to Mars illustrates the maxim that the pen is mightier than the sword and Culpeper's writings were welcomed in the new Commonwealth, born from victory against the King in the Civil War. This aspect signifies his increased mental energy, by which his physical health further suffered, his combative style, sharp tongue and the attacks he made on the abuses which he saw in medicine, the Church and the legal profession. The conjunction of Mercury and Venus provided a mordant charm to his writing style but Mars kept him to the point and he loved brevity. The square from Mars to the three planets in Scorpio gave him a militant and subversive edge, with Scorpio signifying his desire to uncover and communicate the truth as he saw it, especially in medicine and in occult subjects such as astrology.

Culpeper reckoned the Moon 'exceeding weak in my genesis, being in a cadent house and in Gemini, a sign which in my opinion more afflicts the Moon than Capricorn'.[8] This restless position for the Moon is amplified by her opposition to Jupiter which can denote self-indulgence, indifference to money and enforced residence in other countries. Charles Carter wrote of the Moon that 'almost any contact of Jupiter tends to bring the native to some extent in touch with ease, comfort and a certain amount of success'.[9] If Culpeper's own money passed easily through his hands, he gained material benefit from his marriage to Alice Culpeper. Gadbury accepted that the Moon in a 'double bodied sign' such as Gemini might indicate two wives, but he thought the awful condition of Venus in Culpeper's horoscope, which prejudiced a good marriage and healthy children, contradicted it. Perhaps Alice was his 'second' wife, after he lost his first love in such tragic circumstances.

Gadbury cast Culpeper's horoscope for the 'estimate time of the birth' of 'a little after noon' on Friday 18 October (old style) 1616 at the latitude of London. Gadbury established the birth time to be eleven minutes past noon (and with the Moon cadent as Culpeper described it) by a process of astrological rectification according to the following events in Culpeper's life:

- going to university: Sun directed to a conjunction of Mercury
- commencement of his practice of physick: Moon directed to a trine of Mercury

- wounded in the Civil War: Ascendant directed to a square of the Sun and then to a square of Saturn
- death: Ascendant directed to an opposition with Mars, together with an unfortunate solar return for the year 1653–4

Gadbury ascertained that Mercury is by far the strongest planet in Culpeper's horoscope, citing his most famous books as proof of his erudition and learning. Saturn's rulership of the Ascendant (the body) and its affliction of the Sun from the cusp of the 4th house is pertinently activated when Culpeper sustained a wound to the chest 'which he never recovered of till his dying day', at which time, eleven years later, the Ascendant degree itself, directed by some unclear measure, opposed Mars, the other malefic planet, natally placed in the 8th house of death.

This appears to be textbook astrological symbolism. Gadbury cast Culpeper's horoscope for London, perhaps for the sake of ease, when he may have been born at Ockley in Surrey, and some astrologers consider his rectifications of the horoscopes of famous individuals to be sometimes dubious. (Here, for instance, Gadbury gives 1634 as the date of Culpeper's going up to Cambridge University, but Thulesius has shown that Culpeper started as an apprentice apothecary in London that year.) Thus I have wanted to rectify Culpeper's horoscope myself. Given the difference between mean and true solar time at the time of year that Culpeper was born, the sundial time of his birth would always be 'a little after' its clock time. I have rectified Culpeper's natal horoscope for a birth time of 12:00:49 (indeed 'a little after noon') at Ockley, on the basis of a progression of Jupiter to the Ascendant at the time of his death, as I will show. My rectified data gives the horoscope on the page opposite.

Owing to the fact that this horoscope differs substantially from Gadbury's only in the zodiac degrees of the Ascendant and Midheaven, secondary progressions (rather than directions, which Gadbury used) of and to these points are deciding factors. I find that for 1632, when Culpeper went to university, not only the Sun but also the Ascendant progressed to Mercury, by conjunction and sextile respectively. Also, when he and Alice Culpeper tied the knot in 1640, the Moon progressed to a trine of the Ascendant in the October of that year, although, since we do not know in which month they married, this progression does

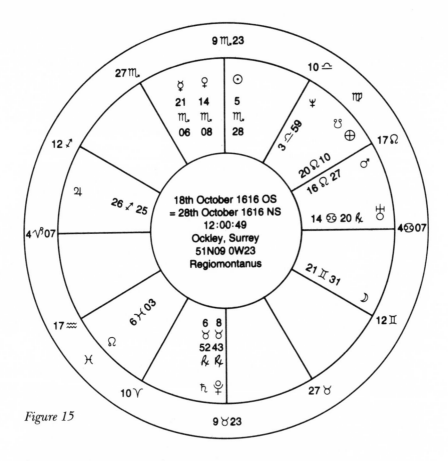

Figure 15

not confirm the rectification.

Culpeper entered a very difficult period two years later. Firstly, he was accused of witchcraft, the case coming to court on 17 December 1642. Secondly, he fought in the war and was wounded in the chest. Thirdly, the Society of Apothecaries hounded Leadbetter to get rid of Culpeper, his unqualified assistant, in the Summer and Autumn of 1643. During these 12 months the progressed Ascendant squared first the Sun and then, crucially, Saturn. Between these contacts, a progressed full Moon occurred, the only one in his life, representing some sort of hiatus. The following year, too, the rectified Ascendant progressed to the square of Pluto. So, leaving Leadbetter on a progression of the Midheaven square the nodes, he famously set up a busy practice at home in Spitalfields. His health was now undermined, as the affliction of the progressed Ascendant by Saturn graphically symbolizes, and eventually he would give up consulting in favour of the less physically demanding occupation of writing. In 1642 progressed Mercury opposed his natal Moon from the 12th house at the time of the witchcraft case. Mercury turned retrograde by progression four years later in 1646, the earliest date I have found in his writings,[10] and made contact with the natal Moon again in 1649, when his first book, *A Physical Directory*, was published. Subsequent busy contacts with the Part of Fortune, a point in a horoscope denoting material gain, and Mars, and the progressed Ascendant and Midheaven, occurred during these last four years of his life, as his other famous works were brought into print.

In this phase of his life, during the Summer and Autumn of 1653, the progressed Midheaven aspected first natal Mars by trine and then progressed Mercury by conjunction. This elevation of Mercury and its own progressed trine to Mars in Leo, in the 8th house and conjunct the Part of Fortune, coincided with his experimentation with the alchemical medicine Aurum Potabile. Apparently assured of its benefits, he made the sale of this cordial (Leo) a legacy (8th house) for his wife just before his death, when the progressed Moon, ruler of his 7th house, sextiled the Part of Fortune. This legacy was subsequently fraught with problems, symbolized by the conjunction of the Part of Fortune with Mars, but the natal reception between Mars and the Sun assured the endurance of his own fame and of the legacy he bequeathed to his fellow countrymen in his life's work, his writings.

Returning now to the Summer of 1634, when I believe the catastrophic loss of his first love occurred, Saturn progressed to the exact opposition of the natal Sun. This once-in-a-lifetime progression symbolizes a great blow to young Culpeper and triggers his melancholic affliction, which accompanied him as a child who never knew his father. The loss of his young love is emphasized by progressed Venus square the nodes and the passage of the progressed Moon, ruler of the 7th house, through and in square to the Sun/Midheaven/Saturn/Pluto opposition. Because the manner of his young love's death – being struck by lightning – was so strange, it would be appropriate to find Jupiter, who rules over thunder and lightning, to be involved. Certainly the natal configuration of Jupiter, ruler of the 12th house of suffering, in the 12th house opposite the Moon, ruler of the 7th house of partners, seems to symbolize this possibility. In May 1634 Jupiter transited the descendant of the natal horoscope. But can we consider Jupiter dignified in his own sign of Sagittarius as a bringer of such loss?

Gadbury identified Jupiter with Culpeper's private enemies,

the 'divines' or churchmen, who 'did disgust him for his studying astrology'. So Jupiter may also symbolize Culpeper's grandfather, William Attersole, who scorned him for not entering the Church and left him with a paltry inheritance at his death in 1640, when Jupiter was transiting Culpeper's ascendant. Furthermore, a Moon-Jupiter opposition signifies quarrels over religion. However, neither of these transits of Jupiter over the natal horizon actually confirms my rectified Ascendant. But progressed Jupiter finally emerges from the 12th house by conjoining this Ascendant in 1654, 4 days after Culpeper died. Since this too is a rare progression, involving a planet already shown to embody loss, I have used it as the basis of my rectification of Culpeper's horoscope. The consolation of Jupiter on the Ascendant now is to free Culpeper from his suffering in the physical world, having carried out God's will, with a hope of life everlasting in the world to come.

7. Regard the Heart, keep that upon the Wheels becauſe the Sun is the Fountain of Life, and therefore thoſe Univerſal Remedies *Aurum potabile*, and the Phyloſophers Stone, cure all Diſeaſes by only ſortifying the Heart.

But that this may appear unto you as cleer as the Sun when he is upon the Meridian, I here quote you an Example, which I performed when I was as far off from my ſtudy as I am now, yet am I not aſhamed the world ſhould ſee how much or little of my Leſſon I have learned without Book.

On *July*, 25. 1651. there came a Letter to me out of *Bedfordſhire*, from a Gentleman (at that time) altogether to me unknown, though ſince well known, who was a Student both in Aſtrologie and Phyſick: The words which are theſe;

Mr. *Culpeper*,

My Love remembred unto you, although I know you not by face; yet becauſe I do much reſpect that pretty little Lark, you ſo lately let fly into the world, which you call Semeiotica Uranica, which I have lately taken into my Cage; I am therefore imboldned to write unto you in the behalf of a Neighbors wife, who is taken with a very violent Diſeaſe which began in the lowr parts of her Body, but is now aſcended upwards, and tormenteth her in her Breaſt, Throat, Tongue, and Lips: This Diſeaſe took poſſeſſion of her (as ſhe relateth to me) about a fortnight before Michaelmas laſt, but the certain day and hour ſhe is not able to nominate; ſhe ſent for me, and enquired whether ſhe were not under an ill Tongue or not, or of what nature the Diſeaſe was: I have ſent you the encloſed Scheam, I could find but one teſtimony of Faſcination or Witchcraft, which was one Sign poſſeſſing the Cuſps of the Twelfth and Firſt Houſes, which to me holds forth no move than a ſtrong ſuſpition of it by the Querent; However I am confident there is a Natural Diſeaſ which hurts much, becauſe the Lord of the Sixt, which uſually gives ſignification of Natural Diſeaſes, is now placed in the Aſcendent; but at preſent I forbear to make any large diſcourſ of mine own Opinions, being deſyrous that you would endeavor your Skill in this Cure, for there is not a Doctor of them all far or near that have been ſo skilful to find out the Diſeaſ, much leſ to effect the Cure. Sr. I expect your Anſwer; mean time bid you farewel, and remain yours in Affection, &c.

The incloſed Scheam.

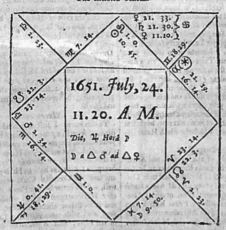

1651. *July*, 24.
11. 20. *A. M.*
Die, ♃ *Hora* ☽
☽ ☌ △ ♂ *ad* △ ♀

Figure 16 A decumbiture chart of 1651 which Culpeper included in the final 'key' chapter of his herbal, The English Physitian *(1652).*

APPENDIX 2

The Horoscope of 1651, from Culpeper's *English Physitian*

This decumbiture appeared at the end of Culpeper's herbal, in a final chapter entitled 'The way of mixing medicines according to the cause of the disease and part of the body afflicted'. This was the 'key of the work' and Culpeper's judgement on the horoscope was intended to teach his readers how to diagnose the cause of the disease through astrology and to treat it with herbal medicines. I reproduce and comment on this astrological teaching below:

> To such as study astrology [who are the only men I know that are fit to study physick, physick without astrology being like a lamp without oil], you are the men I exceedingly respect, and such documents as my brain can give you at present [being absent from my study], I shall give you, and an example to show the proof of them.

- Fortify the body with herbs of the nature of the lord of the ascendant, 'tis no matter whether he be a fortune or infortune in this case.
- Let your medicine be something antipathetical to the lord of the sixth.
- Let your medicine be something of the nature of the sign ascending.
- If the lord of the tenth be strong, make use of his medicines.
- If this cannot well be, make use of the medicines of the light of time [ie the Sun by day and the Moon by night].
- Be sure always to fortify the grieved part of the body by sympathetical remedies.
- Regard the heart, keep that upon the wheels, because the Sun is the fountain of life, and therefore those universal remedies, Aurum Potabile and the Philosopher's Stone, cure all diseases by only fortifying the heart.

But that this may appear unto you as clear as the Sun when he is upon the meridian, I here quote you an example, which I performed when I was as far off from my study as I am now, yet I am not ashamed the world should see how much or how little of my lesson I have learned without book.

On July 25, 1651, there came a letter to me out of Bedfordshire, from a gentleman at that time altogether to me unknown, though since well known, who was a student both in physick and astrology. The words are these.

Mr. Culpeper, my love remembered unto you. Although I know you not by face, yet because I do much respect that pretty little lark you so lately let fly into the world, which you call Semeiotica Uranica, *which I have lately taken into my cage. I am therefore emboldened to write unto you in the behalf of a neighbour's wife, who is taken with a violent disease which began in the lower parts of her body, but is now ascended upwards and tormenteth her in her breast, throat, tongue and lips. This disease took possession of her, as she relateth to me, about a fortnight before Michaelmas last, but the certain day and hour she is not able to nominate. She sent for me and enquired whether she were not under an ill tongue or not, or of what nature the disease was. I have sent you the enclosed scheme. I could find but one testimony of fascination or witchcraft, which was one sign possessing the cusps of the twelfth and first houses, which to me holds forth no more than a strong suspicion of the querent. However, I am confident there is a natural disease which hurts much, because the lord of the sixth, which usually gives signification of natural diseases, is placed in the ascendant. But at present I forebear to make any large discourse of my own opinions, being desirous that you would endeavour your skill in this cure, for there is not a doctor of them all, far or near, that have been so skilful to find out the disease, much less to effect the cure. Sir, I expect your answer, mean time bid you farewell, and remain yours in affection &c.*

My answer to the letter was to this effect: Sir, I received yours, July 25, wherein I find your enclosed scheme, and, I suppose, the nature of the disease, and have sent you such an answer as I could, being far from my study, which I entreat you to take in good part, being *festinanti calamo conscripta* [written in a hurry]. As for the ignorance of your country doctors, they wanting the true judgement of astrology, is to me no ways admirable. I perceive you to be a young man by the time of your genesis, which you also sent me. Beware whom ye trust with that. He that knows your nativity knows when ill directions operate, and if he be an enemy, knows when to do you a mischief. If Cecil had not had Essex's nativity, he had never gotten his head off. But to instruct you, being a young student, I shall give you my judgement methodically.

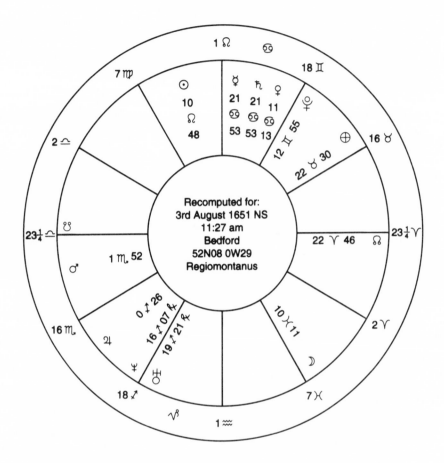

Figure 17

Diacritica you say you can find no arguments of witchcraft, but only one sign possessing the cusps of both twelfth and ascendant. But if you had regarded the propinquity of Venus to Saturn, you would have made another of that. Yet I do not think she is bewitched, because of other more prevalent testimonies. The Moon passing from the beams of Mars to the beams of Venus seem to give some suspicion of honesty, and the disease to come that way, which is increased by Mars' being in the ascendant in Scorpio and the Dragon's Tail upon the cusp. Yet I can hardly believe this, for Cauda in a humane sign usually gives slanders, and not tales of truth. 'Tis a hundred to one if she suffers not in point of good name by the vulgar [this was too true]. Besides, the nearness of Venus to Saturn may well show trouble of mind. And it being in the ninth house, pray enquire whether she has not been troubled about some tenets in religion. [The trouble of mind was true, but it was about a stranger, which the ninth house also signifies.]

Comment Culpeper first of all considers the astrological symbolism to answer the questions 'Is the woman really ill?' and 'Is it a natural illness?' He establishes that the horoscope is describing a natural illness from the position of the ruler of the 6th house of diseases in the most potent part of the chart, the Ascendant. This house and its ruler, Venus in this case because Libra is on the cusp of the Ascendant, always signifies the patient and Venus is an apt significator for a female. Moreover, the fact that the Moon, in separating from a trine aspect of the planet Mars and applying next by the same aspect to Venus, symbolizes the transmission of illness (Mars) to Venus (the neighbour's wife). Thus there is 'some suspicion of honesty' in the woman's complaint and the horoscope is established as radical. Culpeper is further able to determine that there is some gossip going around about this woman and that she is worried (Saturn afflicting the Ascendant) about some 9th house matter, a stranger in this case.

> **Diagnostica** Venus, lady of the twelfth and ascendant, and eighth, shows her always to be her own foe in respect of health. And truly I believe the original of the disease was a surfeit either by eating moist fruits, or else by catching wet when travelling. Venus with Saturn, who is in square to the ascendant, troubles her breast with tough phlegm and melancholy. Besides, there being a most forcible reception between the Moon and Venus from fruitful signs, I question whether she be not with child or not, the Moon being in the fifth house. Mars is lord of the disease, really in the Scorpion, and accidentally in the ascendant, together with Aries on the sixth, show the disease keeps his court in the womb and accidentally afflicts the head from thence, so that heat of the womb must needs be the cause of the present distemper, and Mars in a moist sign in the first, near the second, may well denote heat and breaking out about her face and throat.

Comment Turning to diagnosis, Culpeper argues from the position of Venus and the Moon in the cold and moist signs of Cancer and Pisces that the cause of the woman's disease shared these qualities and was possibly self-inflicted. He suggests the overeating of moist fruits or of catching wet in travelling (travelling is another signification of the 9th house where Venus is posited). The actual manifestation of the disease is shown by hot and dry Mars in Scorpio, the sign associated with the womb, and Culpeper surmises that hot vapours rising from that distempered organ are causing the symptoms in her 'throat, tongue and lips'. The other malefic planet, cold and dry Saturn, is in Cancer and symbolizes the phlegm and melancholy in the lungs. All these planets are in fertile water signs. Added to this, the Moon, already implicated in the transmission of the disease, suggests by her presence in the 5th house of children the possibility to be considered in the differential diagnosis that the woman is pregnant.

Prognostica Whether she will be curable or not, or when the disease will end, is our next point. Truly I can see no danger of death, the Moon being strong in her wane, and applying by trine with a strong reception to the lady of the ascendant. Yet this is certain: Mars strong in a fixed sign will maintain the disease stoutly. Her hopes will be but small when Venus comes to the body of Saturn, viz August 2, for she will be overpressed with melancholy. The time I suppose of her cure may be, if good courses be taken, when Mars leaves the sign he is in and comes to the place where the body of Jupiter is, or at least then it may turn to another disease more propitious. The Sun strong in the tenth shows she may be cured by medicine, and he being exalted in the seventh, and Caput there, I do not know but you are as likely a man to do it as any.

Comment Culpeper now outlines the likely course of the disease and identifies that the Sun, the ruler of the house of medicine in this horoscope, is strong in that angle. This augurs well for medical treatment and for its administration by his correspondent, because the Sun commands a secondary power in the 7th house of the physician or astrologer. More than this, however, the Sun upon the meridian (to repeat Culpeper's earlier phrase) is meant to be understood to represent not just the potential of the astrologer but that of astrology generally in medicine. It is the light which astrology casts onto the healing situation to illuminate the right approach to treatment. Thus in this sense, too, the Sun shows the cure.

Indicationes curativae It is confessed here that the Sun being exceeding strong in the tenth house should naturally signify the curative medicine, and as true that the evil of Mars, viz heat of the womb, and a salt humour in the blood, ought to be removed before you meddle with the tough phlegm in the breast. But yet seeing the disease seems rather to participate of offending heat than any other simple quality, you must have a care of hot medicines, lest you go about ignem olea extinguere [putting out the fire with oil]. The medicines must first be cool; secondly, strengthening the womb; thirdly, repressing the vapours; fourthly of the nature of Sol and Venus.

Comment As for the indications for curing the woman, the medicine must be able to cool the heat of the womb and so repress the hot vapours rising from it. By treating the organ primarily affected, the secondary symptoms of heat manifesting in the head and neck and producing the salt humour in the blood will be removed. Yet there is also the cold condition of the lungs to be corrected and Culpeper warns not to try to do both at the same time. The order of treatment is according to the more prevalent imbalance, heat in this case, and by virtue of the fact that Mars symbolizes more acute disease while Saturn generally indicates a chronic one.

Therapeutice To this intent I first commend unto you Stinking Arrach, a pattern whereof I have sent you here enclosed. You may find it upon dung-hills, especially such as are made of horse dung. It is cold and moist, a herb of Venus in the Scorpion. Also Ros Solis, a herb of the Sun and under the celestial Crab, may do very well, and the better because Venus is in Cancer. It grows upon bogs in untilled places and is in flower about this time. It grows very low, with roundish green leaves full of red hairs, and is fullest of dew when the Sun is hottest, whence it took its name. To these you may add Tansy, which I take to be a herb of Venus in Libra, and Lettuce, if you please, which is a herb of the Moon. Mars having his fall in Cancer, they are all harmless; you may use them according to your own discretion. Also Orpine, another herb of the Moon, is very good in this case.

Comment Culpeper's intention is that the heat of the womb will be treated first with the cooling and moistening herbs stinking arrach, wild lettuce and orpine. This constitutes a treatment of contraries by contraries or allopathy. However, his choice of herbs shows also the use of cosmic sympathy: stinking arrach is a herb of Venus and strengthens the organs ruled by her, in this case the womb. It is also in sympathy with the patient and will strengthen her in the struggle with her disease, because her particular significator in the horoscope is Venus also. Thus like cures like. As to the disease, since the planet Mars does not rule the womb the disease is said to come by antipathy and must itself be treated by antipathy. Thus Culpeper also recommends herbs of the Moon, wild lettuce and orpine, along with a herb of Venus, both planets being in antipathy to Mars. Once this has been effected, the sundew or ros solis, classed as hot and dry in the fourth degree, can be given to cut up the cold, congealed humours in the lungs for their easier expectoration and removal from the body. Again, because Saturn does not rule the lungs, his affliction of that part comes by antipathy and the cure must therefore be by antipathy to Saturn, in this case by a herb of the Sun. Sundew is still used for respiratory diseases today. Finally tansy, another herb of Venus, hot in the 2nd degree and dry in the 3rd, is given to restore her womb and the patient as a whole to a harmony and balance (Libra on the ascendant is the sign of the balance or scales). The greater drying power of tansy is needed to correct the moisture indicated by the quality of the signs occupied by Venus and the Moon in the horoscope. Moreover, Culpeper wrote in his herbal, 'Dame Venus was minded to pleasure women with child by this herb, for there grows not a herb fitter for their uses than this is.' Tansy was said by Culpeper to prevent miscarriage and 'if her womb be not as she would have, this decoction will make it as she would have it, or at least as she should have it'. Thus he clearly recommended it to his correspondent with the woman's possible pregnancy in mind. Today, on the basis of pharmacology, the use of tansy in pregnancy is contra-indicated because of the danger of abortion by it. Culpeper concludes:

> Sir, I wish you well, and if you esteem of my lark above his desserts, I pray trim his feathers from him – correct the errors by the errata – else will he make but unpleasing music. Thus remains yours &c.
>
> I the rather chose this figure to judge of, because none should have just occasion to say of us astrologers that we do as physicians' vulgar practice is, when they judge of piss: pump what they can out of the querent and then judge by his words.

AFTERWORD

While I was working on this decumbiture for a presentation at a conference on astrology and medicine in March 1988, an incident occurred which brought the illumination of astrology in this centuries-old horoscope very much into my life and which reveals, I believe, something of the nature of astrology itself.

One Sunday that February, over lunch, my wife peeled an orange to find a perfectly formed but much smaller orange inside. My sister, who was present, was struck by this and instantly pronounced it a symbol of fertility. I told her later that my wife's period was late and that she was feeling a little off-colour and slightly nauseous. More concerned now about her condition, my wife had a pregnancy test the following week. This proved negative but her 'sickness' continued. I reflected on casting a decumbiture to see if she was pregnant or sick when it suddenly dawned on me that the divination was already in front of my eyes in the 1651 horoscope I was working on.

I decided to compare the decumbiture from Culpeper with my wife's natal chart: Mars in Scorpio was *exactly to the minute* conjunct her 5th house and fertile Jupiter; Venus in Cancer was conjunct her Ascendant (orb 30') and the nodes were conjunct but reversed (orb 30'). Such startling synastry between major significators persuaded me that both women were pregnant! My wife did have another pregnancy test the following week, the morning after a full Moon which fell zodiacally conjunct her natal Venus, ruler of her 5th house of children. This test was positive.

Here then is an example of the power of astrology to be meaningful and revealing in the context in which it arises. The fact that the horoscope in question was cast 337 years earlier only adds testimony to a 'secret mutual connivance' in nature whereby phenomena seemingly unrelated in time or space may be found to have a connection through astrological symbolism, if we have our eyes open to the possibility.

The pregnancy was unremarkable enough, except for a dry, persistent, non-productive cough, paroxysmal at times ('tormenteth her in the breast, throat, tongue and lips'), which began midway through the pregnancy. There was certainly some 'trouble of mind' for my wife due to the stress of negotiating with doctors over a home birth. Her own GP, a female doctor, immediately removed her and our first child from her list of patients for wanting a home delivery and complained about her in front of other patients gathered in her waiting room ('Cauda – the south node – in a humane sign usually gives slanders'). Obstetricians tried to frighten her into hospital with tales of post-partum haemorrhaging and death. I tried to be reassuring here by using Culpeper's prognosis from the decumbiture of 'no danger of death'. Everything turned out well in the end with a smooth birth at home without drugs or stitches on 14 October, when *the Sun was transiting the ascendant* of the 1651 decumbiture. Our new daughter's natal Ascendant fell on the Part of Fortune of Culpeper's chart.

The curious correspondence of events in my wife's pregnancy with those given in Culpeper's judgement may have an apt signature in Neptune. In 1988 this trans-Saturnian planet was transiting over my wife's Ascendant ruler, the Moon, including a station 1' from exact conjunction. Neptune is thought to represent paranormal phenomena. In my wife's natal chart, Neptune is conjunct her 5th house Jupiter.

NOTES

INTRODUCTION

[1] F N L Poynter, 'Nicholas Culpeper and his Books' in *Journal of the History of Medicine* 17 (1962), p153.

[2] Olav Thulesius, *Nicholas Culpeper: English Physician and Astrologer* (Macmillan Press, 1992).

[3] *Journal of the History of Medicine* 49 (1994), pp120–122.

[4] Kerry Bone, 'A Systematic Approach to Western Herbal Therapeutics' in the *European Journal of Herbal Medicine*, Vol 2, no 2 (Spring 1996) pp35–42.

[5] Foreword to *Hildegard's Medicine*, an account of the work of the 12th-century German mystic, written by Dr Wighard Strehlow and Gottfried Hertzka MD (Bear and Co., Sante Fe, 1988).

[6] R Newman Turner, 'Free radicals and disease: the toxaemia hypothesis' in *Complementary Therapies in Medicine*, Vol 4, no 1 (January 1996), pp43–48.

[7] James Hillman, *The Thought of the Heart* (Eranos, 1979).

[8] Roy Porter, 'Trust Me, I'm a Doctor', *Observer Review* (16 June 1996).

[9] Kerry Bone, ibid.

[10] J Tester, *A History of Western Astrology* (Boydell Press, 1987), p18.

[11] Quoted in Thulesius, *op cit*, p165.

[12] Hakim G M Chishti, ND, *The Traditional Healer* (Thorsons, 1988), p1.

[13] Henry E Sigerist, *Civilisation and Disease* (Cornell University Press, Ithaca, 1945), p153.

[14] H J Eysenck and M W Eysenck, *Personality and Individual Differences: A Natural Science Approach* (New York, 1985), p3.

PART 1 A STUDENT OF PHYSICS AND ASTROLOGY: THE LIFE AND DEATH OF NICHOLAS CULPEPER 1616–1654

[1] *The Dictionary of National Biography (DNB)* states that Culpeper was born in London, but this biographical sketch contains errors of which this may be one. Culpeper's natal horoscope was cast by John Gadbury for the latitude of London (J Gadbury, 'The Nativity of Nicholas Culpeper' in *Culpeper's School of Physick* [London, 1659], and in J Gadbury, *Collectio Geniturarum* [London, 1662, p140]), though this may have been done out of convenience. *See* note 3.

[2] '*The Life of the admired Physician and Astrologer of our times, Mr Nicholas Culpeper*' in *Culpeper's School of Physick* (London,, 1659), C1ʳ, hereafter referred to as '*Life of … Culpeper*'. This biographical sketch, considered a contemporary and biased source, was written by Culpeper's amanuensis, William Ryves.

³Thulesius, *op cit*, p1. It is by reason of these two events occurring at Ockley, Culpeper's baptism on 24 October following his father's burial on 5 October, that Olav Thulesius thinks it very unlikely that Culpeper was born in London and rather believes that he was born at Ockley.

⁴Gerald Loder, *Wakehurst Place, Sussex: An Account of the Manor and its Owners* (London, 1907), chapter on the Culpepers.

⁵*ibid.*

⁶The material for this paragraph is largely taken from Thulesius, *op cit*, ch1, and Loder *op cit.*

⁷His parents had wed on Wednesday 25 October 1615 and so had been married less than a year when his father died. Gadbury states that Culpeper 'never gained good' by his kindred, which may apply both to the Culpeper and the Attersoll families. 'The Nativity of Nicholas Culpeper' in *Culpeper's School of Physick*, B5ᵛ–B6ʳ.

⁸*DNB*, entry on William Attersoll. Attersoll complained of 'the poor living living I now enjoy' and 'the poor cottage' he lived in, though he continued there for forty years!

⁹*ibid.* 'The trouble [ie about his poor income] was occasioned by a suspicion on the part of Attersoll's parishioners that the new parson was too much of a scholar and unlikely to be a preacher after the type of their former.'

¹⁰*ibid.*

¹¹*Life of ... Culpeper*, C1ᵛ.

¹²Thulesius, *op cit*, pp12 and 18. Gadbury gives 1634 as the year in which Culpeper started his studies at Cambridge (*The Nativity of Nicholas Culpeper*, B8ʳ) but Thulesius (*op cit*, p28) has found the following entry in the *Apothecaries Society Court Book* (London, 1617–51), dated 14 November 1634 and signed by three wardens of the society : 'Nicholas Culpeper, son of Nicholas Culpeper late of Ockley in the County of Surrey, clerk in holy orders, examined and bound to Simon White for 8 years from that date'.

¹³*Life of ... Culpeper*, C2ᵛ–C3ʳ.

¹⁴*See* for instances Keith Thomas, *Religion and the Decline of Magic* (London, 1971), ch 12, esp pp.369–71.

¹⁵Both Thulesius and Mrs C F Leyel, notable herbalist of the first half of the 20th century, are of the opinion that Culpeper studied some medicine whilst at Cambridge, Leyel stating that at university 'he made a study of ancient Greek and Arabic medicine' (C F Leyel, *The Truth About Herbs* [London, 1946], p23).

¹⁶*Life of ... Culpeper*, C1ᵛ–C2ᵛ. Thulesius asserts that the lady in question is Judith Rivers (born 20 December 1615), that she was Culpeper's childhood sweetheart and that the long absence of Nicholas, when he began his studies at Cambridge, made their hearts so fond of one another that their secret desire to marry became overwhelming. Thulesius, *op cit*, pp22–26.

¹⁷*Life of ... Culpeper*. Culpeper was apprenticed to Simon White on 14 November 1634, see note 12.

¹⁸The *Apothecaries Society Court Book* states that 'Nicholas Culpeper is turned over to Francis Drake 25th February 1636', quoted in Thulesius, *op cit*, p28.

¹⁹Thulesius, *op cit*, pp28, 32.

²⁰Harold J Cook, *The Decline of the Old Medical Regime in Stuart London* (Cornell University Press, 1986), pp46–47, 71–72, 95–97.

[21]Thomas, *op cit*, p 10. 'In the first years of its foundation the college had only a dozen members, whereas London's population was perhaps sixty thousand. By 1589 the college's membership had risen to thirty-eight while the population had more than doubled. Thereafter the number of inhabitants continued to rise spectacularly, but the size of the college remained almost stationary until the Civil War period.'

[22]C F Leyel, *The Truth About Herbs* (London, 1946), appendix II.

[23]Cook, *op cit*, pp94–104.

[24]*Life of … Culpeper*, C3^v; *The Nativity of Nicholas Culpeper*, B8^v. The date (1640) means that this is the earliest mention of Culpeper practising medicine.

[25]Thulesius, *op cit*, p33.

[26]C L Ewen, *Witchcraft & Demonianism* (1933), p434; Thulesius *op cit*, p117. 'Nicholas Culpeper of St Leonard's, Shoreditch, gentlemen, at St L., on 17th December., 18 chas.I, bewitched Sarah Lynge, widow, who languished until 12th January following. Not guilty.' Sarah Lynge recovered.

[27]*The Nativity of Nicholas Culpeper*, B8^v.

[28]*Life of … Culpeper*, C6^r.

[29]William Attersoll was buried on 30 May 1640 (*DNB*).

[30]*Life of … Culpeper*, C3^r.

[31]'The character of Nicholas Culpeper' in *Culpeper's School of Physick*, c1^v.

[32]*DNB*.

[33]C F Leyel, *The Truth About Herbs*, p23.

[34]*Life of … Culpeper*, C4^r.

[35]Culpeper, *A Physical Directory or a Translation of the London Dispensatory* (1649), 'To the Reader'.

[36]*ibid*. When Culpeper issued his *English Physician*, its price was three pence.

[37]Thulesius, *op cit*, p66.

[38]*Life of … Culpeper*, C5^v–C6^r.

[39]*DNB*.

[40]*Mercurius Pragmaticus*, pt ii, no 21 (4–9 Sept. 1649), quoted in *DNB* and Thulesius, *op cit*, p67.

[41]L Fioravanti, *Three Exact Pieces* (1652), prefix addressed to 'Friend Culpeper'.

[42]Culpeper, *A London Dispensatory* (1651), 'A Conclusion'.

[43]Cook, *op cit*, p121.

[44]Culpeper, *A Physical Directory* (1649), 'To the Reader'.

[45]Bernard Capp, *Astrology and the Popular Press: English Almanacs 1500–1800* (London 1979), p59.

[46]*ibid*, p79.

[47]*ibid*, p87. The 'heroic conqueror' refers to Oliver Cromwell.

[48]*ibid*, p79.

[49]*ibid*, pp79–80.

[50]*Black Munday Turn'd White, or the Astrologers Knavery epitomised. Being an answer to the great prognostics of Mr Lillie, Mr Culpeper and the rest of the Society of Astrologers concerning the Eclipse of the Sun on Monday Last* (1652), p7; 'tycho' is Tycho Brahe (1546–1601), the famous astronomer-astrologer.

[51]*A Faire in Spittle Fields, where all the Knick Knack's of Astrology are Exposed to open Sale. Where Nicholas Culpeper brings under his velvet jacket: 1. His Challenges against the Doctors of Physick; 2. A Pocket Medicine; 3. An Abnormal Circle etc.*, written by J B Gent (1652). Quote from p4.

[52]Culpeper, *Catastrophe Magnatum,* p75.

[53]Culpeper, *A Physical Directory* (1650), 'To the Impartial Reader'.

[54]*ibid.*

[55]This last was one of three translations made by Culpeper of leading anatomists of his day, the two other works being Bartholin's *Anatomy* and Riolan's *Encheiridium anatomicum et pathologicum,* published as *A Sure Guide.* These reflected Culpeper's own sound knowledge gained by attending anatomical dissections and demonstrations given by surgeons and doctors he knew. See Thulesius, *op cit,* pp84–85.

[56]Thulesius, *op cit,* p79. It is not surprising that so many of the Culpepers' children died young when, along with Alice's illness, we consider the 36 per cent mortality rate within the first six years for children born in London at this time (see Thomas, *op cit,* p5).

[57]*The Second Book of the Presages of Hippocrates,* ch 5 in *Semeiotica Uranica* (1651); *English Physitian,* under 'Mallows', by which he was cured; *Life of ... Culpeper* c5ᵛ.

[58]Charles E Bodemer, *Materialistic and Neoplatonic Influences in Embryology* in *Medicine in 17th Century England,* ed. A Debus (University of California Press, 1974).

[59]Culpeper, *Astrological Judgement of Diseases* (1655, reprinted AFA 1959), pp53–54.

[60]Culpeper, *The English Physitian Enlarged* (London, 1656), 'To the Reader'.

[61]*DNB.*

[62]Culpeper, *Pharmacopoeia Londinensis* (1653), 'To The Reader.'

[63]*The Nativity of Nicholas Culpeper,* B8ʳ.

[64]*Life of ... Culpeper,* c7ʳ&ᵛ.

[65]*Culpeper's School of Physick,* C8ᵛ-C2ʳ. The other quotations in this section, unless separately referenced, are from this description of Culpeper's character.

[66]Culpeper, *Ephemeris for 1651,* quoted in Capp, *op cit,* p161.

[67]D L Cowen, 'The Boston Editions of Nicholas Culpeper' in *Journal of the History of Medicine* 2 (1965), p156–165. Thulesius, *op cit,* ch 15.

[68]Culpeper, *A New Method of Physick* (1654), 'To the Reader' (dated 12 November 1653), A2.

[69]Peter Cole advertised *Medicaments for the Poor* and *Health for the Rich and Poor, by Diet, without Physick* as separate books, bound together with a third work, his own *Culpeper's Ghost* (1656). Using Poynter's list of Culpeper's works, we find that, by considering *Two Books of Physick,* as indeed two separate works, and grouping together the separate publications of the various books of Daniel Sennert's *Practical Physick* (1662–4) as ultimately one work, the total number of posthumous publications of Culpeper's works by Peter Cole is 17. Thulesius, *op cit,* p 159, gives a different, but unconvincing, breakdown.

[70]Peter Morellus, *The Expert Doctors Dispensatory* (1657), A3ʳ&ᵛ.

[71]Quoted in Culpeper, *The English Physitian Enlarged* (1656), C8ʳ&ᵛ.

[72]Capp, *Astrology and The Popular Press,* p87; Poynter, *Nicholas Culpeper and his Books,* p162.

[73]Thulesius once again doubts that this is a genuine work by Culpeper on the grounds that, since Culpeper was opposed to surgical incision for the removal of stones in the bladder, *The Chyrurgeons Guide* could not have been penned by him. He is way off the mark here and appears not to have actually read the *Guide,* which is subtitled 'the errors of some unskilful practitioners in chirurgery' and

deals substantially with the treatment of hernias, so that his readers would not need recourse to use the 'runners about, called cutters for the stone and ruptures' (ie hernias). Culpeper condemns their savage practice of commonly removing the stone (ie a testicle) in the process of excising a hernia. For Culpeper's treatment of stones in the bladder, see the relevant chapter in his *Urinalia*, London 1658, appended to editions of his *Astrological Judgement of Diseases*.

[74]Thulesius, *op cit*, p157, who suggests the *Treatise* was the brainchild of John Heydon who married Alice Culpeper on 4th August 1656 (DNB).

[75]Culpeper, *Pharmacopoeia Londinensis* (1654), printed for Peter Cole, B4^v, dated January 1st 1653/4 (ie since, in Culpeper's day, the New Year began on 25 March, any day from 1 January to this was attributed, as we see it, to the previous year. Thus our 1 January 1654 was written as 1 January 1653).

[76]Culpeper, *A Physical Directory* (1651), p129.

[77]Capp, *op cit*, p208.

[78]Allen G Debus, *The English Paracelsians* (New York, 1966), pp142–4 and p169 for the method of preparation of *Aurum Potabile*.

[79]Culpeper, *Pharmacopoeia Londinensis* (folio 1653),B1^r.

[80]Culpeper, *Treatise of Aurum Potabile* (London, 1657), p16. F N L Poynter (*Nicholas Culpeper and the Paracelsians*, p214) is convinced that the *Treatise* is a genuine work, since 'the literary style is that of Culpeper with many of the same points in his other writings. When we look at the ideas we find that they are the same as those expressed in a long 'Premonitory Epistle to the Reader' included in the preliminaries to the *Pharamacopoeia Londinensis* of 1653 and signed by Culpeper.'

[81]Anon (Philaretes Tantarara Tantarara), *Culpeper Revived from the Grave, to discover the cheats of that Grand Imposter, call'd Aurum Potabile. Wherein is declared the grand falsities thereof, and abuses thereby, Published to undeceive the people and to stop the violent current of such a mischievous design* (Spittlefields, August 1655), pp2, 4; Poynter, *Nicholas Culpepper and the Paracelsians*, p212.

[82]Poynter (*ibid*) suggests the authorship of a rival printer since Peter Cole, 'the stationer not far from Leaden Hall', comes under attack for the 'specious pretence ... cast over this illegitimate libel to the injury of the dead' and for intending thus to print works in Culpeper's name which he had never written (pp5–6). Peter Cole had his say in *Culpeper's Ghost* (1656).

[83]*Culpeper Revived from the Grave*, p4.

[84]Culpeper, *Treatise of Aurum Potabile* (London, 1657), A8^r.

[85]Cook, *op cit*, p121.

[86]The last of nine essays in *Chymical, Medicinal and Chyrurgical Addresses: Made to Samuel Hartlib, Esquire* (1655), leader of the influential Hartlib circle whose programme was intellectual and social reform and the transformation of medicine, 'predicted that soon a universal medicine would make everyone healthy, end death, and so eliminate the medical profession'! (Cook, *op cit*, p124).

[87]It was dated 1 January 1653/4. A 10-line introduction to *An Astrologo-Physical Discourse*, emphasizing the importance of the concepts of sympathy and antipathy and dated 2 January 1653/54 is the only writing by Culpeper that I have found to be dated later than this. See the *Pharmacopoeia Londinensis* of 1654.

[88]M Mackaile, *Moffet-Well ... As, also, the Oyly-Well... To these is subjoined a Character of Mr Culpeper and his Writings* (1664). Mackaile doubted that Culpeper penned the *Arts Master-piece* of 1660, because the ingredients mentioned were too costly.

[89]Hugh G Dick, 'Students of Physick and Astrology' in *Journal of the History of Medicine* 1 (1946), pp300–315, 419–34. Dick is of the opinion (p312) that 'this outburst' of books on astrological medicine cannot be attributed *altogether* (my italics) to Culpeper's success', since there was a general rise in books on astrological subjects in this period.

[90]Thulesius, *op cit*, p142.

PART 2 SECTION 1 THE SEVEN NATURAL THINGS AND THE CONSTITUTIONAL BASIS OF MEDICINE

[1]It should be pointed out that Galenism is impossible to define precisely since the term covers everything which Galen wrote plus all the modifications on his teachings over 14 centuries. Seventeenth-century Galenism thus represents a particular understanding of this body of knowledge. The interest here is in Culpeper's orientation towards the material.

[2]Culpeper, *Art of Physick*, ch 4. Lester S King, *The Transformation of Galenism in Medicine in 17th Century England*, ed A Debus (University of California Press 1974), p8. Much of the following section on the elements is drawn from this essay.

[3]Why 4 in number? This allowed a division into two pairs of opposites and may have derived from the addition of one, the element Earth, which was never omitted from any popular list of elements amongst the ancient Greeks, to 3, the number of the brothers Zeus, Poseidon and Hades, who as Gods had command over certain aspects of natural law or *moirai*. Early Greek cosmologists may have regarded each of these *moirai* as primary elements. A resulting four-fold division of this kind can be traced in the writings of Homer and Hesiod. *See* John Burnet, *Greek Philosophy: Thales to Plato* (London, 1962), p26.

[4]Thomas Hall, *History of General Physiology, 600 BC to AD 1900* (University of Chicago, 1975), Vol 1, pp85–93, 104–106; O Cameron Gruner MD, *A Treatise on the Canon of Medicine of Avicenna* (London, 1930, reprinted NY, 1970), pp34–56.

[5]Jostein Gaarder, *Sophie's World* (Phoenix, 1995), p30.

[6]Mazhar H Shah, *The General Principles of Avicenna's Canon of Medicine* (Karachi, Pakistan, 1966), pt1, ch 2.

[7]Culpeper, *Treatise of Aurum Potabile*, ch 1.

[8]Culpeper, *Art of Physick*, ch 51.

[9]Polycletus lived during the third century BC. 'He was universally reckoned the most skilful artist of his profession among the ancients ... One of his pieces, in which he had represented a bodyguard of the king of Persia, was so happily executed, and so nice and exact in all his proportions, that it was looked upon as a most perfect model, and accordingly called *the rule*.' (From J Lempriere's *Classical Dictionary*).

[10]Culpeper, *Art of Physick*, ch 51.

[11]*ibid*, ch 51 & 50.

[12]Culpeper, *Pharmacopoeia Londinensis* (1653), 'To The Reader'.

[13]Culpeper, *Art of Physick*, ch 59. *See also* his *Astrological Judgement of Diseases* (1655), republished by AFA 1959, pp109–114 for similar descriptions of simple and compound temperaments.

[14]Francis Packard, *The School of Salernum: Regimen Sanitatis Salernitanum* (New York, 1920), p134. This is the English version by Sir John Harington, a courtier of Queen Elizabeth I, which was first published in 1607.

[15]These images are taken from Levine Lemnie, *The Touchstone of Complexions* (1633), an English translation of L Lemnius, *De habitu et constitutione corporis quam Graeci krasin, triviales complexionem vocant*, 2 vols (1561), bk 2, ch 2.

[16]Culpeper, *Art of Physick*, ch 59.

[17]Packard, *op cit*, p136.

[18]Lemnie, *op cit*, bk 2, ch 5.

[19]Culpeper, *Astrological Judgement of Diseases*, p2.

[20]Culpeper, *Art of Physick*, ch 59.

[21]Packard, *op cit*, p140.

[22]M T Cicero, *On Old Age*, xi, Loeb edn, trans W A Falconer, p45.

[23]Culpeper, *Art of Physick*, ch 59.

[24]Packard, *op cit*, p138.

[25]Lemnie, *op cit*, bk 2, ch 3.

[26]Gruner, *op cit*, pp76–92; Hall, *op cit*, pp64–74, 148–150; Shah, *op cit*, pt 1, ch 4.

[27]Gruner, *op cit*, pp 66–68.

[28]Henry Sigerist, *Civilization and Disease* (Cornell University Press, 1944), p151.

[29]Robin Fahraeus, 'Basic Facts Concerning Humoral Pathology and Relics of These in the Language and in Folk Medicine' in *Papers on Folk-Medicine*, ed Carl-Hermann Tillhagen (Nordic Museum, Stockholm).

[30]Bernard T Donovan, *Humours, Hormones and the Mind* (Macmillan, 1988), p4.

[31]Aristotle's view was that the second concoction took place in the heart as well as in the neighbouring spleen and liver (Hall, *op cit*, p110). Galen accepted that some black bile, the dregs of the first concoction in the stomach, were received in the spleen straight from the mesenteries (Rudolf E Siegel, *Galen's System of Physiology and Medicine* [Basle, 1968], pp258 ff). The vital spirit is formed in the heart from the light and vaporous portions of blood.

[32]Hall, *op cit*, p148.

[33]*ibid*. The pathway for black bile to pass from the spleen to the stomach, according to Galenic physiology, is the 'gastro-splenic anastomoses', the subject of much controversy in the wake of the Vesalian revolution in anatomy. The anastomoses are probably the short gastric veins which drain the fundus and left part of the greater curvature of the stomach, and the left gastro-epiploic vein which drains both its surfaces. These veins are all tributaries of the splenic vein, and since blood was thought to flow outwards, or in some cases in both directions, along the veins in the Galenic system, these blood vessels connecting stomach and spleen were thought of as the pathway for black pile to enter the stomach.

[34]A Brock, *Greek Medicine* (London, 1929), p10.

[35]*ibid*.

[36]Hall, *op cit*, pp106–107, 140–141; Gruner, *op cit*, pp93–106; Shah, *op cit*, pt 1, ch 5.

[37]Culpeper, *Art of Physick* (1652), ch 4. Culpeper uses the word 'member' for the similar parts, Aristotle's *homoiomeres*. Of these similar parts, the arteries, nerves

and veins are called subservient parts because they carry, respectively, vital spirit from the heart, animal spirit from the brain and natural spirit in blood from the liver. The spermatic vessels which carry male semen and female 'spermatical matter' are also subservient to the testes and ovaries.

[38]King, *op cit*, p13.

[39]King, *op cit*, p21.

[40]*ibid*, p23. Once again, as in the remarks about the *physis*, there is an appeal to the mystery of an organism in its unity and the notion that something is more than the sum of its parts, in this case its qualities. Of course there is now an explanation for most of these 'occult' qualities, thanks to the advances science has made over recent centuries: the chemical structure of scorpion poison and the pharmacology of purgative medicines, the rabies virus and so on. Yet the Galenic reasoning about such forces in nature was perfectly logical within its own body of knowledge.

[41]Culpeper, *Art of Physick*, ch 4.

[42]Gruner, *op cit*, pp118–134.

[43]Culpeper, *Treatise of Aurum Potabile*, ch 1.

[44]*ibid*, ch 9.

[45]Culpeper, *Astrological Judgement of Diseases*, p49.

[46]Hall, *op cit*, pp107–119.

[47]Culpeper, *Treatise of Aurum Potabile*, ch 8.

[48]Thomas S Hall, 'Life, Death and the Radical Moisture' in *Clio Medica* 6 (1971), pp3–25.

[49]Peter H Niebyl, 'Old Age, Fever and the Lamp Metaphor' in *Journal of the History of Medicine and Allied Sciences* 26 (1971), pp353–368.

[50]For the Aristotelian teaching, see Hall, *op cit*, pp113ff, also King, *op cit*, p17.

[51]*Culpeper's Midwife Enlarged* (1676) bk 2, sect 2, pp63–64.

[52]Galen's view was that there was a steady decline in innate heat throughout life, while others argued that it increased during youth and then declined. *See* Niebyl, *op cit*, Shah, *op cit*, pt 1, ch 3, sect 3.

[53]Niebyl, *op cit*.

[54]Gruner, *op cit*, p270.

[55]'Doctor Diet's Directory' in *Culpeper's School of Physick* (1659), p280.

[56]L J Rather, 'Old and new views of the emotions and bodily changes', in *Clio Medica* 1 (1965), pp1–25; Gruner, *op cit*, pp143–155.

[57]These are the chordae tendineae of the heart valves which were thought to brace and sustain the heart and which vibrated according to the emotions felt.

[58]Culpeper, *Art of Physick*, ch 85; Gruner, *op cit*, pp212–214.

[59]Gruner, *op cit*, pp10–11.

[60]Seigel, *op cit*, pp221–224.

[61]Donovan, *op cit*, pp11–12.

[62]Richard Lower MD, in his work *De Catarrhis* (On Catarrhs) of 1672, was the first to state that phlegm does not come from the brain but is secreted from the nose itself. Further, he suggested that the effluent from the brain which passes to the pituitary gland is taken back into the blood, thus hinting at the gland's true role as the master hormonal gland. *See* Donovan, *op cit*, p3.

[63]Culpeper, 'An Astrologo-Physical Discourse of the Human Vertues in the Body of Man' in *Pharmacopoeia Londinensis or the London Dispensatory* (London, 1669),

A5ᵛ. The *Discourse* was first published in Culpeper's lifetime, appended to his *Ephemeris for the Year 1651*. All Culpeper's statements quoted in this section come from this discourse.

⁶⁴It was thought that the various components of the intellect were located not in the substance of the brain itself, but in the cavities or ventricles of the brain which are filled with circulating cerebro-spinal fluid. Remember that the brain was considered cold and moist in quality, like the element Water, and ruled by the Moon. It is perhaps in keeping with this symbolism, and in the absence of any way to measure mental activity in the various parts of the brain, that such a view was held. Shah, *op cit*, pt 1, ch 6, sects 5 and 6, states that imagination was held to reside in the first two ventricles, judgement in the middle or third ventricle and memory in the fourth ventricle.

⁶⁵Michael MacDonald, *Mystical Bedlam: Madness, Anxiety and Healing in Seventeenth Century England* (Cambridge University Press, 1988), p180, paraphrasing Burton in *The Anatomy of Melancholy*.

⁶⁶Culpeper, *Art of Physick*, ch 59.

⁶⁷Bernard Capp, *Astrology and the Popular Press: English Almanac 1500–1800*, (London, 1979), p227. Thomas May (1595–1650) was buried in Westminster Abbey.

⁶⁸Hans H Simmer, 'The Beginnings of Endocrinology' *in Medicine in 17th Century England*, ed A Debus (University of California Press, 1974).

⁶⁹Hall, *op cit*, p154.

⁷⁰'Willis [Thomas Willis (1621–75)] replaced immaterial form and hidden quality with a substance which exerts specific actions and thus causes quality.' *ibid*, p231.

⁷¹ *Culpeper's Midwife Enlarged*, bk 1, sect 2, ch 3, pp29–30. Thulesius, *op cit*, p88, has formed the view that Culpeper conceived the seed of a woman to be an egg from the following (unreferenced) quotation: 'Women have a two-fold spermatical matter, the one watery, which moistens and refreshes the womb and fruit in it, the other which is *thick in the tubae* [the egg] which is mixed with the seed of man to make conception.' I assume that both the italics and parenthesis are Thulesius's. The Hippocratic treatise which Culpeper refers to is *On Generation* (c370 BC).

⁷²Thulesius, *op cit*, ch 9, specifically p88.

⁷³Shah, *op cit*, pt 1, ch 6 sect 3.

⁷⁴Culpeper, *An Astrologo-Physical Discourse*, A6ʳ, A6ᵛ. All quotes from Culpeper on these virtues are taken from this section of the *Discourse*.

⁷⁵Shah, *op cit*, p 1, ch 6, sect 3. Anatomically, retention was possible through the activity of oblique or transverse fibres in an organ while both expulsion and attraction, or absorption in Shah's terminology, occurs by means of longitudinal fibres of consecutive segments of organs.

PART 2 SECTION 2 THE PRESERVATION OF HEALTH AND THE PREVENTION OF DISEASE: THE SIX NON-NATURAL THINGS

[1]'Sanitas est quaedam harmonia humorum', quoted in O Cameron Gruner MD, *A Treatise on the Canon of Medicine of Avicenna* (London, 1930, reprinted NY, 1970), p77.

[2]John Burnet, *Greek Philosophy, Thales to Plato* (London, 1962), p50.

[3]Thomas Hall, *History of General Physiology, 600 BC to AD 1900* (University of Chicago, 1975), Vol 1, p35.

[4]Gruner, *op cit*, p560.

[5]Culpeper, *Art of Physick*, ch 4–6.

[6]*ibid*, ch 82.

[7]*ibid*.

[8]*ibid*, ch 83.

[9]*ibid*, p145; Peter Holmes, *The Energetics of Western Herbs* (Artemis, 1989), Vol 1, p16.

[10]L. Lemnie, *The Touchstone of Complexions* (1633) bk 1, ch 2.

[11]Theoharis C Theoharides, 'Galen on Marasmus [Peri Masasmou]', *Journal of the History of Medicine and Allied Sciences* 26 (1971).

[12]Lemmie *op cit*, bk 1, ch 2.

[13]*ibid*.

[14]Mazhar H Shah, *The General Principles of Avicenna's Canon of Medicine* (Karachi, Pakistan, 1966), pt 3, introduction.

[15]Culpeper, *Health for the Rich and Poor, by Diet, without Physick* (London, 1656), 'To the Reader'.

[16]The inclusion of massage reflects the regime of Arab physicians and is quite unknown in Culpeper's writings.

[17]Gruner, *op cit*, pp188–192, 443–4.

[18]L J Rather, 'Pathology at Mid-Century' *in Medicine in 17th Century England*, ed A Debus (University of California Press, 1974), p102.

[19]Robert Burton, *The Anatomy of Melancholy*, pt 1, sect 2, memb 2.

[20]Galen, *Of Protecting the Health*, bk V, from *Medical Quotations* (Collins, 1990).

[21] Burton, *op cit*, pt 1, sect 2, memb 2, subsect 5.

[22]*The Medical Works of Hippocrates*, trans J Chadwick and W Mann (Oxford, 1950), pp90–112.

[23]Culpeper, *Art of Physick*, ch 85, covers the 6 non-naturals. See also L Riviere, *The Universal Body of Physick* (London, 1657), pp295–8; Gruner, *op cit*, pp175–209.

[24]We may recall that there was some argument among certain of the Ancient Greek philosophers over whether respiration and the intake of *pneuma* or digestion or *pepsis*, (as it was for Aristotle) represented the central activity in the living body. *See* Peter H Niebyl, 'Old Age, Fever and the Lamp Metaphor', *Journal of the History of Medicine* 26 (1971), pp353–68.

[25]D Guthrie, *A History of Medicine* (London, 1945), p260. The translated title of the text of Bernardino Ramazzini (1633–1714) is *On the Diseases of Artificers, which by their particular Callings they are most liable to*.

[26]Henry Sigerist, A History of Medicine, Vol 1 *Primitive and Archaic Medicine* (Oxford University Press, 1977), p77.

[27]*ibid*, p114.

[28]Hippocrates, 'Tradition in Medicine', in *The Medical Works of Hippocrates*, p17.

[29]Sigerist, *op cit*, p147.

[30]Keith Thomas, *Religion and the Decline of Magic* (London, 1971), p7.

[31]*ibid*.

[32]*ibid*. See also Samuel Radbill, 'Paediatrics' in *Medicine in Seventeenth Century England*, ed A Debus (University of California Press, 1974).

[33]F N L Poynter and K D Keele MD, *A Short History of Medicine* (London, 1961), pp109–110. *See also* Thomas, *op cit*, pp85–89.

[34]Culpeper, *Health for the Rich and Poor*, pp1–2.

[35]*ibid*, p10.

[36]*Life of … Culpeper*, C4^v. Regarding his feared intemperance, *see* Culpeper, *Health for the Rich and Poor*, 'To the Reader'.

[37]Culpeper, *Health for the Rich and Poor*, p13.

[38]L J Rather, 'Old and New Views of the Emotions and Bodily Changes', *Clio Medica* 1 (1965), p4.

[39]Hippocrates, 'A Regimen for Health' in *The Medical Works of Hippocrates*, p214.

[40]Francis Packard, *The School of Salernum: Regimen Sanitatis Salernitanum* (New York, 1920), p90.

[41]'Doctor Diet's Directory' in *Culpeper's School of Physick*, pp277–342.

[42]Culpeper, *The English Physitian*, under 'fennel'.

[43]The quotations in this section are from Culpeper's *Art of Physick*, ch 59.

[44]Culpeper, *Art of Physick*, ch 85. See also Gruner, *op cit*, pp383.

[45]Riviere, *op cit*, bk 4, ch 27.

[46]*ibid*, and ch 28. Culpeper, *Art of Physick*, ch 85. *See also* Gruner, *op cit*, pp210–212, 417–9.

[47]Packard, *op cit*, p77.

[48]Riviere, *op cit*, bk 4, ch 29; Gruner, *op cit*, pp229–30, 253.

[49]Robin Fahraeus, 'Basic Facts concerning Humoral Pathology and Relics of these in the Language and in Folk-Medicine' in *Papers on Folk-Medicine*, ed Carl-Hermann Tillhagen (Nordic Museum, Stockholm).

[50]Lemnie, *op cit*, bk 2, ch 2. *See also* Howard Haggard, *Devils, Drugs, And Doctors*, (London nd), pp272–3 and ch XI generally for a discussion of the deleterious effects of sexual abstinence or a repression of the sexual instinct.

[51]Hall, *op cit*, p54. *See also* Gruner, *op cit*, p230.

[52]Culpeper, *Health for the Rich and Poor*, ch 14, 10.

[53]*ibid*, ch 8, 11.

[54]Riviere, *op cit*, p303.

[55]*Culpeper's Midwife Enlarged*, bk 3, sect 1.

[56]*ibid*, bk 2, ch 2. It may be argued with the benefit of contemporary knowledge that if a woman's seed is the ovum she releases monthly from the ovaries, then she is naturally restricted in the frequency of release of her seed, unlike a man, and that frequent sexual intercourse should not be debilitating.

[57]*ibid*; Lemnie, *op cit*, bk 2, ch 2.

PART 3 AS ABOVE, SO BELOW: ASTROLOGY, MEDICINE AND HERMETIC PHILOSOPHY

[1]S J Tester, *A History of Western Astrology* (Boydell, 1987), p23. The oft-quoted reference in support of the inclusion of astrology in Hippocratic medicine is from *Airs, Waters, Places*, 2. But here, as in 'Epidemics', bk 1, the author is showing the importance of observing the heliacal risings or settings of the Pleiades, Arcturus and Sirius in order to know how the season is progressing and when to anticipate a change, for 'changes in the seasons produce changes in the mechanism of the body'.

[2]D Pingree, *The Yavanajataka of Sphujidhana* (Cambridge, Mass, 1978), vol 2, p436.

[3]A Bouché-Leclercq, *L'Astrologie Grecque* (Paris, 1899), pp519–20.

[4]An ancient tradition states this same Asclepios to have been originally a native of Memphis in Egypt who emigrated to Greece and introduced into that country a knowledge of medicine. His daughter was Hygieia, the goddess of health (hygiene).

[5]Frances Yates, *Giordano Bruno and the Hermetic Tradition* (London, 1964), p49.

[6]Pingree, *op cit*, p430. The Greek text is in J L Ideler, *Physici et medici graeci minores* (Berlin, 1841), vol 1, pp387–96.

[7]Culpeper, 'A Premonitory Epistle to the Reader' in *Pharmacopoeia Londinensis* (1653).

[8]*ibid.*

[9]*ibid.*

[10]Culpeper, *Semeiotica Uranica*, 'To The Reader'.

[11]Culpeper, 'A Premonitory Epistle to the Reader' in *Pharmocopoeia Londinensis* (1653).

[12]*ibid.*

[13]Culpeper, *Health for the Rich and Poor, by Diet, without Physick*, 'To the Reader'.

[14]Culpeper, *Treatise of Aurum Potabile*, ch 2.

[15]*ibid*, ch 3. This is the only reference I have found in Culpeper's writings to the three Paracelsian principles.

[16]Ptolemy, *Tetrabiblos*, bk 1, ch 3. Quotations are taken from the translation made by Robert Schmidt for Project Hindsight and the Golden Hind Press (1994).

[17]G Cornelius, *The Moment of Astrology: Origins in Divination* (Arkana, 1994), p86.

[18]M Ficino, *Three Books on Life*, a critical edition and translation by Carol V Kaske and John R Clark (New York, 1989), introduction, p51. Ficino credited the Arabs with the origination of the notion of the world spirit.

[19]Culpeper, *Treatise of Aurum Potabile*, ch 8. If minerals, too, have an aerial spirit by which cosmic sympathy can operate, there is no reason to doubt (as Thulesius does) that Culpeper would pen a work on 'the secret virtues of stones': 'The Expert Lapidary' in *Culpeper's School of Physick*.

[20]Tester, *op cit*, p178.

[21]Ptolemy, *op cit*, bk 1, ch 3.

[22]Compare his decumbiture in *Semeiotica Uranica* bk 2, ch 7 with the 1651 'scheme' reproduced in Appendix 2, below. Further evidence is afforded in Culpeper's application of his version of the *Iatromathematica of Hermes Trimegistos* to 'the time of the patient's first lying down or demanding the question:

Culpeper's Astrologicall Judgement of Diseases from the Decumbiture of the Sick much Enlarged (London, 1655), reprinted by the American Federation of Astrologers (1959), p75.

[23]*Anima Astrologiae or, A Guide for Astrologers*, 4th edition, facsimile of the 1886 edition (Regulus, 1989), p1.

[24]See Appendix 2.

[25]*Culpeper's Astrologicall Judgement of Diseases from the Decumbiture of the Sick much Enlarged* (London, 1655).

[26]*ibid, The Third Book of the Presages of Hippocrates*, ch 1. His admission that 'I have been a piss-prophet all my life' only confirms his knowledge that urinalysis does not reveal the presence of all diseases. See also *The Second Book of Presages of Hippocrates*, ch 7, in *Semeiotica Uranica*.

[27]Culpeper, *Semeiotica Uranica*, bk 1, my italics.

[28]*ibid*, bk 2, ch 7.

[29]E A Wallis Budge, *The Divine Origin of the Craft of the Herbalist* (published at Culpeper House by the Society of Herbalists, 7 Baker Street, London W1, 1928), pp51–2.

[30]This is the caduceus, symbolically a staff entwined with two serpents, an emblem of the Sumerian god Ningishzida and possessed by the Greek Hermes, and which today is the logo of the British Medical Association.

[31]*See* Geoffrey Cornelius, *The Moment of Astrology: Origins in Divination* (Arkana, 1994); Maggie Hyde, *Jung and Astrology* (Aquarian, 1992); and their joint work with Chris Webster, *Astrology for Beginners* (Icon, 1995).

[32]Said of Ficino, as the first to do so, in Ficino, *op cit*, introduction, p54. For his part, Culpeper had no problem in accepting the theory of Copernicus, formulated in the century separating Ficino and Culpeper, that the Earth goes round the Sun. Indeed, the implication that the Sun is the centre of the cosmos only confirmed the truth of Hermetic philosophy for Culpeper. *See* his *Treatise of Aurum Potabile*, ch 9.

[33]Culpeper, *Semeiotica Uranica*, bk 2, introduction. The work by Duret, the second part of which deals with medical astrology, is entitled *Novae Motuum Ephemeridis Richelianae* (1641). Culpeper also included a section from Duret containing observations from two other French astrologers, Augerius Ferrerius and Thomas Boderius, in the 2nd edition of his *Astrological Judgement of Diseases* (1655). These were omitted from the first edition because Culpeper found them 'very imperfect'. *See also* Jacques E Halbronn, 'The Revealing Process of Translation and Criticism in the History of Astrology' in *Astrology, Science and Society*, ed Patrick Curry (Boydell, 1987), pp200–202.

[34]Culpeper, *Semeiotica Uranica*, bk 2, ch xi, with additions from *The Coelestial Governours* in *Culpeper's School of Physick*, pp182–5. This short piece, published posthumously in one of Nathaniel Brook's compendia, is undated but must predate the *Semeiotica Uranica* since the latter specifically revises some of the inclusions of the former. As to the correspondences themselves, where two signs are associated with a part, such as Libra and Scorpio with the bladder, this is reminiscent of the innervation of an organ from several adjacent spinal segments.

[35]It was also reckoned that a planet in its own sign, say Moon in Cancer, was in its first sign and therefore could signify the parts of the body associated with the

first zodiac sign Aries, namely the head. Moon in Leo, the second sign from its own, signified the throat, Moon in Virgo the hands and arms, and so on. Planets ruling two signs could count from either place. Lilly produced such a table of significations which Culpeper criticized in *Semeiotica Uranica*, bk 2, ch xi, pt 4. He had fashioned a table of his own in his *Directory for Midwives*, bk 2, sect 2, but this was never brought forward in the *Semeiotica Uranica* or elsewhere.

[36]Dorotheos of Sidon, *Carmen Astrologicum*, trans D Pingree (Teuber, 1976), bk 5.

[37]Culpeper, *Semeiotica Uranica*, bk 2, ch ix.

[38]Lilly, *Christian Astrology* (Regulus, 1985, reprint of the 1647 edition), p259.

[39]Culpeper, *Semeiotica Uranica*, bk 2, ch xi.

[40]*ibid*, bk 2, ch ix.

[41]*ibid*, bk 1.

[42]*ibid.*

[43]*ibid*, bk 2, ch xi.

[44]*ibid*, ch x iii. Culpeper also repeats other indications given in Duret for a disease on the left or right side of the body, in the upper or lower parts, in the front or back and if easily visible or hidden, but his desire is to 'leave them to the approbation of Dr Experience'.

[45]Culpeper, *Semeiotica Uranica*, bk 2, ch xii.

[46]*ibid*, bk 2, ch xiv, parts ii & iii.

[47]Culpeper, *Health for the Rich and Poor, by Diet, without Physick* (London, 1656), ch 8.

[48]M Ficino, *op cit*, bk 3, proem (preliminary discourse).

[49]*Life of ... Culpeper*, C4[r&v].

[50]Culpeper, *Semeiotica Uranica*, bk 2, ch i.

[51]For a brief summary in English, see Cornelius O'Boyle, *Medieval Prognosis and Astrology: A Working Edition of the Aggregationes de crisi et criticis diebus* (Wellcome Unit for the History of Medicine, Cambridge, 1991).

[52]*ibid*, p11.

[53]Culpeper, *Semeiotica Uranica*, bk 2, ch i.

[54]*ibid.*

[55]*ibid*, bk 2,ch xiv.

[56]*ibid*, bk 2 , ch xi.

[57]Culpeper, *The English Physician Enlarged* (1653), 'To the Reader'.

[58]Culpeper, *Semeiotica Uranica*, bk 2, ch xv, 'for the cure of any disease, take these few rules'.

[59]*ibid*, bk 2, ch xi.

[60]*ibid.*

[61]*ibid*, bk 2, ch xv, where this matter is explained.

[62]*ibid*, bk 2, ch iii.

[63]*ibid*, bk 2, ch ii.

[64]O Neugebauer, *The Exact Sciences in Antiquity*, 2nd edition (Dover, 1969), p81.

[65]Culpeper identifies in which of the 12 houses each of the planets 'joy', 'rejoice' or 'delight' in *Semeiotica Uranica*, bk 2, ch ix. He says, 'If you cannot have the planet in the ascendant [or angle, presumably] in his own sign, see to have him in the house he delights in.' Particularly, the Sun delights in the 4th, 9th and 11th houses; the Moon in the 3rd and 7th; Saturn in the Ascendant, 8th and 12th; Jupiter in the 2nd, 9th and 11th; Mars in the 3rd, 6th and 10th; Venus in

the 5th and 12th; and Mercury in the Ascendant and 6th.

[66]See Appendix 1 for the astrological calculation of the temperament.

[67]Culpeper, *Treatise of Aurum Potabile*, ch 2.

PART 4 THE ENGLISH PHYSICIAN: HERBAL MEDICINE AND THERAPEUTICS

[1]Culpeper never clearly and fully laid out this doctrine anywhere in his original works, perhaps for him astrology was so central to the diagnosis and treatment of disease. Consequently, I have drawn on other texts to expound these principles, namely O Cameron Gruner, MD, *A Treatise on the Canon of Medicine of Avicenna* (London, 1930, reprinted NY, 1970); Mazhar H Shah, *The General Principles of Avicenna's Canon of Medicine* (Karachi, Pakistan, 1966); Hakim G M Chishti, ND, *The Traditional Healer* (Thorsons, 1988), and L Riviere, *The Universal Body of Physick*, translated by William Carr (London, 1657).

[2]Chishti, *op cit*, pp17–18.

[3]Shah, *op cit*, p225.

[4]A Brock, *Health and Conduct* (London, 1923), p42.

[5]Gruner, *op cit*, pp257–82, 452–514.

[6]Belching, but not acidic in taste, could also arise from the swelling of burned fatty foods or scorched meat in the stomach of an overheated body.

[7]See Gruner, *op cit*, pp257–282; Chishti, *op cit*, pp92–6.

[8]It was variously thought that black bile was voided by the body via the haemorrhoidal veins and by the intestines.

[9]Riviere, *op cit*, bk 3, ch 6.

[10]Shah, *op cit*, p227; Gruner, *op cit*, pp276–8.

[11]Shah, *op cit*, pp228–9; Gruner, *op cit*, p277.

[12]Riviere, *op cit*, bk 3, ch 11–12.

[13]'Febrilia, or a Treatise of Fevers in General' in *Culpeper's Last Legacy* (1655), pp49–72.

[14]Shah, *op cit*, pt 2, ch 2, sub-chaper B, sect xxix.

[15]Riviere, *op cit*, bk 3, ch 7.

[16]The details of this paragraph are from Alfred White Franklin, 'Clinical Medicine' in *Medicine in 17th-century England* (University of California Press, 1974).

[17]John Fernelius, Abdiah Cole and Nicholas Culpeper, *Two Treatises, The First of Pulses, the Second of Urines* (1662). See Gruner *op cit*, pp283–322 for a detailed study of Avicenna's teaching, which is delivered more plainly in Chishti *op cit*, pp78–87, and comprehensively dealt with in Reuben Amber and Babey-Brooke *Pulse Diagnosis: Detailed Interpretations for Eastern and Western Holistic Treatments*, (Aurora Press 1993).

[18]'Urinal Conjectures' in *Culpeper's School of Physick* (1659), pp222–5.

[19]A full consideration of urinalysis may be found in Gruner, *op cit*, pp323–53 and Chishti, *op cit*, ch 8.

[20]*The Second Book of the Presages of Hippocrates*, ch 7 *Presages by the Urine in a fever*, in *The Astrological Judgement of Diseases*, 1655.

[21]Culpeper, *Art of Physick*, ch 59.

[22]*The Second Book of the Presages of Hippocrates*, ch 7.

[23]Massage was included in the therapeutics of the Arab physicians but was not mentioned at all by Culpeper.

[24]Culpeper, *Pharmacopoeia Londinensis* (1669), pp267–305. The *Key* covers the manifest qualities of herbal medicines, their appropriateness to each part of the body, and their actions.

[25]*ibid*, p267.

[26]Culpeper, *The English Physitian*, 'To the Reader'.

[27]*ibid*, under 'Lesser Celandine'.

[28]These are among the few examples of the doctrine of signatures given by Culpeper. William Cole, a notable doctor of signatures, plagiarised Henry More in his argument that many plants were left without signatures because, if they all possessed one, 'the rarity of it, which is the delight, would be taken away by too much harping on one string'. Quoted in A Arber, *Herbals, Their Origin and Evolution* (Cambridge University Press, 1986), p254.

[29]Culpeper lays out the signs of excess heat, cold, dryness and moisture in each organ in his translation of Galen's *Art of Physick* (1652). The most important signs are included in this section.

[30]Culpeper, *The English Physitian* (1656), pp280 *et seq.*

[31]The two dispensatories are found on pp1–52 and pp54–84 respectively. In a few places in the table I have included details from J Dantz, *Tabulae Simplicium Medicamentorum, quae apud Dioscoridem, Galenum et Plinium sunt* (Basileae, 1543).

[32]'A Key to Galen and Hippocrates, their Method of Physick' in *Pharmacopoeia Londinensis* (1669), p267.

[33]John ab Indagine, quoted in Lynn Thorndike, *A History of Magic and Experimental Science* (NY, 1941), vol 5, p176.

APPENDIX 1 THE NATAL HOROSCOPE OF NICHOLAS CULPEPER

[1]*Culpeper's School of Physick* (1659), B2ᵛ–B8ᵛ.

[2]This is taken from Gadbury's own publication of his judgement of Culpeper's nativity in *Collectio Geniturarum* (London, 1662), p140, because of its clearer presentation of the same horoscope.

[3]Culpeper, *Art of Physick*, ch 59.

[4]William Lilly, *Christian Astrology* (1647), pp532–4, and the example on p743.

[5]The table of the Essential Dignities of the Planets According to Ptolemy is in *Christian Astrology*, p104, and is to be used with the Table of Fortitudes and Debilities on p115, as in Lilly's worked examples on pp178–180 and pp744–5.

[6]Lilly, *op cit*, p533.

[7]Culpeper, *A Physical Directory*, introduction 'To the Impartial Reader'.

[8]Culpeper, *Astrological Judgement of Diseases* (AFA, 1959), bk 2, ch xi, pt 3.

[9]Charles E O Carter, *The Astrological Aspects* (Fowler & Co, 1972).

[10]'Febrilia, or a Treatise of Fevers' in *Culpeper's Last Legacy* (1676), p67.

A Glossary of Some Words Found in Culpeper's Writings

Abstergent	cleansing away thick and corrupt humours
Adust	burned
Adventitious	not natural, but coming from external causes
Ague	malarial or intermittent fever
Alexipharmical	medicines resisting plague, poison and venomous diseases
Alteratives	medicines which alter the qualities of the body and humours by heating, cooling, drying and moistening, as opposed to purging or sweating medicines, etc
Apoplexy	stroke
Atrobilious	of black bile or melancholy
Balneum Mariae	a water bath, used for certain preparations of medicines
Bilious	choleric
Black jaundice	hepatocellular or cholestatic jaundice
Bloody flux	haemorrhage, dysentery
Cacochymy	the abounding of ill humours
Chin-cough	whooping cough
Clyster	an enema
Courses	menstrual flow
Crude	raw, undigested
Defluxion	a flow of humours into a part, causing pain or swelling
Diathesis	disposition
Discuss	to dispel invisibly, eg a swelling
Distillation	a trickling down of thin humours from the brain to a part
Dropsy	a watery swelling in the tissues or cavities of the body
Emulgent veins	veins carrying blood to the kidneys
Emulsions	milk of almonds and of the cold seeds

Emunctuaries	lymph nodes
Epitheme	medicines applied in bags, commonly to the heart, liver, spleen, etc
Errhines	medicines to be sniffed to purge the brain
Falling sickness	epilepsy
Felon	whitlow
Fits of the Mother	hysteria
Flux	an excessive flow of any body secretion
Fuliginous	smoky, misty
Fundament	anus
Gate-vein	portal vein
Glutinous	clammy like glue
Habit	the whole bulk and substance of the body
Horrors	shivering
Iliac passion	volvulus
Impostume (Apostume)	purulent swelling or abscess
Incrassate	to thicken
Kernels	hard swellings
Kibes	chilblains
King's evil	cervical tuberculosis, scrofula
Laevity	smoothness
Lenitive	a gentle, refreshing, cordial medicine
Marasmus	a consuming fever, eg consumption
Matrix	womb
Megrim	migraine
Morphew	morphoea, scleroderma
Mother	womb
Nidorous	smelling of burned fat, scorched meat or fried oil
Peccant	an offending humour, causing disease
Phthisis	consumption (TB), corruption
Pituitous	phlegmy
Porraceous	green, of the colour of leeks
Pugil	an amount of a herb held between thumb and 3 fingers
Purblind	myopic
Rarity	thinness
Reds	menstrual flow
Reins	kidneys
Repletion	overabundance and fulness of blood or humours
Rheum	watery or catarrhal discharge, cf *rheumatic*
Rotten	proceeding from infection
St Anthony's fire	erysipelas, possibly ergot poisoning

Scirrhus	a hard swelling without pain
Secundines	afterbirth
Siccity	dryness
Spagyric	a 'chemical physician'
Stopping	an obstruction
Surfeit	an excess of food, drink or sex
Swimming in the head	vertigo
Tenesmus	a continual desire to go to stool and voiding nothing but slime or bloody matter
Tensive	stretching out
Terms	periods, menstruation
Tetters	a form of herpes, ringworm or eczema
Venery	lechery, sexual intercourse
Ventricle	cavity of the stomach or brain
Water-gate	the private parts in women
Wen	sebaceous cyst
Whites	leucorrhoea

USEFUL ADDRESSES

Australia

Federation of Australian Astrologers
PO Box 159
Stepney
SA 5069
Australia

National Herbalists Association of Australia
Suite 14, 247–249 Kingsgrove Rd. (PO Box 65)
Kingsgrove
NSW 2208
Australia

UK

The Company of Astrologers
PO Box 3001
London N1 1LY
Tel: 01227 362427

The National Institute of Medical Herbalists
56 Longbrook Street
Exeter
Devon EX4 6AH
Tel: 01392 426022

Urania Trust
396 Caledonian Road
London N1 1DN

(for nationwide information on tuition and consultations with astrologers)

USA

American Botanical Council
PO Box 201660
Austin
Texas 78720–1660
USA

Astrological Federation of America
PO Box 22040
6535 South Rural Road
Tempe
Arizona 85285–1040
USA

INDEX